Biological Rhythms, Sleep, and Performance

Wiley Series on Studies in Human Performance

Series Editor

Dennis H. Holding

University of Louisville
Kentucky, USA

Biological Rhythms, Sleep, and Performance

Edited by

Wilse B. Webb

Sleep Laboratory
Department of Psychology
University of Florida

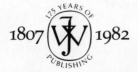

JOHN WILEY & SONS

Chichester · New York · Brisbane · Toronto · Singapore

Library of Congress Cataloguing in Publication Data:
Main entry under title:

Biological rhythms, sleep, and performance.

  (Wiley series on studies in human performance)
  Includes indexes.
  1. Biological rhythms.   2. Sleep — Physiological
aspects.   3. Work — Physiological aspects.
4. Performance.   I. Webb, Wilse B.   II. Series.

OP84.6.B564   612'.022   81-14754

ISBN 0 471 10047 1   AACR2

British Library Cataloguing in Publication Data:
Biological rhythms, sleep and performance.
   — (Wiley series on studies in human performance)
   1. Human biology
   I. Webb, Wilse B.
   612'.015   QP34.5

ISBN 0 471 10047 1

Phototypeset by Dobbie Typesetting Service, Plymouth, Devon and printed by the Pitman Press Ltd., Bath, Avon.

List of Contributors

MICHAEL BONNET, Ph.D.   Research Associate, Veteran's Administration Hospital, Cincinnati, Ohio, *USA*.

W. P. COLQUHOUN, Ph.D.   Director, MRC Perceptual and Cognitive Performance Unit, University of Sussex, Brighton, *England*.

LAVERNE C. JOHNSON, Ph.D.   Chief Scientist, Naval Health Research Center, San Diego, California, *USA*.

PERETZ LAVIE, Ph.D.   Senior Lecturer, Faculty of Medicine, Technion —Israel Institute of Technology, Haifa, *Israel*.

TIMOTHY H. MONK, Ph.D.   Scientist, MRC Perceptual and Cognitive Performance Unit, University of Sussex, Brighton, *England*.

CHESTER A. PEARLMAN, M.D.   Veterans Administration Hospital, Boston, Massachusetts, *USA*.

DONALD I. TEPAS, Ph.D.   Professor and Chair, Department of Psychology, Illinois Institute of Technology, Chicago, Illinois, *USA*.

WILSE B. WEBB, Ph.D.   Professor of Psychology, University of Florida, Gainesville, Florida 32611, *USA*.

Contents

Series Preface

Research on human performance has made considerable progress during the past forty years, reaching a respectable depth of analysis in several areas while, at the same time, becoming broader in scope. As a result, there have emerged a number of theoretical ideas which impinge on the general development of experimental psychology and, moreover, a great deal of knowledge has been obtained in ways which encourage direct, practical application. The series of *Studies in Human Performance*, well represented in this volume, is intended to explain these ideas and their applications in adequate detail.

Approximately half of the books in the series are monographs, while the remainder, like the present text, are edited volumes. Although writing a monograph is often regarded as the more difficult assignment, producing an edited volume presents a considerable challenge. On the hand, it provides an opportunity to bring to bear a concentration of expertise which is otherwise unattainable; on the other hand, the multiplicity of contributors carries with it a risk that the overall result may be disorganized or, literally, incoherent. In the *Human Performance* series, every effort has been made to counter the disadvantages attendant on using the edited format, while preserving the advantages of drawing upon special knowledge. The chapters have been commissioned in accordance with an integrated plan for each volume, information about each chapter has been circulated among the contributors in order to ensure cohesion, and editorial control has extended to the level of difficulty as well as to the format of each text.

The result of these preparations should be a series of books which combine readability with high standards of scholarship. The aim has been to supply a good deal of content, but within an expository framework which emphasizes explanation rather than mere reporting. Thus, although each volume contains sufficient material for the needs of graduate students or advanced under-graduates in experimental psychology, the books should provide readily accessible information for applied psychologists in many areas. In addition, it is hoped that the books will be useful to practitioners in ergonomics, to persons with interdisciplinary interests in production and industrial engineering, in physical education and in exercise physiology, and to psychologists in other fields.

The present volume succeeds in meeting the special challenge of integrating research areas which have developed independently for some time. It seems unfortunate that the histories of sleep research and biological rhythm research have been largely disparate since, as the book demonstrates, there can be no doubt that these areas share theoretical and methodological concerns in common. The recognition of a common basis in concepts like the fluctuation of arousal makes for a significant advance.

The most important findings concerning biological rhythms are clearly presented, as part of a sustained interleaving of sleep and chronobiology issues. At the same time, sleep represents much more than one extreme in the daily arousal curve. To help understand the relation of sleep to human performance the book offers a great deal of specific information on the stages and characteristics of sleep, and on the consequences of shifting sleep schedules. It also delineates the ways in which loss of sleep, perhaps by inducing fatigue, affects different kinds of performance; those whose interests in fatigue extend beyond the loss of sleep should note the companion volume in this series on *Stress and Fatigue in Human Performance*. The book also makes a strong methodological contribution. The difficulties in quantifying rhythmic trends are squarely faced, although the necessary mathematical concepts are all explained with clarity and care. The result seems compatible with the overall objective of the series, that each book should be within the grasp of any educated person who has the motivation to study its subject matter.

DENNIS H. HOLDING
Series Editor

Preface

It would be very nice if Prefaces could be made a required reading part of a book by other than book reviewers. Sometimes, admissably they are filler materials before the often coy expressions of gratitude to faithful typists, patient wives, and subdued children. More often they are heartfelt expressions of hopes and fears by the author or editor about the book in hand. As such, prefaces are good ways to gain perspective on what the book is all about.

I reluctantly agreed to edit this book relating sleep, biological rhythms, and performance in the *Human Performance* series. A part of that reluctance stemmed from an inherent laziness which has become increasingly manifest with age and the blunting of the goad of ambition. This problem was exacerbated by the knowledge that the book would not be an easy one. The interrelationships between the areas were, to use a few appropriate descriptive terms, generally emergent, amorphous, accidental, unrecognized, ill-defined, and, at best evolving. In short, the task was not one of reviewing a coherent set of data about performance but to seek coherence within disparate but related enterprises. And most critically such a state of affairs calls for expertise. Although I may immodestly claim such in sleep research, that is by no means the case in the area of biological rhythms. While I have been increasingly drawn to that area's constructs and techniques in my attempts to better comprehend sleep, my learnings have been hard won, hand wrought, and relatively recent. As for performance, my training and background as a psychologist have provided me with the fundamentals, and experimentation with behaviour over the years has given practice. However, this is the expertise of a worker in the vineyard not a philosopher thereof.

But in spite of these good reasons not to proceed I have done so. My reasons are these.

The series, as I understand it, is to cover 'the entire range of human performance'. I am aware that each person's interests magnify the importance of that interest as an important determinant of behaviour (e.g. astrologists, endocrinologists, behaviour modifiers). However, I have lived long enough with sleep research, and, more recently with biological rhythms, to be reasonably sure from the data that they are (sleep and biological rhythms) salient and often neglected determinants of human performance. One of my reasons for agreeing to proceed was to increase that awareness in others. In an early letter to the General Editor for the Series I wrote: 'I was glad to see sleep and biological rhythms recognized as determinants of performance.'

The most crucial element, however, was a sense from the literature that I was reading that three largely independent areas — performance measurement, biological rhythms, and sleep — were increasingly interactive with each other. The performance variations resultant from sleep variations were increasingly emphasized. Both biological rhythm researchers and researchers were measuring changes in performance relative to time of measurement. Sleep researchers and performance measurements were displaying increased interest in and use of biological rhythm concepts and analysis techniques in interpreting and analysing their data.

The general impression one received of these interactions, however, was that they were often casual, accidental, and idiosyncratically determined. Sleep and biological rhythm researchers often chose performance measures from limited perspectives relative to their complexities and appropriateness. Performance measurements and sleep variables, wrapped in intensities of techniques and particular issues, were treated in isolation and ignorance of profound rhythmic influences. At least that was my perception of the interrelations between the three areas.

It was this impression that provided the primary positive motivation for proceeding with this volume. There was the belief that each field could become more comprehensive and enriched by the others and that a review and an attempt to integrate the data from these perspectives could serve that purpose.

The final determinant was the availability of expertise in trying to accomplish the task. Led by Peter Colquhoun who edited the earliest book relating human performance and biological rhythms (*Biological Rhythms and Human Performance*, 1972), the Medical Research Unit at Sussex, England has provided leadership and active research in these interactions. Tim Monk of that Unit has written a chapter on the analytical methods of the biological rhythm research area (Chapter II) and Colquhoun has reviewed the issues and data of performance measurement in a biological rhythm framework (Chapter III). I have similarly provided a chapter reviewing sleep in a biological rhythm perspective (Chapter IV). The following three chapters consider the effects on performance of three major rhythm changes in sleep. Laverne Johnson, from an extensive background of sleep research and sleep deprivation experiments, has written the chapter on performance changes and sleep deprivation (Chapter V). Chester Pearlman, who has had an extensive and leading role in the exploration of the performance effects relative to sleep structure changes has reviewed these data in Chapter VI. Chapter VII discusses performance in a significant and growing societal pattern — shifted work/sleep schedules. This has been done by Donald Tepas who is currently doing research on these problems in both field and laboratory settings.

Chapters VIII and IX are concerned with two special aspects of these areas. At first blush Chapter VIII, by Michael Bonnet, on performance during sleep is puzzling. Doesn't performance stop with the onset of sleep and begin with awakening? Isn't sleep really non-performance? Bonnet examines that critical interface between sleep and waking; the capacities of the organism to respond to sensory input, to adapt to signals, the potential for integrative performance. By such explorations of the ongoing process of sleep and the performance capacity of the subject, both our understanding of sleep and performance are enhanced. Peretz Lavie in Chapter IX brings us to an area of research in which the three fields clearly, of necessity, merged. The question explored: are there ultradian (less than 24 hour rhythms) in performance and if so do they reflect an extension of sleep rhythms? Combining high skills in chronobiology techniques and a comprehensive understanding of sleep, Lavie, in this chapter on ultradian performance variations, exemplifies the fruitfulness and necessity of an interactive approach.

I have provided an introductory chapter reviewing the background, terms and procedures of sleep, biological rhythms, and performance and a brief envoi.

I have had the advantage of reading the book closely. I believe it accomplishes the useful purpose of explicating the status and exciting presence of the healthy interaction occurring across and within each area. This should promote and facilitate further exchanges. Yet more critically I hope that this attempt to take a more coordinate and comprehensive approach drawn from generally independent perspectives may serve our common purpose — a better understanding of the behaviour of man.

Biological Rhythms, Sleep, and Performance
Edited by Wilse B. Webb
© 1982 John Wiley & Sons Ltd.

Chapter 1

Sleep, Biological Rhythms, Performance Research: an Introduction

Wilse B. Webb

Sleep research, chronobiology or biological rhythm research, and performance research are three elaborate and largely independent enterprises. There have been, of course, interactions between them. For example, the measurement of performance following sleep deprivation, measures of variations in performance as a function of time of day, changes in rhythmic biological systems during sleep compared to waking have all been studied. However, these typically have been isolated importations of experimental variables or techniques in the service of the primary interest of the researcher. The chrono-biologist or the sleep researcher selects a convenient performance measure; the performance researcher explores whether his particular measure is stable across time; or the chronobiologist assesses changes in a biological variable during sleep.

The recent literature of each field provides evidence that this interplay between these fields is increasing both in amount, in sophistication, and in beneficial ways. At the same time each research area has increased in its complexities and its spread of interests. To facilitate a continued cross-fertilization of the fields, more information about the interests and dimensions of the 'non-primary' areas of research within each enterprise can be useful.

The purpose of this first chapter is to provide a general background of each area and a foundation for the succeeding chapters. These latter serve as elaborations and reviews of particular findings and procedures. Because this chapter is devised primarily for the 'non-area' researcher, the strokes are intentionally broad and non-technical. Each researcher in a primary area may readily skip the description of that area.

SLEEP RESEARCH

Background

Attempts to explicate sleep can be found in the early Greek writings. Hippocrates wrote extensively on sleep and Aristotle devotes three chapters of his *De Natura* to sleep and dreams.

The background of sleep research, however, parallels the history of life science research. Pieron in his 1913 book, *Le Problème Physiologique du Sommeil*, extensively reviewed research related to sleep to that time. A count of his cited references reveals a limited but increasing presence of such research. The average number of papers or books cited per year from the 1800s were as follows: 1801-20 = 0.3; 1821-40 = 1.1; 1841-60 = 3.5; 1861-80 = 8.5; 1881-1900 = 16.5; 1901-10 = 35.0. When Kleitman (1963) revised his 1939 book, *Sleep and Wakefulness*, his bibliography contained 4337 items.

A surge of contemporary sleep research, however, occurred in the late 1950s and early 1960s. Through the 1920s, 1930s, and 1940s articles and books on the subject were averaging about 100 per year. In the five year period from 1963 to 1967 this output increased fivefold, and by the late 1970s the annual sleep bibliography published by the Brain Research Institute of UCLA exceeded 1500 articles.

This explosion of sleep research is attributable to at least two factors. First there were rapid advances in central nervous system research during this period, and sleep represented a major state change and challenge. Second, and

Table 1 Percentage of all articles in five year periods

	1926–30	1946–50	1963–67	1968–72	1973–77	1978–79
Neurophysiology	10	14	24	16	12	11
Physiology	15	13	5	4	5	7
Biochemistry	13	15	13	20	6	7
Pharmacology*					12	13
Endocrinology*					4	3
Sleep disturbances	26	19	14	16	20	22
Ontogeny/Phylogeny	10	7	7	8	9	9
Sleep deprivation	3	1	13	6	4	3
Dreams	4	6	6	5	5	4
Biorhythms	**	**	**	4	5	4
Others	19	25	18	21	18	16
N/year	50	100	450	650	1500	2066

*Separate coding introduced in 1973.
**Not coded.

more particular, there was the identification of a 'third state' within sleep. There were periods of activation during sleep, in both humans and animals, which, in humans, was closely associated with dreaming.

Table 1 displays the distribution of published articles by sub-areas across selected five year periods. Clearly, the search for physiological mechanisms and correlates has constituted the centre of the effort and comprises at least a third of the research effort. Throughout the recent era, the place, role, and characteristics of 'activated' sleep within each area has been the dominant focus. For example, the increased publication rate in sleep deprivation seen in the 1963–67 period is primarily attributable to specific deprivation of this type of sleep.

One may readily infer from this table a further characteristic of the area; its interdisciplinary scope. Research and researchers are drawn from at least the following disciplines: neurosciences, neurology, physiology, biochemistry, pharmacology, endocrinology, psychiatry, clinical psychology, paediatrics, zoology, comparative psychology, psychoanalysis, and biomedical engineering. In short, it has been a stepchild of many disciplines but a favoured child of none.

Terms and Variables

Sleep is measured in three dimensions:

(1) patterns of sleep (sleep/waking relations);
(2) structures of sleep (within sleep characteristics); and
(3) subjective evaluations of sleep ('good', 'deep', etc).

Sleep patterns. The patterns of sleep are measured by sleep onset and termination and the resultant placements of sleep in time. The usual time unit is the 24 hour period. The major summary variables are total sleep time, the number and length of episodes, and the placement of sleep within the 24 hours. Thus a rat's sleep pattern would be described as averaging beteen 12 and 13 hours of total sleep time, in 120 episodes with an average length of about 6.5 minutes. The sleep occurs in a 60–40 ratio relative to a light/dark cycle. The typical young adult human would have a pattern of 7–8 hours of total sleep, a single sleep episode of about 7–8 hours and a nocturnal placement. These figures would be modifed by age, individual differences, naps, and such change variables as shift work schedules.

Sleep structure. The structure of sleep is conventionally indexed by electro-encephalographic (EEG) measures. The onset and the occurrence of sleep results in systematic changes in EEG recordings. The EEG records can be reliably, visually categorized in the 'stages', each displaying distinctive characteristics. In scoring records for stages of sleep, records are reviewed in one minute or 30 second epochs. Each epoch is scored into stages using the following criteria:

Stage 0—An epoch 50% of which shows 8–12 cps (alpha) activity with a minimum amplitude of 40 microvolts (μV) (peak to peak). This is waking, resting, eyes-closed state in an alpha dominant subject.

Stage 1—An epoch containing less than 50% 8–12 cps of 40 μV activity, and no more than one well defined spindle or K-complex (below). This is a low voltage desynchronized record.

Stage 2—An epoch with at least two well defined 'sleep spindles' brief 12–14 cps activity (circa 2 sec), or two K-complexes (sharp spontaneous rises with a slow descent), or one of each.

Stage 3—An epoch containing at least 20% but not more than 50% 0.5–3 cps activity of at least 40 μV (microvolts) amplitude.

Stage 4—An epoch containing at least 50% of 0.5–3 cps waves which are 40 μV or higher in amplitude. Stages 3 and 4 are often designated slow wave sleep (SWS).

Stage REM—An epoch of stage 1 plus evidence of conjugate rapid eye movements (REMS).

Figure 1 schematically presents the various sleep stages described above.

These data can be indexed in a large number of ways for a given sleep period or group of such periods. Major components of analysis are:

(1) Total sleep time (sleep onset to termination);
(2) sleep latency (time from 'lights out' to sleep onset);
(3) awake time (awake time within total sleep);
(4) stage totals (percentage or absolute time of individual sleep stages);
(5) stage changes (number of stage events or number of individual stages);
(6) temporal distributions (stage latencies, stage lengths, interstage intervals, per hour distribution of stages).

Subjective measures. Self-reports about sleep may be obtained from question-naires ('How long do you usually sleep?') or in a sleep 'diary' form ('When did you go to bed—When did you get up?'). The questions may be qualitative ('Was your sleep restful?') or quantitative ('How long does it take you to get to sleep?'). The responses may range from open ended ('Tell me about your sleep') to Likert-type scales ('Rate your motility on a scale from 1 to 7').

These measures have the usual difficulties associated with subjective measures. While they add a rich and vital dimension to the sleep process, their reliability and validity hinge heavily on the form of the question, the accessibility of the information to the subject, and modulator variables such as personality, mood, and willingness to respond. For example, the question, 'How many

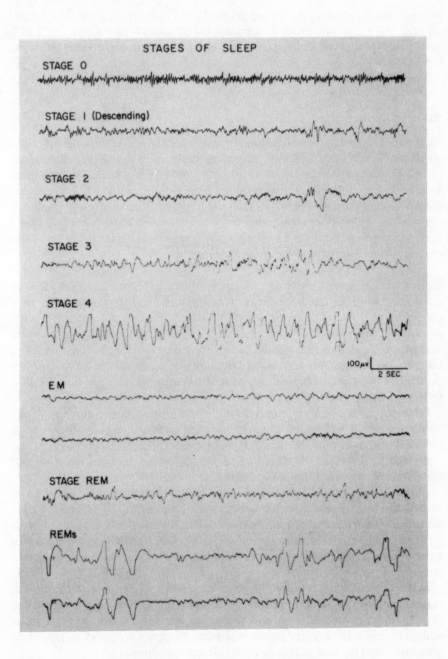

Figure 1   Schematic characteristics of the electroencephalographic stages of sleep. EM, eye movement recordings for stages 0 through 4; REM, rapid eye movement recordings

minutes does it usually take you to get to sleep?' is different from 'How many minutes did it take you to get to sleep last night?', and both differ from 'Did it take you a longer or shorter time to get to sleep last night than the night before?'

The special area of dream content requires subjective responses.

Research Methodology

Contemporary sleep research has focused on the EEG criteria of sleep structure. These measures have served as both independent and dependent measures. EEG variations in sleep structure have been studied as dependent variables, e.g. the effects of presleep exercise on sleep EEG measures. Deprivation of various stages and their effect on performance are examples of sleep as an independent variable. In addition, there have been studies of concomitant variations of behaviour, physiological and electrophysiological measures associated with the presence of sleep.

Sleep as a dependent variable. As noted above in Table 1, a considerable portion of research has been concerned with the neurophysiological control mechanisms of sleep and particular emphasis has been given to the 'activated' or REM sleep phase. The experimental methods have been the classical extirpation and electrical stimulation procedures and, more recently, biochemical stimulation and assays. In addition, much of the work has been descriptive or correlative in nature, such as single nerve cell activity in relation to sleep, waking, and sleep stages.

Because of substantial commercial and therapeutic interests, the pharmacological studies of sleep have been extensive. These studies have included studies of pharmacological effects on sleep latencies, awakening, and sleep length, as well as the effects of various drugs on the sleep structure and the effects of drug withdrawal on sleep.

Large differences in both sleep patterns and sleep structure are apparent in association with age and between species. These data and effects of time schedules on sleep are reviewed in Chapter IV.

The presleep environment, as well as behavioural variations prior to sleep, have been less widely investigated, although such variables as exercise and stress have received attention.

Increasing emphasis has been given to the relationship between pathological states such as physical illnesses, psychopathology, and sleep variations. Studies of insomnia and sleep disorders such as sleep apnoea, hypersomnia, and narcolepsy have been considered both as dependent and independent variables. That is, their causes and their effects are considered.

Concomitant relations. These studies measure and compare variations in a wide range of redundant and psychological conditions in the presence of sleep. Such studies constitute a primary overlap between sleep research and biological rhythm research. For example, variations of endocrine output and temperature during sleep have been extensively measured. A recent emphasis has been in the interactive effects on other physiological systems such as the pulmonary system and its role in sleep apnoeas.

Of particular import for this book are the effects of sleep *per se* on aspects of behaviour which fall in the performance domain. Chapter VIII reviews performance variations in the presence of sleep in the areas of sensory perception, adaptation, and learning.

Sleep as an independent variable. In these studies, variations in sleep are considered as modifier variables. In essence, sleep may be varied by its presence or absence, its structural components, or variations in the scheduling of sleep. These latter involve variations of prior wakefulness, length of sleep, and placement of sleep.

Certainly, the variation which has been studied over the longest time span is the absence of sleep or sleep deprivation. The relations of total and partial deprivation of sleep to performance are reviewed in Chapter V.

In 1960 the REM deprivation design was introduced. This involved the selective deprivation of this stage by awakenings at REM onset, with opportunities to continue all other sleep stages. Selective deprivation of REM and other sleep stages have studied effects on subsequent performance variables such as recall, acquisition, and motivation. These studies of selective deprivation are reviewed in Chapter VI.

While Chapter IV explores the effects of variations in time schedules of sleep on sleep *per se*, the effects of variations in timing of sleep on performance measures are reviewed in Chapter VII. These have centred on the shiftwork or jet lag studies, and, in addition, include non-circadian sleep/wake schedules.

The Search for Determinants

As noted in Table 1, a substantial portion of sleep research has been concerned with the search for the internal determinants of the presence or absence of sleep, i.e. the central nervous system as an independent variable. This has been a search for the efficient or proximal 'cause' of sleep—the sleep 'centre' or sleep 'button'. The attributions have been various and many, extending from a cooling of 'vapours' (Aristotle) or 'blood' (Hippocrates) to the current biochemical attributes of the monoamines and, more recently, peptides. Hypnotoxins have been posited (Kleitman lists some 18) and there has been a plethora of central nervous system inhibitory theories. It has been increasingly clear that the sleep system is unlikely to yield to a single and simple 'centre' concept.

The research continues apace. Two somewhat dated but remarkably comprehensive reviews are found in *Reviews of Physiology*, Volume 64 (Jouvet and Moruzzi, 1972). This volume is entitled 'Neurophysiology and neurochemistry of sleep and wakefulness': and is written by two of the giants of the research area—Giuseppe Moruzzi and Michel Jouvet respectively. More recent reviews are by Morgane and Sterne (1974) on the neurochemistry of sleep systems and McGinty, Harper, and Fairbanks (1974) on the neurophysiology of sleep. An historical approach and overview may be found in Webb (1973).

Relevant Readings

For more extended background information about sleep a number of resources can be recommended:

Chase, M. and Walter, P. (1970–80). *Sleep Research*, Vol. 1–8. Los Angeles, Brain Research Institute. This is an annual bibliography of the sleep research literature, a KWIK and author index and the abstracts from the Association for the Psychophysiological Study of Sleep meetings.

Webb, W. B. (1975). *Sleep, the Gentle Tyrant*. New Jersey, Prentice-Hall. This is a general and non-technical presentation about sleep and dreams.

Webb, W. B. and Cartwright, R. D. (1978). *Annual Review of Psychology: Sleep and dreams*. This is a summary of research on sleep and dreams.

Williams, R. and Karacan, I. (1978). *Sleep Disorders*. New York, John Wiley. This is an up-to-date review of the sleep disorder area.

BIOLOGICAL RHYTHM RESEARCH

Background

Like observations about sleep, the synchrony of behaviour and physiology with time extends into the history of man. The seasons, the moon phases, and the tides, the daily beat of night and day have formed the rhythmic warp of existence in gathering of plant and animal foods and movement across space. However, organized and systematic research on the biological synchrony within the organism relative to time is a recent development.

Systematic observations of rhythmic responses, independent of environmental determinants, began to emerge in the eighteenth century. For example, de Mairan, a Dutch astronomer, reported in 1724 a regular pattern of leaf movement in a constant environment. From at least this point can be traced a spreading of discovery of persistent rhythms which were apparently internally determined.

However, like sleep research, the emergence of an organized research discipline and an intensive growth period is of recent origin. While the Society for Biological Rhythms was organized in 1937, the late 1950s and 1960s can be identified as the period of contemporary vigorous growth of biological rhythm research into a discipline. A few landmarks of this beginning were the publication by Harker in 1958 of *The Physiology of Diurnal Rhythms*, the introduction by Halberg in 1959 of the term 'circadian rhythm' and, in 1960, a major international symposium on biological rhythms (Cold Spring Harbor).

From this point the pace quickened. Between 1960 and 1970 major books on biological rhythms by Bunning, Cloudsley-Thompson, Reinberg, and Gata, Richter and Sollenberger appeared. Two journals were founded in 1970 and 1973. A sharp and steady increase in the articles has occurred. In short, both sleep research and biological rhythm research can be viewed as newly developed disciplinary areas.

The areas share another characteristic: their interdisciplinary character. It was noted that sleep research reflects a broad range of disciplines. In this area one finds biologists, botanists, endocrinologists, biochemists, microbiologists, physiologists, neurologists, gynaecologists, pharmacologists, ethologists, comparative psychologists, aerospace physicians among a group of other disciplines. While drawing more heavily from the biological field, one can also say that, like sleep research, it has emerged from many disciplines but has found centrality in none.

There is a further similarity between these research efforts that is shared with sleep research—a heavy emphasis on the search for mechanisms. In biological rhythm research this is metaphorically described as 'the clock and the hands', where the 'hands' are considered the measured manifestation of the rhythm and the 'clock' as the underlying timing system. The analogy in sleep research is the search for the 'sleep centre'.

Terms and Variables

A biological rhythm can be described as a measurable change in a biological event which displays a tendency to reoccur in a systematic time schedule. This is complicated, however, by noting that such temporally ordered changes occur as a function of:

(1) systematic, timed changes in the external environment, e.g. light, temperature, and learned signals;
(2) homoeostatic systems in which a depletion (or excess) results in a counter response, e.g. eating or drinking; or
(3) internal or endogenous timing systems, e.g. bird migration or the oestrus cycle.

It is clear that the third category gets at the core meaning of a biological rhythm. As we shall see, biological rhythm research involves not only defining the presence of timed change but the establishment of the change as a function of endogenous temporal control.

The terms used to describe the characteristics of the change in time have been frequently drawn from mathematics and engineering. The detailed procedures for defining these parameters as well as the core definitions of the designated terms are considered in Chapter II.

A few of the terms help to specify the nature of the enterprise. The *cycle* and *period* refer to the time interval between a designated point in the reoccurring variable being measured. The *phase* of a rhythm is designated at a real time point, e.g., 12 noon or 12 midnight and the *acrophase* is the point where the rhythm is maximum. The term phase is a crucial one since rhythm may be in or out of phase, e.g. occurring or not occurring at the same time interval. A *phase shift* refers to the change of variable in its time of occurrence.

A few other frequently used terms are in order. *Exogenous* is used to refer to environmentally determined timing variables and *endogenous* to refer to the intraorganismic timing systems. Time cues, either internal or external, are called *synchronizers* or *Zeitgebers* (time givers), a term introduced by Aschoff (1981). The demonstrated relationship between a biological change and a Zeitgeber is called *entrainment*. This term does not imply a causal relationship since, for example, activity may proceed or lag behind actual light changes.

The term *circadian* was introduced by Halberg to identify those rhythms that approximate a 24 hour period; circa (about) and dies (day). The term *ultradian* is used to refer to periods shorter than circadian, and *infradian* for those which are longer, despite their apparent inappropriateness.

Research Issues

Problems and procedures of chronobiology involve:

(1) the establishment of a recurring temporal order for a biological variable;
(2) the relations to or absence of correlates external (exogenous) to the organism; and
(3) the determination of internal (endogenous) determinant variables.

The presence of rhythms. The particular variables studied in biological rhythms have ranged extensively. An illustrative listing includes migrations, spawning, hibernation, mortality rates, time estimates, sensory–motor responses, accidents, drug susceptibility, activity levels, sleep, moods, menstruation, leaf movements, insect pupation, temperature, gonadal changes, cardiovascular response, endocrine responses, metabolism, mitosis, and cellular responses. In short, any biosystem which exhibits measurable change properties holds potential as a variable.

The time scales also have shown a wide range. The more obvious infradian rhythms are annual (e.g. hibernation), seasonal (e.g. migration) or circalunar (e.g. tidal and menstrual). The circadian rhythm includes not only the 24 hour period but also the free running (time-free) rhythms which may be somewhat longer or shorter than 24 hours (below). The ultradian rhythms include the 'basic rest/activity cycle' (circa 90 min) as well as such short responses as single nerve cell firing.

Given the variable of interest and the possible temporal interval being exhibited by that variable, the first step is to establish the presence of a temporal order in the data. There are two general procedures of data collection. In the *transverse* method measures are taken across a fixed time span on independent subjects. For example, temperature measures may be taken at six selected times across a 24 hour period for a number of subjects. An alternative is the *longitudinal* method in which repeated measures on a single subject are obtained in repeated time intervals.

Clearly, the number of observations required and the time points of measurement are sharply dependent upon the amplitude differences in the functions, the frequency characteristics present, and the complexities of the wave forms resulting from 'noise', i.e. the components of the wave forms (number and interdependence and stationary character). Consider here the difference between the problems of migratory times and some such continuously changing variable as metabolism or endocrine secretions.

At the heart of biological rhythm research has been a continuous concern with the development and application of methods of 'microscopic' analyses of its time ordered data. Indeed, it is commonplace to begin consideration of biological rhythms with methodological reviews because these procedures often are not familiar to the performance and sleep research workers. Such a review of analytical techniques is given in Chapter II.

Endogenous and exogenous determinants. The defined presence of a timed sequence of a biological event, of course, does not define the timing source of the rhythm displayed. Such timing sources may be time cues external to the organism or time sources contained with the organism. Further, an endogenous system may be entrained or coordinate with external Zeitgebers. The determination of these relationships constitutes the essential research of this area.

Before outlining the general strategy of this process it is important to emphasize a distinction between this model of response determination and other classical concepts of response variation. The nature of biological systems requires that they show changes in time. In the realm of behaviour or performance, five major sources of behaviour change generally cited are:

(1) reflex responses: these are responses which are patterned and inherent in the organism in response to distinct stimuli such as salivation, pupillary responses to light or withdrawal responses to pain. These are also identified as unconditioned responses.

(2) instinctive responses: these are complex patterns of inherently determined responses which are 'released' by specific environmental cues.

(3) learned responses: these are responses which have been systematically associated with cue and reinforcement histories.

(4) Homoeostatic responses: these are responses which are associated with the maintenance of a constant state, such as blood sugar, oxygen levels, or hunger and thirst.

(5) maturation or development changes: these are response changes which are identified with growth or aging. These generally involve the development of capacities (or incapacities) to respond, such as walking, talking, sexual reproduction, etc.

All of these may show time characteristics. Further, their relations to exogenous and endogenous control variables are different. The time order of the first three (reflex, instinctive, and learned) are directly a function of the time sequence of the environmental variables. The latter two (homoeostatic and maturation) are endogenously controlled mechanisms but may be organized in a time sequence.

The biological rhythm model differs from these. Although the other response determinants may modulate or even override biological rhythms, these are conceived of as endogenous, inherent systems whose sole phase determination is the passage of time *per se*. Simply, a mature organism in a physiologically 'balance' (homoeostatic) state in a constant stimulus environment would, in a biological rhythm model, continue to display a rhythmic response at repeated time points.

Prime examples of biological rhythms can be readily cited: animal migration patterns, hibernation, ovulation, the rise and fall of body temperature, various haematological and endocrine rhythms, and wheel running. Variation in these have all been demonstrated in presumably constant environments and stable energy conditions.

There are grey areas of overlap and competitive explanations among the models. For example, single event changes, such as moulting and pupation, lend themselves to 'maturational' explanations. Yet, more difficult to clearly differentiate between are homoeostatic systems and biorhythmic systems, since in a constant environment 'loss–recovery' systems may be organized in repetitive time schedules. Thus it is argued that systems as diverse as sleep or refractory periods in nerve cell responses are 'depletion–recovery' periods. (see Chapter IV). Relative to external stimulus control, Brown has urged that biological rhythms in presumably constant environments are 'evoked' by unrecognized geophysical variables (1977). 'Hard core' behaviourists would argue that most behavioural responses are best understood as learned adaptive habit in response to regularly occurring environmental cues. Thus sleep may be considered a learned adaptive system in response to changing cues of light and dark or 'fatigue' precursors.

Research Methods

As noted, the initial requirement in biological rhythm research is the establishment of the presence of a rhythmic event. The purpose is to establish a measurable association between the variable of interest, e.g. glandular secretion rate, migratory tendencies, performance efficiency, sleep or activity onset, and a time period. Simply, at the same time period (either across subjects or repeatedly within subjects) does an identifiable or measurable difference occur? This can be called the *identification* design.

However, the critical task for the biological rhythm researcher is to determine whether this variation is under the control of time *per se*. To this end three major experimental designs have been developed.

'Time-free' designs. In this design an effort is made to eliminate all environmental cues of time by holding such cues constant. For example, light, temperature, and noise levels are kept at a constant level across the 24 hours. If the change in a variable is maintained in a systematic schedule a strong case may be made for an endogenous timing system.

Desynchronous designs. In this design the environmental cues are arranged in a time sequence different from that in which the change variable appears. Assume that the change is in a circadian, or approximate 24 hour sequence. These experiments would then order the primary environmental or exogenous time cues in an other-than-24 hour sequence. For example, for lower animals, the light/dark sequence may be modified to an 18 hour schedule of light and dark; with human subjects, isolated from time cues, clocks may be modified to display 18 hours in 24 hours of real time. In these modified schedules, if a sequence continued on a 24 hour rhythm, an endogenous system could be readily inferred.

Phase change designs. In these designs a presumed exogenous determinant of the change variable is 'changed' in the time schedule. There are three sub-variations in this paradigm. These may be illustrated with sleep as the phase change variable. In the 'mimic' design sleep behaviour may be introduced into or across the waking period by bed rest. In the 'deletion' design, sleep may be replaced in part or totally by continued waking behaviour. In the 'displacement' design the time period of sleep may be shifted to another period within the 24 hour sequence. These designs are shown schematically in Figure 2.

The purpose of the phase shift design is clear. If the change variable immediately 'tracks', i.e. remains entrained to the shifted variable, in the

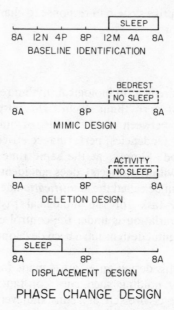

PHASE CHANGE DESIGN

Figure 2   The various phase change designs in biological rhythm research with sleep as
a variable of change. A = a.m.; p = p.m.; N = noon; M = midnight

'mimic' or the 'displaced' designs, or fails to vary in the 'deletion' design, an exogenous control may be inferred. If, on the other hand, there is a continuation of the change in the time sequence an endogenous component is a reasonable assumption.

Particular strengths of these phase shift designs are that the role of a particular determinant is tested and, further, the time sequence of readaptation or 're-entrainment' may be studied.

The application of these designs has been extensive, and detailed reviews of these studies can be found in the books and reviews cited at the end of this section. An overall perspective is presented in Figure 2 of Chapter II. This figure classifies the papers published in the two chronobiological journals. Using roughly the designs described here we can see that, after subtracting the non-experimental categories ('theoretical', 'methodological', and 'other'), of the remaining 81% of articles some 37% of the articles can be classified as 'identification' experiments (circadian detection). Without doubt a substantial, if not majority, number of the 'infradian and ultradian' designs also fall within this matrix.

The Search for Determinants

As with sleep research, a significant portion of biological rhythm research has focused on attempts to determine the underlying control mechanisms of established rhythms. These attempts are often metaphorically described as the search for the 'clock' (in contrast to the observation of the 'hand' or the observed rhythm).

Assuming the research has indicated that the 'clock' is endogenous, there are then three general approaches. The first is the search for phase relationships between rhythms. If precise phase relationships are noted between two or more rhythms one may infer a common clock system. If there is a precedent of one in relation to another in time, one may infer that one served as the 'trigger', or timer, for the other. In this procedure the phase shift experiments are particularly crucial. In these experiments presumably coordinate rhythms may shift or be re-entrained at different rates. For example, sodium excretion and potassium excretion show a close linkage in a stable rhythmic environment but show marked differences in re-entrainment to phase shift schedules.

The second procedure is the more classical 'intrusive' approach in which a presumed coordinative 'centre' or 'clock' is surgically (or chemically) removed or modified and the course of the rhythm is observed.

Reading

For more extended reading in this area a number of recent books can be recommended:

Aschoff, J. (Ed.) (1981). *Handbook of Behavioral Neurobiology. Vol. V. Biological Rhythms.* New York, Plenum. A complete and detailed review.

Colquhoun, W. P. (Ed.) (1971). *Biological Rhythms and Human Performance.* New York, Academic Press. An older revision focused on performance.

Conroy, R. and Mills, J. (1970). *Human Circadian Rhythms.* Baltimore, Williams and Wilkins. An excellent brief review of human circadian rhythms.

Luce, G. (1970). Biological Rhythms. In: *Psychiatry and Medicine.* Washington, D.C., National Institutes of Health, US Dept. HEW. Written at a lay level.

Saunders, D. (1977). *An Introduction to Biological Rhythms.* London, Blakie. An introductory graduate level text which emphasizes zoological findings.

PERFORMANCE RESEARCH

Background

Certain landmarks and trends in the measurement of performance can be cited. There have been four major tributaries: sensory–discriminatory performance, learned performance, mental abilities measurement, and skill performance.

The first of these, sensory based performance, falls in the general matrix of psychophysics with foundations in the early work of Weber and Fechner in the 1860s. The methodology centres on methods of stimulus presentation and measurements of effects. Learned performance focuses on changes in measured behaviour as a function of experience and can be dated from the early work of Ebbinghaus in the late 1800s using nonsense syllable learning. This area dominated psychological research in the 1930s and 1940s and included verbal learning, animal maze learning, and classical conditioning. The mental abilities area stemmed from interests in ability or capacity measurement and has clear roots in the individual differences and testing traditions initiated by Galton in the late 1800s and Binets 'intelligence' testing in the 1890s. These efforts are generally subsumed under the term psychometrics. The skills and motor performance area has a less clear background and pattern. Certainly the early works of Bryan and Harter on telegraphy performance (1896) and the laboratory experiments of Woodworth (1899) could be cited as early and noble precedents.

These broad areas have tended to develop independently and their adjunctive relations to other interests have been different. The sensory area is often related to receptor organs and the central nervous system on one hand and human engineering on the other. The mental abilities measurement has been incorporated into assessment testing for cognitive capacities and personality testing and has been extensively applied in industrial, school, and clinical settings. The learning area has focused on theoretical issues with limited application. Motor skills research has been linked closely with development in applied psychology and human engineering.

A core problem in performance measurement has been the organization of the various measures, and such efforts, initiated by Spearman in the early 1900s, have been associated with significant developments in correlational procedures and factor analysis.

Two emergent developments are apparent. During and after World War II the human factor or human engineering area emerged. This involved the study of man–machine relations involving 'man' as an 'operator' between 'machine' produced 'information' or 'display' and a response which frequently involved continuous adjustment (or 'motor skill'). This resulted in an integration of the sensory and motor skill areas. A related development was 'information processing'. While this area has generally focused on the internal processing of complex information and its utilization, the developments in this field have begun to feed back into the heretofore independent areas of sensory input and learned performance.

Unlike sleep and biological research, the performance measurement then is no newcomer. It has had a long, continuous, and complex history across the twentieth century.

A second difference is notable. Performance measurement has been, almost exclusively, the domain of a single discipline–psychology. This has advantages for developmental purposes. Although *the aims* within a discipline may have independent interests, their language tends to be common and their communications are facilitated. There is, however, a disadvantage. The transfer of developments to other disciplines such as biology or physiology is less likely, due to the insularity which results from a comfortable disciplinary boundary.

Terms and Variables

The extensity and complexities of the terms and variables which have developed over the long history of performance measurement may be recognized by the fact that this is a single volume in a ten-volume series concerned with performance.

Some of the problems of defining the various aspects of performance may be illustrated by listing some of the components involved in presenting a simple learning task. At least the following components must be considered:

    a, instructions;
    b, stimulus presentation;
    c, sensory reception;
    d, perception;
    e, memory;
    f, learning;
    g, abilities;
    h, activation;
    i, response output.

Each of these components has complex and contextually dependent interactive relations to each other component. Further, each contains a wide range of subconsiderations. The issues have merged, changed, and seen different emphases across time. For example, the term 'activation' contains the entire tangle of concepts such as attention, motivation, drive, and emotions. 'Abilities' incorporate such broad categories as intelligence and cognitive abilities, as well as narrowly focused motor skills or mathematical ability. In short, slightly modifying the term 'performance' to that of 'behaviour', one may readily recognize that the measurement, understanding, and prediction of such behaviour constitutes the history and domain of experimental psychology.

In the process of experimentation, significant advances in performance measurement have been made. The citation of a few examples should give pause to the casual measures of performance.

On the stimulus input side, under the rubric of psychophysical methods, a number of standard procedures for stimulus presentation have been developed e.g. the method of limits, the method of constant stimuli, and the method of equal appearing intervals. Rate of stimulus input, which may be measured in terms of interstimulus interval, units of information input, or time for stimulus input, have all been extensively studied relative to other aspects of the behaviour sequence, e.g. perception, learning, and retention. The reception characteristics of the various sensory systems (particularly vision and audition) alone and in combination, have been extensively evaluated.

On the response side of the continuum there is an extensive literature. Performance measures have been variously subdivided into areas. Again, the complexity of the field can be indicated by listing some of these subdivisions:

> state measures and trait measures;
> aptitudes, skill, and achievement measures;
> learning, memory, and problem solving measures;
> cognitive and motor skill measures;
> personality measures;
> sensory and perceptual measures.

These are, of course, not orthogonal dimensions nor are they exhaustive.

The range and character of particular measures is enormous. For example, a 'simple' measure of memory may involve varying times of introjection; varying interpolated events; prompted, free recall or relearning; various criteria of accuracy or speed. The selectivity of any example can be exemplified by noting that the Buros' *Handbook of Mental Abilities Tests* contains more than 1000 tests of mental abilities.

In spite of the particulars and diversities, continued confrontations with common problems have yielded generalized issues and solutions. Consider the psychometric domain and three sub-areas therein: scaling, test development and standardization and, for want of a better term, test categorization.

Scaling is concerned with degrees and kinds of differentiations. This involves both issues associated with stimulus presentations and the differentiation of the obtained responses. As noted above, the area of psychophysical methods has become highly developed relative to the presentation of discrete signals. The units of response may utilize such molar measures as supervisor ratings or latency measures in the microsecond range. The problems involved with the choice of stimulus categories, the treatment of ordinal *vs* nominal scales or corrections for skewness, and the treatment of pretest–post-test measures are examples of prominent concerns in particular designs.

The use of performance measures extends well beyond the evaluation of a particular effect of an experimental variable on individual performance. They may be used to determine an individual's status within a given population for selective or diagnostic purposes. This requires the 'standardization' of such tests on a normative population. In turn, such standardized tests may be used to determine the effect of some variable on a selected sub-sample. This permits 'cross-sectional' studies which may ask, for example, 'Does a population of workers on a night shift show reduced short term memory when administered a standardized short term memory test on the night shift?'

In addition to scaling problems, the standardization of performance measures involved three central problems: the definition of and extensive sampling from a normative population, and assessment of reliability and validity.

The development of population norms requires the careful application of sampling procedures relative to such variables as age, sex, and socioeconomic variables and a resultant careful explication of sampling characteristics and significant performance variations. The application of the tests requires strict adherence to these parameters for appropriate application. Simply, the match between the sample to which the *sample* is applied and the normative sample determines the inferences which can be made about the sample scores and the normative scores.

Reliability of test scores refer to their consistency. A reliable test is one which yields scores in which individuals are ranked in an identical or similar level from testing period to testing period. Elaborate means for assessing and improving reliability have been developed. These problems become more complex when they extend beyond presumably stable traits or achievement measures. Many measures presume variations between measurement periods. These are state variables such as moods, learned responses, or fluctuations in vigilance.

Validity refers to the presumed relationship between the measure used and the intent of the measure. In short, if a scale is purported to measure, say, 'sleepiness', does it reflect a hypothetically *true* measure of sleepiness? Since this question is at the core of effective measurement, the literature is extensive. Several of the more common approaches to validity are 'content validity', 'concurrent validity', and 'predictive validity'. The measure must be considered valid on 'common sense' grounds. If a person reports on a scale that he is 'very sleepy', he may be considered 'sleepy' (content validity). Or, if the measure agrees with other measures of 'sleepiness' taken at the same time, it is declared valid (concurrent validity). Or, if it predicts 'sleepiness' in expected circumstances, such as sleep deprivation, predictive validity is considered established.

Psychometric methods have long struggled with the problems of systematically organizing or categorizing behavioural measures. As noted earlier, the possibilities of measuring performance are limited only by the ingenuity and imagination of the experimenter. While not infinite, human curiosity is nearly boundless. The problem then becomes one of organizing these wide ranging measures. Fundamentally, the issue is, 'What goes with what' and the basic procedures of approach have generally emerged from correlational procedures. At the experimental level, these have involved the use of multiple and partial correlations. The more complex levels of organizing a number of measures have resulted in elaborate developments in factor analysis and discriminant function procedures.

Finally, research in performance measurement has been the fertile soil for ever-increasing sophistication in experimental designs and statistical inference. Experimental designs and statistics are applied to specific empirical events. As the philosopher, Feigl, said of philosophy of science, abstract rules must sell their 'birthrights' for a 'pot of messages'. Each book in experimental design and statistics, in fact, contains a catalogue of lessons derived from performance measurement.

Research Methods

Performance research involves three general aspects: the selection of performance measures, experimental control, and data analyses.

The selection of performance measures naturally is dictated by the purpose of the measurement. Two of the more general purposes are application to solutions of practical behaviour problems or hypothesis testing. Typical of the former would be the effect of a shift work regime on performance. An example of the latter would be the effect of REM sleep deprivation on memory consolidation.

In the applied experiment, three general strategies are available, measurements of the specific tasks required in work performance, a dimensionalized battery, or task sensitive measures. The first two strategies would employ a job analysis of the work production requirements. Then, one may choose to develop measures to measure specific work aspects of the particular job, usually in the work setting. In a classical Swedish study of shift work effects on telephone operators, the number of errors in completing telephone connections and their latencies were obtained. An alternative would be to select standardized reaction time or short term memory tasks, or some other general requirements of the task. The third alternative would be to select tests which have been shown to be sensitive to the independent variable. In a shift worker study, for example, one may choose a vigilance task which has been shown to be sensitive to sleep loss or sleep variations.

Hypothesis testing is specifically directed by the presumed effect. The dependent variable of performance is selected to permit inferences about the effect of an independent variable on a specifically hypothesized performance variation. For example, one may hypothesize an effect of REM deprivation on short term memory. In such an experiment then, one would select a short term memory task to be used in the presence of REM deprivation.

Experimental control involves effective input of the independent variables, the accurate measurement of the dependent variables and elimination of measurement of concomitant 'extra' determinative variables. The purpose of the experiment often determines the context of the measurement which, in turn, imposes limits and problems of measurement. At one extreme are 'real life' or field studies in work settings and, at the other, laboratory settings. In the former, control of the independent variable and covariables is more often limited and measurement of the dependent variable often difficult. For control, one must often resort to statistical, in contrast to experimental control (see Chapter VII).

A core problem inherent in performance measurement needs noting. Performance measures are 'outcome' variables and the measured behaviours reflect a complex of subcomponents of 'motivation', 'capacity', 'individual differences', and 'learning'. If, for example, there is a decrement in performance, say, a reduction in number of additions in one half hour after a given period of sleep deprivation, the degree to which change is a function of an inability to perform, a change in willingness, or 'offsetting' degrees of learning are problems for resolution by analysis and design procedures. These problems are given more elaborate treatment in Chapter III.

The interactions of performance measurement with the area of biological rhythms and sleep has added unique and severe complexities to the problems of measurement. These are treated in detail in Chapters II, III, and VII. For illustrative purposes consider three emergent problems: repeated measurement, sleep period measurement, and *the* course of a performance rhythm.

By its design, the longitudinal procedure used in biological rhythm research requires repeated measurement. In a simple experiment, for example, one may administer a performance test across a ten day period at two times during the day to determine if there is time of day effect. Clearly, the subject's 'motivations' and their level of 'learning' are not comparable on the first day and the tenth day. While the use of the transverse procedure can offset some of these problems, these procedures also bring their own complexities (see Chapters II and III).

The measurement of a possible rhythmic effect on performance during the subject's usual sleep period poses considerable problems. While the subject is asleep he is not available for testing. One must either resort to sleep deprivation across the sleep period or arousing the subject from sleep. Both procedures are clearly confounding (see Chapter III). One may 'avoid' these problems by shifting the sleep period to another point (the displacement design) and measure performance in the preshifted period. Indeed, this is the basic procedure of time schedule studies of 'shift work' and 'jet lag' considered in Chapter VII. However, as discussed in detail in that chapter, the adequacy of the shifted sleep, the timing of sleep, and the social and physical surround of both the new sleep period and the measurement period constitute major control problems.

The evolving research relative to the chronobiology of performance has begun to emphasize the early simplistic notion that there was *a* biological rhythm form relative to performance. This resulted in the arbitrary choice of a performance measure to establish *the* circadian rhythm. So strong was this assumption that the transfer was not only presumed across the performance domain. It was further presumed that by measuring a physiological function, such as temperature, one could thereby infer similar performance variations. Contemporary performance research has begun to emphasize the specific shape of temporal variations in performance of different tasks and the necessity to match the task to the issue at hand. This is discussed in Chapters III and VII.

INTERDISCIPLINARY RELATIONS

Problems

Interdisciplinary research is *de facto* in contemporary science. However, as a *de facto* phenomenon, it is a largely unguided process mediated by happenstances of time, place, and individually generated needs and interests. Over time, some formalization occurs by incorporation of cross-discplinary developments into texts and training programmes. These interactions are facilitated by symposia, new journals, new societies, and even centres.

In some instances this amounts to direct important of technical developments into a field. The infusions of engineering and physics into radiology or computer developments into artificial intelligence designs come to mind. In other instances, research developments in one area become foundation materials in emergent areas. Biochemistry is a clear example. Complex interdisciplinary developments such as the neurosciences, must, of necessity, include a range of disciplines from pycology to biochemistry.

This protean process has inherent problems. Stephen Leacock dramatically gave some sense of the problem:

> 'The broad field of human wisdom has been cut into a multitude of
> little professional rabbit warrens. In each of these a specialist digs
> deep, scratching out a shower of terminology, head down in an
> unlovely attitude which places an interlocutor at a grotesque
> conversational disadvantage.'

A first problem is vocabulary. Engels notes that: 'In science, each new viewpoint calls forth a revolution in nomenclature.' It is a common experience in interdisciplinary meetings or seminars to have the significant part of those events consciously or unconsciously devoted to vocabulary exchange.

The complexity of each area has created the necessity that each discipline digs deeply and busily. As a result, added extradisciplinary concerns involve new complex learning and may be viewed as a waste of valuable time relative to the work at hand.

There is a psychological problem. As a scientist enters another disciplinary area he takes on vulnerability and often must display less competence than a recent graduate student. Worse, if he attempts to achieve and maintain expertise in both areas he courts becoming a 'jack-of-two-trades' and an expert in neither.

With such dire concerns the call for enhanced interdisciplinary activity needs strong justification. Some of these are apparent.

Potential Contributions

Sleep research. Sleep research has intensively measured and extensively studied variations of the sleep process. There is substantial evidence that sleep serves as a determinant or modulator variable of both performance and biorhythmic systems. In short, it could be considered as a viable independent variable for many performances and biological rhythm variables.

In particular, sleep has a long history as an effective 'phase change' variable in chronobiological research and, further, has been shown to be a significant modulator variable for a broad spectrum of biological systems. Its continued usage is certain. Studies focused on sleep *per se* often included concomitant and informative measures of additional variables such as temperature, endocrine and other physiological measures. The transfer of these measurements and the increasingly refined measures and understanding of sleep hold rich potential for chronobiology. Relationships between the variations in the structure and patterns of sleep and performance have been established. Where such variations may be present — particularly in field settings associated with extended performance and modified work schedules — the fruits of sleep research must be incorporated into appropriate performance measures. As with chronobiology, sleep oriented studies often, within their designs, include performance measures and the findings can be used to extend our understanding of performance.

Biological rhythms. The research on biological rhythms, beyond its description of particular systems and the search for determinants of these systems, has developed both procedures of analysis and conceptual schema of significance. As noted in Chapter IV, the biological rhythm area of research has already begun to have a significant impact on sleep research. This has occurred in four particular ways.

First, there has been an increased attention to the temporal organization of the sleep process. Second, the measurement of change in sleep parameters in varied time schedules has been a substantial part of sleep research. In this instance sleep has been an independent variable among the other biological systems. In both of these instances the advanced methods of analysis developed by the biological rhythm area have been crucial. A particular intersection of these areas has been in the exploration of the potential presence of the ultradian activated sleep cycle across the 24 hours and its manifestation in the waking state. Finally, at a conceptual level, application of the biological rhythm model as a theoretical construct in which sleep is conceived of as an inherent, adaptive evolutionary derived system may serve as an alternative to homoeostatic, motivational, or acquired systems.

In the performance area it is increasingly demonstrated that time *per se* serves as a significant variable relative to a wide range of variation in performance. Furthermore, the increasingly sophisticated measurements of performances have served to emphasize and enhance our understanding of the multidetermined, independent, and complex patterns of biological rhythms. Specifically, the demonstrated dependent/independent relationships of an increasing variety of performance measures to other systems such as temperature further our comprehension of chronobiology and must be comprehensibly incorporated. As with sleep research, the sophisticated time series measure procedures are critical tools in this research.

Certainly, a minimum transfer from the biological rhythm area is the increasing awareness of time of testing as a crucial control variable to reduce 'noise' in experimental designs, when this is not a part of the experimental design.

Performance research. Performance research has elaborately considered measurement aspects inherent in such research. These involve highly sophisticated developments in presentation of stimuli, experimental controls, response measures and dimensionalizations, and data analysis procedures. Whenever performance becomes a variable of choice, these hard won developments must form the bedrock of sound experimentation in both chronobiology and in sleep research.

SUMMARY

This chapter has introduced the development and characteristics of essentially independent disciplines; sleep research, biological rhythms research or chronobiology, and performance measurement. Background, basic terminologies, and research methods have been presented. The increasing and necessary convergence of the fields is noted and the potentials for future interaction are discussed.

REFERENCES

* Aschoff, J. ed. (1981). *Handbook of Behavioral Neurobiology, Vol. V. Biological Rhythms*, New York, Plenum.
* Brown, F. A. (1977). Interrelations between biological rhythms and clocks, pp.215–234.

In: *Aging and Biological Rhythms.* H. Samis and S. Cupobianco (Eds.). New York, Plenum.

Chase, M. and Walter, P. (1970-80). *Sleep Research*, (Vol. 1-8). Los Angeles, Brain Information Services (UCLA).

Cold Spring Harbor Symposium in Quantitation Biology (1960). Long Island Biological Association, New York.

- Conroy, R. T. and Mills, J. N. (1970). *Human Circadian Rhythms.* Baltimore, Williams and Wilkins Co.

- Harker, J. E. (1958). *The Physiology of Diurnal Rhythms.* Cambridge, Cambridge University Press.

Jouvet, M. and Moruzzi, G. (1972). Neurophysiology and neurochemistry of sleep and wakefulness. *Reviews of Physiology*, Vol. 64. New York, Springer-Verlag, 357pp.

Kleitman, N. (1963). *Sleep and Wakefulness.* Chicago, University of Chicago Press.

- Luce, G. (1970). Biological rhythms. In: *Psychiatry and Medicine.* Washington, D.C., National Institutes of Health, US Dept. HEW.

McGinty, D. J., Harper, R. M., and Fairbanks, M. (1974). Neuronal unit activity and the control of sleep states. In: *Advances in Sleep Research*, Vol. I., W. D. Weitzman, (Ed.). New York, Spectrum Publications, Inc., 424pp.

Morgane, P. and Sterne, W. (1974). Chemical anatomy of brain circuits in relation to sleep and wakefulness. In: *Advances in Sleep Research*, Vol. I., W. D. Weitzman, (Ed.). New York, Spectrum Publications. Inc., 424pp.

- Saunders, D. S. (1977). *An Introduction to Biological Rhythms.* London, Blackie.

Webb, W. B. (1973). *Sleep: An Active Process.* Glenview, Ill., Scott, Foresman.

Webb, W. B. (1975). *Sleep: The Gentle Tyrant.* New Jersey, Prentice-Hall.

Webb, W. B. and Cartwright, R. D. (1978). Sleep and dreams. *Annual Rev. Psychol.* **29**, 223-252.

Williams, R. and Karacan, I. (1978). *Sleep Disorders: Diagnosis and Treatment.* New York, John Wiley, 417pp.

Biological Rhythms, Sleep and Performance
Edited by Wilse B. Webb
©1982 John Wiley & Sons Ltd.

Chapter 2

Research Methods of Chronobiology

Timothy H. Monk

The measures taken by chronobiologists have an immense range of complexity, covering everything from the concentrations of a particular ion in a leaf, to the logical reasoning efficiency of a man. Similarly, the time scale that is considered also varies enormously, ranging from heart rates with periods of under a second, to seasonal and life cycle rhythms having a period of a year or more. In short, chronobiology is concerned with almost any regular periodic fluctuation of behaviour or physiology in almost any sort of organism.

Clearly, such a universal definition of chronobiology encloses much too much for its methodology to be comprehensively covered in a single chapter. Indeed, even if it were, much of it would be of very little interest to the average reader of a book on *Biological Rhythms, Sleep, and Performance*. The present chapter will thus limit its examples to a small subset of the field of chronobiology and focus on the circadian (having a period of about 24 h) rhythms of the physiology and/or behaviour of mammals (especially man).

This limitation is not as extreme as it may initially sound. First, it coincides with the maximal area of involvement by workers in the field, covering about 85% of the papers published in the two journals *International Journal of Chronobiology* and *Chronobiologia* which are specifically dedicated to chronobiology. Second, nearly all of the research methods are equally applicable (and are indeed applied) to the areas of interest that have been excluded. Thus, in limiting the present discussion to this small subset of chronobiology, very little generality has been lost.

In writing this chapter, the author has sought to keep it comprehensible, and relevant to workers in other disciplines. It is certainly not the aim of this chapter to provide a comprehensive guide to the methodology of the area for the benefit of either chronobiologist or statistician. Although a standard work of that type is indeed sorely needed, it would clearly be out of place in the present chapter. The aim is rather to provide a helpful guide to the research method of chronobiology for those coming into the area from other disciplines, particularly those of sleep and/or human performance.

There are two compelling reasons why such a guide is necessary. First, there is a fairly pronounced schism in the area, with chronobiologists divided into two methodological 'camps'. These camps can be characterized as being either pro- or anti- the Minnesota Cosinor method (see later section), and the method recommended to any newcomer to the area will often depend radically upon which particular brand of chronobiologist he happens to run into first. Moreover, the wealth of information acquired by the other 'camp' may well be lost to him. Second, the area has spawned a bewildering variety of jargon and illustrative tools that often make the literature rather difficult to understand.

Thus in trying to steer the newcomer around all the various pitfalls, the chapter must have as its first aim the bridging of the gap between the two approaches to chronobiology. Only by accepting the validity of both views, and describing the methods used by each, can a genuinely useful guide be constructed.

Apart from the problem of bias mentioned above, there is a further reason why a reasonably comprehensible guide to the methodology is needed. With a few honourable exceptions (e.g. Orr and Naitoh, 1975), most methodological papers appear to have been written for the benefit of the statistician, rather than the experimenter, and thus tend to lurch into a mass of alarming equations at the slightest excuse. This is a symptom of the tendency in chronobiology for data to be passed on to a statistician for analysis, rather than being analysed by the researcher himself. Since the researcher is often only rather dimly aware of what the statistician is doing, and the statistician probably vague about the exact hypotheses and techniques of the researcher, this inevitably leads to some inappropriate analyses and conclusions. Thus a major aim of this chapter is to give the researcher a much clearer indication of what the various statistical techniques actually involve. Obviously, this cannot be done in any but the most superficial way without equations, but the present chapter will use them only as necessary.

BASIC TERMS AND DEFINITIONS

Chronobiology is primarily concerned with the fluctuation of some particular measure over time. Thus the basic unit of measurement is a temporal sequence of observations, with each observation indexed by the time at which it was made. This temporal sequence is referred to as a *time series*. Very often the hypothesis to be tested is that the time series exhibits some sort of predictable regularity or *periodicity*, such that after a certain interval of time the sequence of measurements or observations starts repeating itself. This periodicity is referred to as a *rhythm*. The label given to a rhythm indicates its temporal domain. Thus periodicities of less than a day are referred to as *ultradian rhythms*, of about a day as *circadian rhythms* and of more than a day as *infradian rhythms*. Infradian rhythms can be further categorized as *circaseptan* (weekly), *circatrigintan* (monthly) or *circannual* (yearly).

The rhythm that is apparent in the time series may stem either from an oscillator that is internal to the organism (in which case it is *endogenous*) or from regular fluctuations of the external environment (whence it is *exogenous*). Very often the rhythm is a mixture of the two.

Many of the statistical techniques that are used by chronobiologists have been borrowed from a field of communications engineering. Several methods are thus based on the principles of Fourier analysis, relying upon a resolution of the apparent rhythm into one or more sinusoids. The *cosinor method* relies upon fitting a single cosine curve to the time series, and is probably the most frequently used form of Fourier analysis. One particular version of this technique ('the Minnesota cosinor') has become widely used throughout the world. Strictly speaking, that method is the only one that should be called 'cosinor', but the label has also been used for other, less sophisticated, sinusoid fitting techniques. The various types of Fourier analysis in general, and the cosinor method in particular, are described in detail in later sections.

A principle aim of chronobiologists is often the characterization of the whole time series by a single rhythm of a particular periodicity, size, and shape. When such a rhythm is repeated through the time period, the aim is to have a satisfactory fit to the whole time series, i.e. acceptably small residual differences between the individual data points and the curve. The process is thus one of information reduction, so that the whole time series can be accurately described by a small number of parameters. The major parameters of a rhythm are the *period* (time between successive repetitions of the cycle), *amplitude* (half the difference between peak and trough values), and *phase* (whereabouts in time the rhythm is, in relation to a time standard). The phase is usually expressed in terms of the *acrophase* which represents the time at which the rhythm achieves its maximum. This time is usually expressed either in ordinary time units or as an *angle*. The angle measure derives from the trigonometric origins of Fourier analysis. Basically, the duration of the period of the rhythm is considered to be 360° (or 2π radians) since it is then that the cycle repeats itself. The acrophase is then expressed as so many degrees past the time reference (often midnight or half-way through the sleep period ('mid-sleep')). Thus in a 24 hour time schema, if 'midnight' is designated as 360° (or 0°), 6 a.m. (0600) is 90°, 12 noon (1200) is 180°, and 6 p.m. (1800) is 270°.

The main interest in phase derives not only from comparisons between the rhythm and the environment routine, but also between two or more rhythms that can be *in phase* (having the same acrophase) or *out of phase* with each other. The final major parameter is the *mesor* which represents the level of the curve (i.e. the 'centre line'). Note that if sampling is irregular, the mean and mesor of the time series may not be equal. The five major parameters are illustrated in Figure 1.

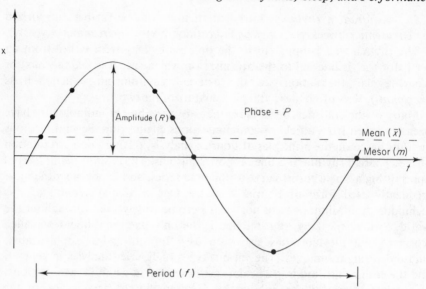

Figure 1   The five major parameters of a rhythm. Note that when sampling is irregular,
the mean and mesor may not coincide

If the whole series is to be predicted from a single cycle, it is obviously important that the rhythm is not changing either phase, shape, or amplitude as the time series progresses. Such changes are collectively referred to as *non-stationarity*. Chronobiologists generally tend to try and keep to stationary rhythms because of the enormous problems that otherwise result. Sometimes, however, the non-stationarity is the major component of interest, particularly in studies of transmeridianal flight ('jet lag') or shift work, where the organism is trying to adjust to a new set of time cues. These cues are referred to as either *synchronizers, entraining agents,* or *Zeitgeber.* They may be either *physical,* such as the timing of sunrise and sunset, or *social,* such as meal times, working routines, etc. In any case where there is an endogenous component to the rhythm, there will be an interval of non-stationarity before the rhythm adjusts to the new time schedule. This process of adjustment is referred to as *re-entrainment.* Much work has been done on the rate of re-entrainment of various rhythms, and what happens to the rhythms while re-entrainment is taking place (see Aschoff *et al.*, 1975, for a comprehensive review).

The other way that non-stationarity can be induced is by the total elimination of all Zeitgeber. This is accomplished by isolating the subject from all time cues, leaving it in permanent light or darkness. Under such conditions the circadian rhythms *free run* to a period that is often different from the 24 h that is characteristic of the world outside. In man, for example, although there are marked individual differences, the circadian rhythms often free run to a period of about 25 h. Thus the subject becomes more and more out of step with the world outside, until after about three and a half weeks he has effectively 'lost' a day. When an organism is free running, the rhythms that were previously *entrained* by the Zeitgeber to a strict 24 h routine, often start to separate out, thus indicating which oscillators, or groups of oscillators, are responsible for them. Clearly, rhythms that are free running at different periods (referred to as *internal dissociation*) cannot come from the same oscillator. Alternatively, the periods of two rhythms may still be equal, but their normal phase relation breaks down (when they are referred to as *internally desynchronized*). These aspects are discussed in more detail by Wever (1973).

The preceding discussions have assumed that the data has been collected in the form of a long time series covering several cycles of the rhythm under investigation. Such an approach can be labelled *longitudinal* in that the accuracy of estimation is enhanced by increasing the length of the experiment, rather than the number of subjects under investigation. An alternative approach is the *transverse* one, where the duration of the experiment is short (perhaps only one cycle), but the accuracy is enhanced by increasing the number of subjects under investigation.

In using the transverse approach, it is vital that the subjects comprising the sample are equivalent in rhythm amplitude and phase, if a meaningful result is to be obtained. Likewise, in the longitudinal approach, stationarity of the rhythm is important.

RESEARCH AREAS

A good metaphor for the field of chronobiology and its development is provided by likening it to a young political movement, battling for acceptance by an establishment that is intent on preserving the status quo. Initially, the movement was not persecuted, but rather ignored, with a massive indifference by an establishment convinced of its own righteousness. Later would come grudging acceptance, but often only in the form of mere 'lip-service'. Within the metaphor, the 'establishment' represents the concept of homoeostasis, which has been the bane of chronobiologists. This concept of a static self-regulatory organism has for many years dominated biological ideas to the exclusion of the regular temporal changes studied by the chronobiologist. Due mainly to the vigorous work of pioneers such as Halberg and Aschoff, physiologists have started grudgingly to accept the validity of the chronobiological cause. However, in the fields of medicine and psychology, very little ground has been made, and doctors are still largely content to adminster drugs and psychologists to run experiments without controlling for, or making use of, circadian effects.

Thus one major preoccupation of chronobiologists has been simply to demonstrate that rhythms do indeed exist, that they are predictable, and that they are not of trivial magnitude. This is the basic groundwork that must be covered before the more complex topics of entrainment and free running can be considered. Hence much of the published work has taken the form of 'There *is* a rhythm in X and these are its parameters'. Chapter I referred to this as the 'searching for the hands of the clock', i.e. finding the external, observable consequences of the oscillator in the organism.

To obtain a rough idea of how much work has been taken up with this 'searching for hands' type of activity, the author surveyed all papers that had been published in the two journals specifically dedicated to chronobiology (*The International Journal of Chronobiology* and *Chronobiologia*) since their inception. Papers were arbitrarily classified into eight groups:

A *Circadian rhythm detection.* Demonstrating a circadian rhythm in a particular measure or set of measures from a particular set of subjects or patients, and listing its parameters.
B *Drug effects.* (1) The circadian rhythm of X has this effect on the effectiveness or toxicity of drug Z; (2) the diagnosis of disease Y will depend on the circadian rhythm of X; (3) drug or disease Y will have this effect on the circadian rhythm of X.
C *Schedule effects.* (1) The effects of changing light/dark cycle, or time zone, or work pattern, on the circadian rhythm of X; (2) the effects of a constant environment on the circadian rhythm of X (free running).
D *Theoretical.* Discussions and models of the way in which various oscillators or systems of oscillators might be producing the circadian rhythmicity (or changes thereof) that are observed.
E *Methodology.* Discussing the use and validity of old statistical methods, and introducing new ones.
F *Sleep.* (1) The effects of sleep and/or sleep deprivation *per se*; (2) ultradian rhythmicity in sleep parameters.
G *Ultradian and infradian.* Any study primarily interested in an ultradian or infradian rhythm.
H *Other.* Primarily these are introductory and proselytizing articles about chronobiology.

The results of the survey are summarized in Figure 2. From this figure it is clear that, in these journals at least, studies involved in the basic groundwork of circadian rhythm demonstration (i.e. 'searching for the hands') form by far the largest category. Thus in the description of methodologies that is to follow, most emphasis will be given to the basic mechanism of discovering a rhythm, and finding out what it looks like.

The second largest category in Figure 2 (drug effects) is of clinical studies that investigate the interaction between circadian rhythms and disease and its treatment. This category broadly corresponds to the fields of chronopathology (disease/rhythm interactions) and chronopharmacology (drug/rhythm

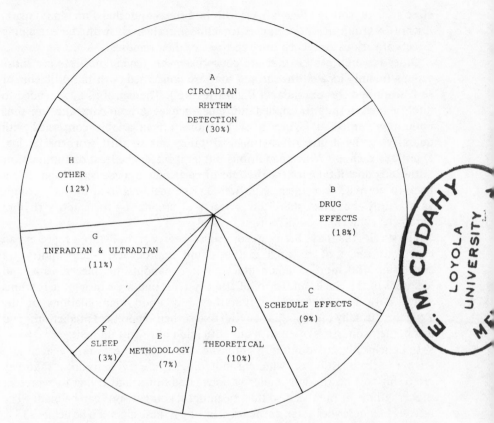

Figure 2   Percentages of papers published in the journals *Chronobiologia* and *International Journal of Chronobiology* devoted to various research questions (see text)

interactions) as defined by Halberg *et al.* (1977) in their glossary. Studies of this sort have formed a vigorous, and in many ways, distinct branch of chronobiology. The methodology of this branch has often tended to involve the simple comparison of survival or recovery rates under different treatment conditions, and thus requires comparatively little need for further description and explanation, apart from that of the basic rhythm detection methods.

The number of studies of schedule free running and re-entrainment effects (category C) is undoubtedly underestimated by this sample. In terms of actual research effort, this category is as important as category A (circadian rhythm detection). The reason for the under-representation is that the major research groups that have been concerned with such effects have been located outside the United States, and have published their work in journals other than those surveyed for Figure 2.

The most eminent of the research groups working in the field of schedule effects is, of course, that of Aschoff in Erling-Andechs. For many years, Aschoff's group has been concerned almost exclusively with the entraining effects of various Zeitgeber, and the effect of their removal.

Other research groups that are concerned with schedule effects are those groups (mainly located in Europe) that are concerned with the problems of shift work and transmeridianal flight ('jet lag'). These groups have tended to publish their results in applied journals such as *Ergonomics* and are thus under-represented in Figure 2. Such studies are invariably concerned with quantifying the degree of rhythm disruption due to shift work or jet lag. Questions such as 'Which conditions/subjects suffer the least disruption?' or 'How long does it take for the rhythms of particular subjects/conditions to get back to normal?' can then be answered. The methods used by such groups vary greatly, but most share the property of attempting to quantify rhythm parameters and changes thereof.

The studies that have been categorized as theoretical in Figure 2 represent an enormous range of research methods and approaches. Such studies are addressing the more fundamental questions about the mechanisms and locations of the clocks and/or oscillating systems that are causing the rhythms which have been observed. Often they rely upon manipulations of the Zeitgeber (usually the light/dark cycle) to test their theoretical predictions, and again, their concern is often with quantification of re-entrainment.

In conclusion, an admittedly simplistic (though not necessarily inaccurate) answer to the question of 'what chronobiologists are trying to do' is that they are trying to find rhythms under various conditions, and trying to represent these rhythms by numbers, so that meaningful comparisons can be made. The next section describes some of the ways in which these aims can be achieved.

STATISTICAL METHODS

In this section, the various statistical techniques are described and evaluated. The text follows a (hopefully) logical path from the comparatively simple 'macroscopic' techniques that give an overall impression of a rhythm, to the more complicated microscopic techniques, which are more powerful in detecting rhythms, and which provide estimates of the rhythm's parameters.

Throughout this section a consistent convention with regard to concepts and symbols has been maintained. The time series is presumed to be a set of n measurements or observations, each measurement being indexed by the time at which it was recorded. Thus x_t denotes the tth measurement to be taken, and $(x_1, x_2, \ldots x_n)$ the complete time series. When talking about the measurements themselves, the author refers to the 'x values of the time series'. When talking about the reading 'at time t', the author is actually referring to the tth observation, rather than some particular clock time represented by t.

'Eyeball' Techniques

The most obvious analytical technique is, of course, simply to look at a plot of the whole time series and pick out the maxima and minima. Known as the 'eyeball' or 'naked eye' technique (Poppel, 1975), this has been much favoured by Aschoff and his associates. The main precondition to this form of analysis is that the sampling interval is not too big, or the data too noisy, for the timings of the maxima and minima to be readily apparent. Thus, the eyeball technique is much more satisfactory when continuous records are taken (e.g. of cage activity, or of body temperature from telemetry) than when sampling is comparatively infrequent (e.g. for urinary electrolytes). In fact, if the preconditions mentioned above are fulfilled, the 'eyeball' technique is probably the best one for time series that are non-stationary (e.g. shift work, free running), since in such cases most microscopic methods can give erroneous results. The eyeball technique is, of course, almost mandatory when studying the time series of a binary valued variable (such as asleep/awake).

The usual method of displaying such data is to have each subjective day appearing below the last, with bars representing periods of activity (solid) and rest (open). The x axis consists of more than one cycle of 24 hours, to account for observed periods that are not exactly equal to 24.0 h (as, for example, in free running). The maximum and minimum of the temperature rhythm (estimated by the eyeball technique) are illustrated by upward and downward pointing triangles, respectively, and the timing of darkness represented by overall shading. An artificial example, showing dissociation between temperature and activity rhythms, is illustrated in Figure 3.

An elaboration of this technique is described by Webb and Agnew (1974) who fitted a straight line to the set of sleep onset times (left-hand end of each solid bar) using a 'least squares' procedure. This line could then be used to give a 'predicted' sleep onset time for each day. Also, its slope gave a measure of the degree to which the 'free running' rhythm differed from 24.0 hours. The slopes of different groups of individuals could then be compared using normal statistical tests (e.g. the 't' test).

Buys-Ballot Tables

The second macroscopic technique relies on an *a priori* specification of the rhythms period (e.g. 24.0 h in the circadian case). The first step is to cast the data into a 'Buys-Ballot' table (Enright, 1965; Williams and Naylor, 1978). In the circadian case, this simply involves casting the data into an $h \times m$ matrix where the m columns represent 'times of day' and the h rows 'days'. The general specification of the Buys-Ballot table is given in Table 1.

The average of each column represents the 'time of day' effect of the variable, which can be plotted to illustrate the shape and amplitude of the

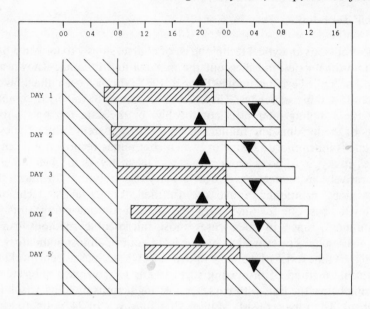

Figure 3   'Aschoff bars': artificial data to illustrate the technique. Note that the right-hand end of one bar represents the same point in time as the left-hand end of the next. See text for an explanation of the symbols

'average' rhythm. Such a plot is known as a *chronogram* or *plexogram* (for more precise definitions, see Halberg *et al.*, 1977). For convenience, all such plots will be referred to as chronograms throughout this chapter (and cosinor displays will *not* be referred to as chronograms). Clearly, the chronogram is an essential step in most macroscopic techniques, particularly that of analysis of variance (considered in the next section).

Apart from the chronogram, there is further information that can be obtained from the Buys-Ballot table. Any lack of 'goodness of fit' of the

Table 1   General form of the Buys-Ballot table

	Time of day			
	t_1	t_2	. . .	t_m
Day 1	x_1	x_2	. . .	x_m
Day 2	x_{m+1}	x_{m+2}	. . .	x_{2m}
Day 3	x_{2m+1}	x_{2m+2}	. . .	x_{3m}
.	.	.		.
.	.	.		.
.	.	.		.
Day h	$x_{(h-1)m+1}$	$x_{(h-1)m+2}$	. . .	x_{hm}
Mean	x_{t_1}	x_{t_2}	. . .	x_{t_m}

rhythm results in both a reduction in amplitude of the chronogram and an increase in the variance of the sample (column) used to estimate each point (of the chronogram). Thus a Buys-Ballot table can be cast iteratively for different lengths of period, and various measures of either variability or amplitude (Enright, 1965; Williams and Naylor, 1978) used to determine the 'goodness of fit' of that period. These measures can then be plotted against period to give a *periodogram*, the peaks of which would indicate periods with comparatively good fits.

Analysis of Variance

A main point to emerge from the above discussion is that, whatever the method, the longer the time series the better will be the accuracy of parameter estimation. However, there are many situations, particularly in psychology, where long time series are simply not feasible. The most obvious of these is human performance, where prolonged practice may either radically change the nature of the task (and thus parameters of the rhythm) or exhaust the test material. An example of the former is provided by Colquhoun (1971, p.82, Figure 9, bottom panel) who inadvertently demonstrated that the rhythm of performance efficiency at an 'additions' task can gradually change its acrophase by up to 6 hours with extended practice. Partly because long time series are too difficult or costly to obtain, and partly because of their natural statistical predilections, psychologists have tended to concentrate on analysis of variance as their major statistical tool.

In using analysis of variance, the research question being answered is very often rather different from those of the other methods being discussed. The main areas of interest are usually:

(1) Is there a consistent time (of day) effect? and
(2) Does that effect change under manipulation X?

The former is tested by the main effect of time, the latter by the interaction between time and manipulation. Thus, although the timing of the peak (acrophase) is often of importance, the main emphasis is on the shape of the chronogram (time of day function), and whether or not that changes under the experimental manipulation. Thus although confidence intervals can be constructed around the points of the chronogram, these are drawn in the dimension of the variable, rather than the time dimension.

The simplest analysis of variance design is that in which time is considered as a between subject factor. For convenience, it, and all subsequent designs, will be described in terms of time of day effects (i.e. circadian rhythms), since they are the major area of application. A 'between subject' design simply involves running a separate group of subjects at each time of day of interest. Clearly the groups must be equally matched and care must be taken to avoid self-selection (e.g. 'larks' (morning types) choosing to attend in the morning, and 'owls' in the evening). The advantages of this type of design are that it is essentially 'open ended' in that further groups can be added later on to 'fill out' the finer detail of the time of day function, that only a single version of the test material need be prepared, and that possible carry-over effects (Poulton, 1973) are avoided. The main disadvantages are in lack of power and in the large number of subjects (at least 15 per group) that are consequently required. In the detection of time of day effects, power is an important attribute, since as Gale, Harpham, and Lucas (1972) remark, 'It would appear that (time of day) effects are delicate plants which flourish only under certain critical conditions' (p.270).

The experimental design becomes more complicated when the more powerful within subjects design is employed. Each subject attends at every time of day, and the main problem is to ensure that any apparent time of day effects are not contaminated by simple improvements due to practice, or differences in test material. Thus, if one was testing at 0900, 1500, and 2100, for example, it would be pointless merely testing everyone in that order, since improvements due to practice would produce a spurious peak at 2100. Ideally, every one of the six possible orderings of testing time should be used, with a different group of subjects having each and each group being tested only once per day. This, however, gets unmanageable when more than three testing times are considered (for six testing times, for example, 720 groups would be required).

To avoid this problem, the latin square is used. This ensures that each time of day has a session from each level of practice, and that possible contamination from 'carry-over' effects is minimized, whilst still only requiring k groups of subjects, where k is the number of times of day studied.

A useful version of the latin square technique is the 'rolling latin square' described in detail by Folkard (1975). In this design a 'staggered start' reduces the number of testing days. An example of how the design would be used to study six times of day is given in Table 2. In this design, 'groups' is taken out as a 'between subject' factor, thus reducing the error variance.

The main problem associated with any analysis of variance techniques is that it takes no account of any 'well orderedness' of the time of day function. Thus, as far as the significance of the time of day effect is concerned, a sensible, well ordered time of day effect is no more likely to be significant than a wildly erratic one. This is illustrated by Figure 4, where both functions would have identical F ratios (and thus levels of significance) for the time of day effect, because function B is simply a permutation of the points defining function A.

Analysis of variance is thus a rather conservative (i.e. weak) test of whether reliable time of day effects are present. Paradoxically, it also becomes weaker the more times of day there are being considered. Thus, given that one has a fixed number of subjects to work with and is not too unlucky with choice of

Table 2   Example of how a rolling latin square design might be used to measure performance at six different times of day. The subscript to each time tabulated denotes either the 1st or 2nd day of testing for that group

	\multicolumn{6}{c}{Testing session}
	1st	2nd	3rd	4th	5th	6th
Group 1	0800_1	1100_1	1400_1	1700_1	2000_1	2300_1
Group 2	1100_1	1400_1	1700_1	2000_1	2300_1	0800_2
Group 3	1400_1	1700_1	2000_1	2300_{11}	0800_2	1100_2
Group 4	1700_1	2000_1	2300_1	0800_2	1100_2	1400_2
Group 5	2000_1	2300_1	0800_2	1100_2	1400_2	1700_2
Group 6	2300_1	0800_2	1100_2	1400_2	1700_2	2000_2

testing times, one is more likely to obtain a statistically significant time of day effect with two times of day than with six. Since statistical significance continues to be the criterion for publishing acceptability, there is consequently a dearth of studies in the psychological literature that have tested at more than two times of day. One solution to this problem would be to test the significance of linear and/or quadratic trends in the data. However, unless the trend can be specified on *a priori* grounds, a significant trend without a significant main effect (of time of day) is of dubious statistical validity.

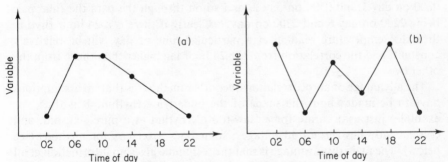

Figure 4   Artificial example to show how two very different time of day functions (A and B) can have an identical *F* ratio, and thus significance of the time of day effect, when tested by analysis of variance

From the above discussion it is clear that analysis of variance techniques are primarily of advantage when the study is transverse (i.e. many subjects but few days) rather than longitudinal (i.e. few subjects but many days). There is, though, no reason why analysis of variance cannot be used in the longitudinal case, with 'replications' (i.e. days) replacing 'subjects' as the variable associated with the error term.

Autocorrelational Techniques

The essence of autocorrelation is that a rhythm is something that repeats itself after a given period of time. Thus if one finds (or happens upon) that period of time, and correlates the time series with a duly delayed version of itself, a perfect ($+1$) correlation will result. The technique thus involves trying out various delays or *lags*, and in calculating the appropriate correlation of the time series with itself for each lag. The values so calculated can then be plotted against lag to give an *autocorrelogram* which is analogous to the power spectrum described later.

The underlying mechanism of the technique is most easily explained by an example taken from a circadian rhythm study. Suppose a measure (say temperature) is taken every hour around the clock for a week, and that lags of 23, 24, and 25 hours are to be considered (though usually, of course, many more days and lags would be considered). The lag of 23 hours would be equivalent to evaluating a 23 hours periodicity in the data. The pairs contributing to this correlation would be the temperatures at 0000 with 2300 on day 1, 0100 on day 1 with 0000 on day 2, 0200 on day 1 with 0100 on day 2, 0300 on day 1 with 0200 on day 2, and so on all the way through the data (the final pair being 0000 on day 7 with 2300 on day 7). For the 24 hour lag the correlation pairs would be 0000 on days 1 and 2, 0100 on days 1 and 2, 0200 on days 1 and 2, and so on through the data (the final pair being 2300 on days 6 and 7) with a total of $24 \times 6 = 144$ pairs in all. For the 25 hour lag, the pairs would be 0000 on day 1 and 0100 on day 2, 0100 on day 1 and 0200 on day 2, 0200 on day 1 and 0300 on day 2, and so on through the data the final pair being 2200 on day 6 and 2300 on day 7. Clearly if there *is* a 24 hour rhythm then the temperature reading at a particular time of day will be relatively constant, and the correlation from the 24 hour lag higher than those from the other two.

The advantage of autocorrelation over other methods is that no assumptions have to be made about the shape of the underlying rhythm. It is thus, for example, just as accurate for a 'saw-tooth' rhythm as a pure sinusoid, and consequently has certain advantages, sometimes, over cosinor methods (see below). The main disadvantage is that the technique gives no information at all about phase, and only relative information about amplitude. It also requires equally spaced samples, and prefers comparatively long time series.

The autocorrelogram can either be used as an end in itself, or considered merely as a 'cleaning up' step, which enhances any periodic components and gets them into phase with each other before a Fourier (harmonic) analysis (see below) is applied. To that end the autocorrelogram is ideal, since the auto-correlogram of a sinusoidal trace remains sinusoidal, with its amplitude decreasing with increased noise, and except for changes in vertical scale, the autocorrelogram of the sum of two unrelated rhythms is often equal to the autocorrelogram of their sum (Walter, 1963, p.158).

The mathematics of the technique are very simple. The first stage of analysis is the transformation of the time series so that it is centred on zero. This is simply accomplished by subtracting the mean of the whole time series from each point. If no other normalization takes place, the technique is known as *autocovariance* (otherwise following identical procedures). Autocorrelation is, in fact, a special case of autocovariance in which each point is further transformed by dividing it by the standard deviation of the time series. Thus in autocorrelation, both 'level' and 'spread' are standardized.

The *autocorrelation* at a particular lag (say L) is then simply the averaged product of pairs of terms. Thus one multiplies each term in the time series by the term that is L items after it in the time series, and takes the average of all the products that one gets. (The *autocovariance* is similarly defined.)

Values of the autocorrelation at particular lags can then be plotted against lag, to give the autocorrelogram, which can then either be used to indicate lags (and hence periodicities) of interest, or passed on for further analysis to give the power spectrum.

Many of the data manipulation techniques described in later sections for ensuring a good spectrum are also used in autocorrelational analysis; another is that of *prewhitening*. Prewhitening simply involves smoothing out sequential dependencies in the data to make the resultant spectrum less erratic (i.e. 'white', using the analogy of the colour spectrum). A technique often employed (e.g. Dixon, 1976) is to add or subtract a certain proportion of the adjacent points in the time series. If such a transformation is applied, the resulting power spectrum has to be *recoloured* by applying a duly transformed inverse of the prewhitening function.

Clearly, the technique of autocorrelation can be as complex or as simple as the researcher wants to make it. If searching for a periodicity in a comparatively noise-free time series, autocorrelation can provide a simple method that does not rely on specifying a particular shape of rhythm. Alternatively, the technique can be applied in a fairly sophisticated way in conjunction with Fourier analysis (see below) in order to look for rather more hidden periodicities. A further use of autocorrelational techniques is in searching for mutual periodic dependencies between different time series. These procedures involve calculating the cross-correlation between two time series in addition to further, more detailed, measures. They will not, however, be considered here; the interested reader is referred to Orr and Naitoh (1975) and Walter (1963).

General Fourier Analysis

Fourier analysis is a widely used technique in science and engineering which has been adopted by the chronobiologist. Its basic unit of operation is the *sinusoid*. The sinusoid is merely the graph that one gets when one takes the cosine (or sine) of a set of increasing values, plotting the cosine on the 'y axis' and the increasing values on the 'x axis'. In a time series the time values are, by definition, increasing, and it is thus possible to take the cosine of these time values and get a sinusoid.

As Bloomfield (1976) points out in his introduction, Fourier analysis has both broad and narrow definitions. In its narrowest sense, Fourier analysis is the complete decomposition of a time series into the sum of a set of sinusoids. These sinusoids specify the time series, and their parameters form its *discrete Fourier transform*. In a wider sense, the term can be used to describe any analytical technique that relies upon quantifying or estimating the time series by resolving it into one or more sinusoids. It is this second, broader, definition that is adopted here.

Since the cosine of any real number must lie between -1 and $+1$, and repeats itself every 360° (or 2π radians), sinusoids are inherently rhythmic, with a period of 360° and an amplitude of 1. The essence of estimating a time series by a sinusoid thus involves multiplying the cosine by a constant (R) to get the right amplitude; multiplying the time variable t by a constant (f) to get the right period; and by adding a constant (P) to the product ft to get the right phase. Thus one ends up with the following equation for x_t (the value of the variable at time t):

$$x_t = R \cos (ft + P) \tag{1}$$

In equation (1), the parameter R represents the amplitude of the rhythm, which varies between $-R$ and $+R$. The parameter f is the angular velocity of the rhythm, and is a measure of how quickly the angle (and hence the cosine value) changes for a given increment in t. Indirectly, it is thus a measure of the *frequency* of the rhythm, since the cosine values will repeat themselves every time the $(ft + P)$ part of the equation moves through 360°. In this chapter, f will thus be referred to as frequency, although it is more accurately described as angular velocity.

Without the parameter P, equation (1) would require that the first point of the time series (at time zero) would be given by $R \cos 0$ which, because $\cos 0 = 1$, is simply R. Thus from these first principles, it is clear that P is merely the appropriate angle for the first point of the time series to be accurately estimated by $R \cos P$ (since at time zero, ft is, of course, zero). Clearly, at an angle of P 'behind' that zero, as it were, the rhythm will be at its peak, and $-P$ (or P as a negative angle) thus represents the *acrophase* of the rhythm. As a methodological concept, however, it is probably easier to accept the first principle's definition of P, regarding its potential for indicating the time of peak as a happy accident. To that end the parameter P will be referred to in this chapter as the phase rather than the acrophase.

For computational and algebraic reasons, equation (1) is often rewritten in a different form, namely:

$$x_t = A \cos ft + B \sin ft \tag{2}$$

where $A = R \cos P$ and $B = -R \sin P$.

These two forms are, in fact, identical, representing *exactly* the same thing, and readers should not be confused by the fact that some authors use equation (1) and others equation (2).

In general, one has to add a term representing the mesor, or mean level, of the time series (see Figure 1); this is represented by the letter M. In fitting the sinusoid, the main interest, of course, is the 'error' of mismatch between the fitted sinusoid and the actual time series. At each sampling time t this can be represented by e_t. Thus the general form of equations (1) and (2) become:

$$x_t = M + R \cos (ft + P) + e_t \tag{3}$$

and

$$x_t = M + A \cos ft + B \sin ft + e_t \tag{4}$$

Thus in equations (3) and (4) one has the description of a time series by a single sinusoid, with allowance made for a mismatch between the fitted and observed curves. Clearly the essence of the problem is to choose values of mesor, amplitude, and phase $(M, R, \text{ and } P)$ that minimize the 'error' or mismatch (e_t). Since one requires to minimize the total mismatch, and one is uninterested in sign, this problem can be thought of as one of minimizing the sum of the squared 'error' (i.e. $\sum\limits_{t=1}^{n} e_t^2$).

The algebra of the situation requires that the period or frequency (f) of the rhythm be either chosen on *a priori* grounds (e.g. as equivalent to a period of 24.0 h in a circadian rhythm study) or be found by trial and error. This can be tedious when there is no *a priori* value (e.g. in free running or ultradian rhythm experiments) but there are techniques (see Bloomfield, 1976, p.18, and Sollberger, 1970, p.66) for improving one's current estimate of frequency, and many iterative ('trial and error') techniques exist. In most cases, though, the problem facing the chronobiologist is one of estimating mesor, amplitude, and phase $(M, R, \text{ and } P)$ for a given period or frequency.

The process of estimation of phase and amplitude is done via the parameters A and B of equation (4) (which is why they have been introduced). The problem is thus one of finding numerical estimates of M, A, and B which, for a given frequency, will minimize the sum of the squared error between the time series and the sinusoid. These numbers in fact correspond to the 'least squares' estimates of M, A, and B and are derived in a way very similar to that for the more familiar equations for the slope and intercept of fitted straight lines. Basically, the problem resolves into that of solving three simultaneous equations for the three unknowns.

If sampling is regular and an integral number of cycles are taken, the whole process is simplified considerably, giving three easy formulae for the required estimates (the notation ^ merely indicates that we are talking about *values*, now, rather than *variables*):

$$\hat{M} = \bar{x} = \sum_{t=1}^{n} x_t/n \tag{5}$$

$$\hat{A} = (2/n) \sum_{t=1}^{n} (x_t - \bar{x}) \cos ft \tag{6}$$

$$\hat{B} = (2/n) \sum_{t=1}^{n} (x_t - \bar{x}) \sin ft \tag{7}$$

Equation (5) merely confirms that under these conditions the mean ($\bar{x}$) and mesor ($\hat{M}$) are the same. It should be remembered, however, that usually this is not the case (see Figure 1, for an example).

Broadly speaking, the methods of Lewis and Lobban (1956), Fort and Mills (1970) and Colquhoun, Paine, and Fort (1978) are applications of the above methods to simply provide least squares estimates of mesor, amplitude, and phase. The method of Ware and Bowden (1977) is more complex in that further steps are made in order to construct confidence intervals around the obtained estimates. One of the procedures suggested by Fort and Mills (1970) differs slightly in taking an *area* measure of mismatch rather than a simple difference measure; the area measure being more appropriate, they suggest, when irregular sampling (e.g. of urinary electrolytes) occurs.

Hitherto, this discussion has been limited to the case where a time series can be adequately (though not perfectly) fitted by a single sinusoid. Clearly, in many (some would say, most) cases other sinusoids need to be included to make the goodness of fit more acceptable. By adding other sinusoids one can change the shape of the rhythm, getting a closer approximation to that of the actual time series. For example, Colquhoun, Paine, and Fort (1978) were concerned with the circadian rhythm of oral temperature in man. They found that 88% of the variance due to time of day could be explained by the single 24 h sinusoid. However, when a second sinusoidal component, corresponding to the first harmonic (i.e. a 12 h component) was also included, a much better fit, accounting for over 99% of the variance, was obtained.

Thus, as one would expect, by resolving the time series into two components rather than one, a better fit to the data was obtained. This result has been pursued by Naitoh, Lubin, and Colquhoun (1979) who compared single sinusoid and dual sinusoid fits to human circadian body temperature data. They concluded that when the data set was small, the single sinusoid fit was preferable, but with a larger data set, the dual sinusoid fit gave more accurate estimates of time of peak and time of trough.

Assessment of Significance

Unless the time series has been resolved perfectly into its discrete Fourier transform, the question of the statistical reliability of the fitted sinusoid (or combination of sinusoids) clearly arises. There are several ways in which this statistical reliability can be tested; most use the F ratio, and none is entirely satisfactory. That used by the Minnesota cosinor method will be considered in a later section.

The particular F ratio that is chosen will depend upon the null hypothesis (H_o) that is to be tested. The most obvious choice of H_o is that the sinusoid (or set of sinusoids) provides no better a description of the time series than its simple mean. Thus, in this case, the F ratio tests whether the residual variability around the mean is significantly greater than that around the fitted sinusoid (or combination of sinusoids). The sum of squared deviations about the mean ($\Sigma(x_t-\bar{x})^2$) and about the cosine curve (Σe_t^2) are thus calculated, and divided by their respective degrees of freedom (Fort and Mills, 1970). These variance estimates are then divided to give an F ratio. Thus:

$$F = \frac{\displaystyle\sum_{t=1}^{n} (x_t-\bar{x})^2/(n-1)}{\displaystyle\sum_{t=1}^{n} e_t^2/(n-3)} \tag{8}$$

where $e_t = x_t-\hat{M}-\hat{R} \cos (ft + \hat{P})$ and for statistical significance, one requires that $F > F_{0.05}(n-1,n-3)$.

An alternative F ratio is that used by Colquhoun, Paine, and Fort (1978) who compare the 'explained' and 'unexplained' sums of squares, testing the null hypothesis that the former is not greater than the latter. Thus, in this case, the denominator remains the same ($\Sigma e_t^2/n-3$)) but the numerator is the difference between the sums of the squares about the mean and that about the cosine curve, i.e. the amount of variance explained by the cosine curve. This the explained sum of squares is $\Sigma(x_t-\bar{x})^2-\Sigma e_t^2$ and its degree of freedom is $(n-1)-(n-3)$, i.e. 2. Again the variance estimates are divided to give an F ratio. Thus:

$$F = \frac{\sum\limits_{t=1}^{n} (x_t-\bar{x})^2 - \sum\limits_{t=1}^{n} e_t^2 \, /2}{\sum\limits_{t=1}^{n} e_t^2/(n-3)} \tag{9}$$

and for statistical significance one requires that $F > F_{0.05}(2,n-3)$. This approach is similar to one suggested by Walters and Curtis (1976).

Other choices of F ratio are possible, but all suffer from the drawback of a rather artificial (and easily 'knocked down') choice of H_o. Thus in using the F ratio to assess the 'goodness of fit' of a sinusoid (or set of sinusoids) it is probably better to regard the obtained F ratio as a comparative, rather than absolute standard. Indeed, although there is no computational reason for avoiding the use of F ratios in the single subject, single cycle case, problems do arise when one tries to relate that to a particular hypothesis test.

Probably the least unsatisfactory method of assessing 'goodness of fit' is provided by the percentage variability accounted for (PVA). The PVA is calculated by simply dividing the explained sum of squares by the sum of squares about the mean and multiplying by 100. Thus:

$$\text{PVA} = \frac{\left(\sum\limits_{t=1}^{n} (x_t-\bar{x})^2 - \sum\limits_{t=1}^{n} e_t^2\right) \times 100}{\sum\limits_{t=1}^{n} (x_t-\bar{x})^2} \tag{10}$$

Although the PVA gives no actual test of significance, it does give a much better idea of how successful the sinusoid (or set of sinusoids) has been in describing the time series. The fact that fits which have a 5% level of significance can still have a PVA of only 35% or less, underlines the remarks made earlier about the unsatisfactory nature of the F tests conventionally used.

The Minnesota Cosinor Technique

Strictly speaking, this technique is the only one that should be referred to as 'cosinor', but because the term has been used to describe other single sinusoid fitting procedures, the prefix 'Minnesota' will be used throughout, to avoid confusion. The Minnesota cosinor is, as Halberg *et al.* (1977) point out in their glossary, actually three techniques, the one used being dependent upon the time series to be analysed. The present discussion will not, however, be concerned with the fitting of a sinusoid to a single short time series. Instead, it will give a general overview of the basic mechanisms underlying the 'sample mean cosinor' and 'group-mean cosinor' techniques.

The first stage of the Minnesota cosinor technique involves the creation of a set of short time series, and the fitting of a sinusoid to each. Second and third stages of analysis then enable confidence intervals to be constructed around the final estimates of phase and amplitude that are produced. The method has achieved widespread acceptance, and the 'cosinor display' has become a useful standard way of presenting the parameters of various rhythms. Confusingly, the cosinor display is sometimes referred to as a 'chronogram', but that usage will not be followed here.

The technique is described in detail in Halberg, Tong, and Johnson (1967) and it is to that publication that the interested reader should initially be referred. A good detailed description (with a critical evaluation) is also given by Van Cauter and Huyberechts (1973). The technique is inherently computer-based, copies of the program being available at various centres around the world.

Earlier in the chapter it was pointed out that studies in chronobiology could be either *longitudinal*, in that a long time series is obtained from relatively few subjects, or *transverse*, in that a large number of subjects each contributes rather short time series. The first stage of the procedure involves creating a set of k short time series, either by 'chopping up' a long time series from a longitudinal study, or by considering each of the short time series from a transverse study. This set of short time series forms the basic data set on which subsequent stages of analysis are performed.

The first step involves fitting a single sinusoid to each of the short time series, using the procedures described above. The estimates of phase and amplitude are calculated for each of the k sets of short time series, yielding k pairs of parameters $(\hat{R}_h, \hat{P}_h)$, $h = 1,2 \ldots k$), to be carried forward to the second stage.

The k pairs of parameters are then transformed from polar to rectangular coordinates (simply by calculating $y_h = \hat{R}_h \sin \hat{P}_h$ and $x_h = \hat{R}_h \cos \hat{P}_h$) as illustrated in Figure 5. This procedure results in a set of pairs (x_h, y_h), $h = 1,2, \ldots k$) of values that are carried forward to the next stage. Essentially this step can be considered as one of plotting the k pairs of points on polar coordinates, and reading them off on normal x and y axes.

The next stage of analysis considers the values (x_h, y_h) to have come from a bivariate normal distribution, and calculates estimates of their mean $(\bar{x}, \bar{y})$ and confidence interval (in the x and y dimensions). Thus the mean point is represented by the average of the xs and the average of the ys.

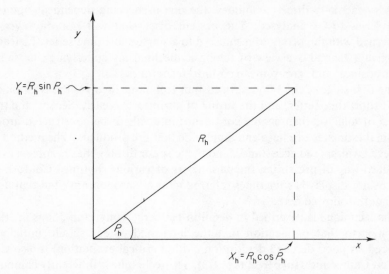

Figure 5   The mapping of a vector representing a phase of P_h and R_h onto x and y
coordinates, as required by the Minnesota cosinor method

Having discovered the mean point $(\bar{x}, \bar{y})$ on rectangular (x and y axes)
coordinates, this point can be 'read off' in polar coordinates to give a final
estimate of phase (angle from base line) and amplitude (distance from origin).
This is equivalent to the transformations:

$$\hat{R} = \sqrt{x^2 + y^2} \text{ and } \hat{P} = \arctan(\bar{y}/\bar{x}) \tag{11}$$

Clearly (as Halberg *et al.* point out), for such estimates to be valid, it is vital
that the k short time series be true estimates of the final time series. As Figure 6
shows, any non-stationarity in terms of phase, can result in a very small final
estimate of amplitude, even if the amplitudes of the contributing short time
series are all large. Thus *any* 'weakness' of the short time series as estimates of
the 'true' series will result in a reduced final estimate of amplitude, and in that
sense, phase, and amplitude are not independent. Hence in comparing two
time series one cannot speak of one having a larger amplitude than the other,
without ensuring that both are equally stationary.

The confidence interval around the mean $(\bar{x}, \bar{y})$ of the bivariate normal
distribution in each dimension indicates an 'area of significance'. This area
corresponds to an ellipse on the polar plot, with the point representing the
final estimates of phase and amplitude at its centre. The rhythm is held to be
statistically reliable if this ellipse does not contain the zero point (i.e. centre) of
the polar coordinates. Since any 'weakness' of the rhythm (see above) is

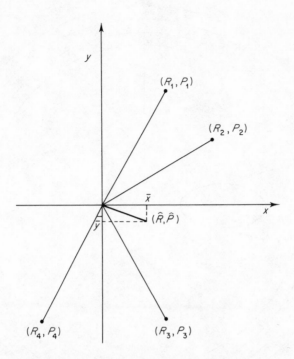

Figure 6   The Minnesota cosinor method: an illustration of how a set of vectors with large amplitudes (R_h), but differing phases (P_h) can combine to give a final vector with a comparatively small amplitude ($\hat{R}$)

represented by a reduction in final amplitude, this statistical test incorporates aspects of both phase and amplitude.

The polar plot used to present the results of the Minnesota cosinor is of a standard form (the 'cosinor display'). This form differs from standard mathematical conventions in two respects:

(1) angles are measured in a clockwise, rather than an anticlockwise, direction; and

(2) the zero point is taken at 'north' rather than 'east'.

These modifications are required to make the cosinor display more comprehensible, when labelled with clock time, for displaying circadian rhythms. They mean, however, that care must be taken when attempting to relate values of phase obtained from the equations presented in this chapter (and the non-biological texts) to those of the standard Minnesota cosinor plot. Usually, however, common sense (and/or a look at the chronogram) will indicate whether the phase has been plotted correctly or not. The standard cosinor

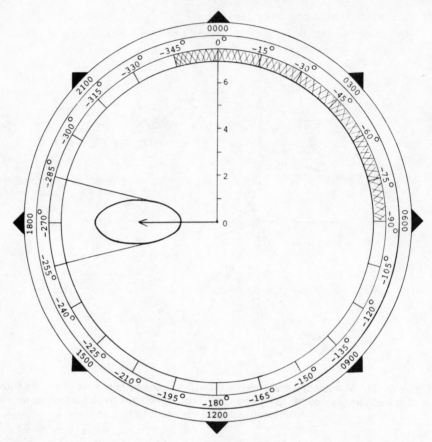

Figure 7   The 'cosinor display' conventionally used to describe the results of the
Minnesota cosinor technique (see text) (artificial data)

display is illustrated in Figure 7 which illustrates an (artificial) rhythm having
an acrophase of 270° (1800) and an amplitude of 4 units, with a confidence
ellipse also plotted.

The computational techniques used for constructing the confidence ellipse
are rather complicated, and unfortunately there are very few helpful
publications in the literature. Tong (1976) gives some of the background, but
requires a knowledge of matrix algebra.

As mentioned above, Van Cauter and Huyberechts (1973) give a description
and critical evaluation of the Minnesota cosinor method, pointing out the
various pitfalls, and suggesting an alternative method to avoid them. The main
dangers of using the Minnesota cosinor inappropriately are cases when the
time series is non-sinusoidal, non-stationary, or insufficient in extent (either
longitudinally or transversely) for meaningful estimates to be made. Although

such violations should cause the confidence ellipse to overlap the pole of the plot (and thus indicate non-significance) the extreme power of the technique may mean that an entirely inappropriate fit still achieves significance. When used correctly, however, the Minnesota cosinor technique and the cosinor display provide extremely useful research methods for the chronobiologist.

'True' Fourier Analysis

In moving to the strict definition of Fourier analysis as the complete decomposition of the time series into a large set of sinusoids, the type of question answered by the statistical technique changes somewhat. Instead of answering the question 'Is there a rhythmic component with a particular frequency?' this technique answers the questions such as 'Are there rhythmicities within a particular range?' or 'Are there any rhythmicities at all?' Thus the results of this procedure enable one to plot the comparative importance of the various sinusoids, i.e. the *spectrum* of the time series.

The method is most easily considered as a generalization of the simple single sinusoid case considered above. For each frequency of sinusoid that is considered, one has to calculate estimates of amplitude and phase. When a sufficient number of frequencies is considered, such a decomposition can exactly describe any time series.

A subset of Fourier analysis is *harmonic analysis* where the frequencies used (known as the *Fourier frequencies*) are taken to be $\frac{2\pi}{n}, \frac{4\pi}{n}, \frac{6\pi}{n} \ldots$ etc., where n is the number of points in the time series.

In the case we have been considering, i.e. a discrete time series with n (presumably equally spaced) data points, it can be shown that:

(1) the number of components that needs to be taken is about $n/2$ (depending upon whether n is odd or even);
(2) the highest frequency that can be detected (known as the *Nyquist frequency*) is $1/2d$, where d is the sampling interval (thus nd is the duration of the whole time series); and
(3) the fineness of resolution of the harmonic analysis (i.e. the 'width' of the frequencies — such that one frequency is distinct from its neighbour) is $1/nd$.

More detailed explanation (in an admirably readable form) can be obtained from Orr and Naitoh, 1975.

Having performed the Fourier analysis using the required number of Fourier frequencies, and obtained estimates of phase and amplitude for each component, the next task is to present the results in such a way that the importance (or *power*) of each frequency can be seen. This is accomplished by calculating the square of the amplitude of that sinusoid. The plot of squared amplitude (*y* axis) against frequency (*x* axis) is known as the *raw spectrogram* or *periodogram* of the time series. By looking for the peaks in such a plot, one can determine the periodicities that are dominant in the time series.

The main problem with the raw spectrogram is its instability, and thus one often *smoothes* the spectrum by collapsing over several adjacent frequencies, taking the average of these points as the number to be plotted. Depending upon whether equal or unequal weights are given to the points making up the average, this procedure is known as *hanning* or *hamming* (see Blackman and Tukey, 1958, p.14). The disadvantage of this procedure, of course, is the lack of frequency resolution that ensues. Thus, for example, if three adjacent frequencies were averaged to smoothe the spectrum, the range of frequencies would increase threefold. This range of frequencies is known as the *resolution* or *bandwidth*. The bandwidth that is required will depend on the proximity in frequency of the periodicities that are to be detected.

Other ways of ensuring a more comprehensible power spectrum involve manipulating the time series prior to applying the Fourier analysis. If a set of time series is available (from different subjects, for example), then computing and 'average time series' for the set can give a much more stable power spectrum, without the increased bandwidth that results from smoothing across frequencies (Orr and Naitoh, 1975). *Detrending* involves the removal of a linear trend in the data by fitting a straight line (by least squares) to the time series, and performing all subsequent analyses on deviations from this line. This technique is often encountered in measures of performance efficiency, where improvements due to practice can occur (see Chapter IV). Another technique is *tapering*, which involves placing correspondingly less emphasis on the first and last 10% (or between 5% and 25%) of the time series. A transformation is applied which leaves the middle portion untouched, but multiplies the first and last portions by a function (often the rising and falling halves of a cosine bell), that ensures the time series smoothly approaches zero at either end (see Tukey, 1967).

Clearly, the computational load in calculating the individual phases and amplitudes of all $n/2$ Fourier frequencies is enormous, even with an electronic computer. However, there is now a technique known as the fast Fourier transform (FFT) developed by Cooley and Tukey (1965) that substantially reduces the number of computations that have to be performed. Indeed, the savings obtained are so dramatic that most computer implementations of Fourier analysis (e.g. Dixon, 1976) use the FFT, and very few studies would now use any other method.

The essence of FFT is in the selection of the Fourier frequencies that are considered. This selection requires that the length of the time series (n) be an integer power of 2 (e.g. 16, 256, 1024), or, at least a number having integer powers of 2, 3, and/or 5 as factors. To accomplish this, most FFT computer programs automatically pad out the time series (usually at the 'far' end) with zeros up to the nearest power of 2 above n. As with conventional Fourier analysis, values of phase and amplitude are obtained, and the square of the amplitude calculated for plotting as the power spectrum.

Problems and Precautions in Using Fourier Analysis

The major problems encountered with Fourier analysis stem from the fact that the technique was not developed for the type of time series conventionally gathered by the chronobiologist. As Sollberger (1970) and Van Cauter and Huyberechts (1973) point out, chronobiological time series are usually much too short, and the sampling intervals too infrequent or too unevenly spaced for Fourier analyses to be accurately applied. Orr and Naitoh (1975) advise that a 200 point time series should be considered as a minimum for the computation of power spectra, and warn that serious problems can arise when n falls below 80. For the fitting of a single sinusoid of known period, conditions can be relaxed slightly, but Naitoh (personal communication) has determined that for a longitudinal study, *at least* 5 cycles' worth of reading are needed to give sensible estimates of mesor, amplitude, and acrophase. Also, Sollberger has shown that inaccuracies can occur when sinusoids are fitted to unevenly spaced data points, although these would probably amount only to less than one hour in phase and 7% in amplitude, for a 24 h rhythm. For a transverse study, of course, the problem becomes one of ensuring that there are enough subjects, and that they are 'in phase'.

In general, the best advice would seem to be to use the Fourier techniques wherever possible, but to bear in mind that assumptions *are* being violated, and that extreme caution should be exerted when presenting and interpreting the results. A useful check that can be applied is to randomly 'shuffle' the x values of the time series and reapply the whole analysis. If a similar spectrum to the original is obtained (rather than an essentially flat spectrum), then one should conclude that one's results are merely artifactual and should be discarded. If, however, different spectra are obtained, and renewed reshuffling of the time series results in a consistent spectrum, it might be possible to obtain the 'true' spectrum by a subtraction technique. This method of checking the validity of an analysis is probably worth doing, whatever the particular method being used.

COMPARATIVE ADVANTAGES AND DISADVANTAGES

The discipline of chronobiology is too young for a definitive list of research methods to be made. The area is in a state of flux; research methods are usually chosen on an *ad hoc* basis, and new techniques are being introduced and developed all the time. Thus even if that were its aim, this chapter could

Table 3 Summary of the various requirements and benefits of the seven major techniques

Method	Requirements				Benefits				
	period known	sinusoidal shape	long series[1]	equal spacing	period found	significance of rhythm	phase found	amplitude found	parameter confidence intervals
Eyeball	No	No[5]	No[5]	No[5]	Yes	No	No[6]	No[6]	No
Buys-Ballot	Yes	No	Yes	No	No[2]	No	No[6]	No[6]	No
Analysis of variance	Yes	No	No	No	No	Yes	No[6]	No[6]	No
Autocorrelation	No	No	Yes	Yes	Yes	Yes[3]	No	Yes[4]	No
'Ordinary' cosinor	Yes[2]	Yes	Yes	No	No[2]	Yes	Yes	Yes	No
Spectral analysis	No	No	Yes	Yes	Yes	Yes[3]	No	Yes	No
Minnesota cosinor	Yes[2]	Yes	No	No	No[2]	Yes	Yes	Yes	Yes

Notes: 1, if not longitudinal a transverse study is assumed; 2, unless used iteratively; 3, but not directly; 4, but only relative to other frequencies; 5, but must have very frequent sampling and lack of noise; 6, but calculable from chronogram.

never hope to be truly comprehensive, and indeed, large areas of research methodology have been entirely left out. Limitations of space have, for example, meant that techniques such as those of complex demodulation (Orr, Hoffman, and Hegge, 1976) and cross-correlation (Orr and Naitoh, 1975) have been omitted. Likewise, quantification of re-entrainment has largely been ignored, and the reader is referred to Winget *et al.* (1975), Monk (1977) and Mills, Minors, and Waterhouse (1978) for a description of some techniques that are available for that particular area of study.

Eventually various standard research methods will evolve and become the accepted techniques for the study of chronobiology. At the moment, the Minnesota cosinor seems a likely candidate as one of those accepted techniques, but its various limitations and weaknesses do demand that other techniques also become standard practice. There is a real danger that for the sake of uniformity or convenience, researchers stick dogmatically to one technique to the exclusion of all others. If this results in violations of the method's assumptions, and consequently in the erroneous reporting of results, then (at the risk of sounding pompous) such researchers will have done science in general, and chronobiology in particular, a grave disservice. If this modest review only serves to draw attention to some of the wide variety of techniques that *are* available, then its presence in this book has been justified. To that end, this chapter finishes with a Table summarizing the various requirements and advantages of the seven major techniques that have been considered.

SUMMARY

This chapter presents the basic terms and concepts used in chronobiology. It describes the research, as a whole, by systematically surveying the studies published in the area. The main body of the chapter describes and evaluates the major analytical methods used in defining and describing the presence of biological rhythms. Simple macroscopic techniques are first considered. These are followed by autocorrelation procedures and the variations involving Fourier analyses are detailed. Particular attention is given to the widely used cosinor method. Finally, a discussion of the advantages and disadvantages of the procedures is presented.

REFERENCES

*Aschoff, J., Klotter, K., and Wever, R. (1965). Circadian vocabulary. A recommended terminology with definitions. In: *Circadian Clocks.* J. Aschoff (Ed.). Amsterdam, North Holland.

Aschoff, J., Hoffmann, K., Pohl, H., and Wever, R. (1975). Re-entrainment of circadian rhythms after phase-shifts of the Zeitgeber. *Chronobiologia* 1, 23–78.

Blackman, R. B. and Tukey, J. W. (1958). *The Measurement of Power Spectra.* New York, Dover.

Bloomfield, P. (1976). *Fourier Analysis of Time Series: an Introduction.* New York, Wiley.

· Colquhoun, W. P. (Ed.). (1971). *Biological Rhythms and Human Performance.* London, Academic Press.

Colquhoun, W. P., Paine, M. W. P. H., and Fort, A. (1978). Circadian rhythms of body temperature during prolonged undersea voyages. *Aviation, Space & Environmental Medicine* 5, 671-678.

Cooley, V. A. and Tukey, J. W. (1965). An algorithm for the machine calculation of complex Fourier series. *Mathematics of Computation* 19, 297-301.

Dixon, W. J. (Ed.). (1976). *BMD — Biomedical Computer Programs.* Berkeley, University of California Press.

Enright, J. T. (1965). Geophysical rhythms and frequency analysis. In *Circadian Clocks.* J. Aschoff (Ed.). Amsterdam, North Holland.

Folkard, S. (1975). Diurnal variation in logical reasoning. *British Journal of Psychology* 66, 1-8.

Fort, A. and Mills, J. N. (1970). Fitting sine curves to 24h urinary data. *Nature,* 226, 1-8.

Gale, A., Harpham, B., and Lucas, B. (1972). Time of day and the EEG: some negative results. *Psychonomic Science,* 28, 269-291.

· Halberg, F., Carandente, F., Cornelissen, G., and Katinas, G. S. (1977). Glossary of chronobiology. *Chronobiologia,* Supplement 1.

Halberg, F., Tong, Y. L., and Johnson, E. A. (1967). Circadian system phase — an aspect of temporal morphology; procedures and illustrative examples. In: *The Cellular Aspects of Biorhythms.* H. Von Mayerback (Ed.). Berline, Springer-Verlag.

Lewis, P. R. and Lobban, M. C. (1956). Patterns of electrolyte excretion in human subjects during a prolonged period of life on a 22-hour day. *Journal of Physiology,* 133, 670-680.

Mills, J. N., Minors, D. S., and Waterhouse, J. M. (1978). Adaptation to abrupt time shifts of the oscillator(s) controlling human circadian rhythms. *Journal of Physiology,* 285, 455-470.

Monk, T. H. (1977). A likelihood ratio method for studying the re-entrainment of circadian rhythms. *Chronobiologia,* 4, 325-332.

Naitoh, P., Lubin, A. and Colquhoun, W. P. (1979). Comparisons of monosinusoidal with bisinusoidal (two-wave) analysis. In: *Proceedings of the XIV International Conference of the International Society* (in press).

Orr, W. C. and Naitoh, P. (1975). The coherence spectrum: an extension of correlation analysis with applications to chronobiology. *International Journal of Chronobiology* 3, 171-192.

Orr, W. C., Hoffman, H. J., and Hegge, F. W. (1976). The assessment of time-dependent changes in human performance. *Chronobiologia* 3, 293-305.

Poppel, E. (1975). Parameter estimation or hypothesis testing in the statistical analysis of biological rhythms. *Bulletin of the Psychonomic Society* 5, 511-512.

Poulton, E. C. (1973). Unwanted range effects from using within-subject experimental designs. *Psychological Bulletin* 2, 113-121.

Sollberger, A. (1970). Problems in the statistical analysis of short periodic time series. *Journal of Interdisciplinary Cycle Research* 1, 49-88.

Tong, Y. L. (1976). Parameter estimation in studying circadian rhythms. *Biometrics* 32, 85-94.

Tukey, J. W. (1967). An introduction to the calculations of numerical spectrum analysis. In: *Spectral analysis of Time Series.* B. Harris (Ed.). New York, Wiley.

Van Cauter, E. and Huyberechts, S. (1973). Problems in the statistical analysis of biological time series: the cosinor test and the periodogram. *Journal of Interdisciplinary Cycle Research* **4**, 41–57.

Walter, D. O. (1963). Spectral analysis for electroencephalograms: mathematical determination of neurophysiological relations from records of limited duration. *Experimental Neurology* **8**, 155–181.

Walters, D. E. and Curtis, R. J. (1976). The combination of results from Fourier analysis in the investigation of biological rhythms. *International Journal of Chronobiology* **3**, 263–276.

Ware, J. H. and Bowden, R. E. (1977). Circadian rhythm analysis when output is collected at intervals. *Biometrics*, 566–571.

Webb, W. B. and Agnew, H. W. (1974). Sleep and waking in a time-free environment. *Aerospace Medicine* **45**, 617–622.

Wever, R. (1973). Internal phase-angle differences in human circadian rhythms: causes for changes and problems of determinations. *International Journal of Chronobiology* **1**, 371–390.

Williams, J. A. and Naylor, E. (1978). A procedure for the assessment of significance of rhythmicity in time-series data. *International Journal of Chronobiology* **5**, 435–444.

Winget, C. M., Bond, G. H., Rosenblatt, L. S., Hetherington, N. W., Higgins, E. A., and De Roshia, C. (1975). Quantitation of desynchronosis. *Chronobiologia* **2**, 197–204.

Biological Rhythms, Sleep, and Performance
Edited by Wilse B. Webb
©1982 John Wiley & Sons Ltd.

Chapter 3

Biological Rhythms and Performance

Peter Colquhoun

BACKGROUND

This chapter is concerned with circadian rhythms in human performance, and with the various factors that can affect such rhythms. In this context, 'performance' is defined in terms of scores of efficiency at various tasks which require the use of cerebral processes in responding to specified sensory information by appropriate motor actions.

The complexity of both the sensory and motor components of a task may vary, as can the 'difficulty' of performing it; however, in general, the tasks so far studied for evidence of circadian periodicity have been relatively 'simple' ones. There are two very good reasons for this: the first is that it is normally only in the simple case that one can obtain correspondingly 'simple' scores readily amenable to analysis; the second is that, by looking at variations in the efficiency with which simple tasks are performed, we are hoping to observe the outward manifestations only of variations in those (relatively) simple underlying 'mental' processes which, in the case of complex tasks, must presumably combine or interact in a manner which is clearly beyond our present capacity to determine. However, it must be admitted at the outset that even the most apparently simple task is, in truth, extraordinarily complex, and that we are not at all certain what particular underlying mental processes are in fact being indirectly measured by the scores we obtain.

Early Research

Variations in performance during the waking day appear to have been first studied systematically at the end of the last century. This earliest work was much concerned with the relationship between 'mental fatigue' and diurnal changes in mental efficiency. Thus Ebbinghaus (1885) reported a consistent tendency for learning (of nonsense syllables) to be more rapid in the morning, an effect which he assumed to occur because 'in the later hours of the day mental vigour and receptivity are less'. On the other hand, Bechterew (1893) maintained that 'the speed of the psychic processes is retarded in the morning and accelerated in the evening. The lowest speed occurred in the afternoon.' This afternoon trough was also commented on by Kraeplin (1893), who related it to the midday meal. Kraeplin, who conducted extensive research on the 'work-curve', also mentioned a 'warm-up' period in the morning, and concluded, in apparent contradiction of Ebbinghaus, that the decrements (and associated phenomena) he observed were 'no indication of (work) fatigue', since they 'disappear after 2–3 hours, even when work is continued'.

Thus, even in this earliest work, there are suggestions of two differing overall time of day trends, and also of a 'post-lunch' effect. The degree to which fatigue was responsible for the observed variation was the subject of dispute. Gates (1916b) notes that the separation of fatigue effects from those due to an underlying temporal trend is extremely difficult. Addressing himself primarily to the question of school time-tabling, Gates conducted a comprehensive series of experiments of his own, using a variety of tests; he concluded that 'as far as the morning is concerned (the curves of efficiency) are identical' (i.e. performance improves up till about noon). But in the afternoon 'certain characteristic differences were found', which, he supposed, were most likely to be caused by a 'difference in the effectiveness in the assault of . . . fatigue, ennui, meals, etc. . . .'. Gates found that 'more strictly mental' processes reached their maximum in the later forenoon, and showed a greater post-lunch decrement; whereas the more 'motor' functions showed 'a continuous increase in efficiency during the (school) day'. He noted that his work confirmed the conclusions of workers such as Winch (1913) and Heck (1913) in this respect; the findings on motor tasks are also similar to those of Hollingworth (1914) who maintained, in addition, that the timing of the 'peak' in such tasks is partly dependent on the subject's customary hours of work.

Laird (1925) reported results which he held were at variance to those obtained by Gates. He found an almost continuous fall over the day in *averaged* performance at tests on several different mental functions, including memory, given in a carefully controlled experiment to college students (but this averaging conceals considerable differences in trend in the different tests). Laird was highly critical of previous laboratory studies, attributing the disagreement among them to 'lack of experimental insight'. Freeman and Hovland (1934) in their review of the area, were also critical of earlier work, mainly on methodological grounds. These authors claimed to be able to classify all the diurnal efficiency curves in the papers they surveyed into four basic shapes: a continuous rise; a continuous fall; a rise followed by a fall; and a fall followed by a rise. It would seem quite possible that these different diurnal trends arose from the particular nature of the different tasks that had been used in the various studies, rather than (as Freeman and Hovland appear to imply) from shortcomings in the experiments themselves (present though they may have been in some).

In his review published originally in 1939, Kleitman (1963), like previous writers in this area, tended to discount most earlier work, and preferred to present, in detail, the results from his own carefully controlled studies. Kleitman found that all the curves he and his co-workers obtained were of the third 'shape' distinguished by Freeman and Hovland, performance rising from early morning to a peak in the middle of the waking period, i.e. somewhere during the afternoon, then declining towards evening. Kleitman took concurrent readings of body temperature in his experiments, and concluded that 'most of the curves of performance can be brought into line with the known 24-hour body temperature curves, allowing for individual skewing of the curves towards an earlier or later, rather than a mid-afternoon, peak'. In the case of 'motor' tasks Kleitman implied that this parallelism is mediated by the underlying relationship between body temperature and muscular tonus. Where the task is predominantly mental in character he suggested two possible interpretations:

'Assuming that the effect of body temperature indicates that one is dealing with a chemical phenomenon (then) either (a) mental processes represent chemical reactions in themselves or (b) the speed of thinking depends upon the level of metabolic activity of the cells of the cerebral cortex, and by raising the latter through an increase in body temperature, one indirectly speeds up the thought process' (p.160).

Although Kleitman's explanation for the phenomenon has not been generally accepted, his emphasis on the relation between temperature and performance (which he found especially marked in the case of reaction time) was important, since it has influenced much of the later work on variations in efficiency with time of day. It is true that, if any afternoon 'dip' is assumed to be a specifically post-prandial phenomenon, and thus to be 'discounted', most observed circadian performance curves could be argued to show some degree of parallelism with the body temperature rhythm. This argument can even be extended to results such as those obtained by Baade (1907) (which were strikingly confirmed 50 years later by Rutenfranz and Hellbrugge, 1957). In a study of speed of simple computation in schoolchildren, two clear performance peaks were found, one before lunch, and one in the late afternoon, the intervening 'trough' occurring 4 hours after the first peak. The proponents of the parallelism hypothesis would describe such a function in terms of an especially protracted meal effect, masking what is basically a single curve. Further suggestions of parallelism appear in recent studies, which will be described later.

The Problem of Measurement

At this point it is necessary to point out that the investigation of possible circadian periodicity in human performance is an undertaking which is beset by a number of problems which do not exist in, for example, corresponding investigations of physiological processes. Perhaps the most obvious of these problems is that task performance is a voluntary activity. This immediately raises the question of the subject's motivation, which basically means 'how hard he is trying'. Since this cannot be measured, it has to be assumed that, on any occasion of testing, the subject is trying to perform at the same level of efficiency as on any other. This is a major assumption, and all that can be done in an attempt to ensure its validity is to make every effort to encourage a constant attitude throughout an experiment. However, since the success of such efforts cannot be assessed, there always remains the possibility that any apparent periodicity in efficiency of performance at a particular task is in fact to some extent (or even entirely) a reflection of fluctuations in motivation which are themselves exhibiting the periodicity observed.

The confounding of diurnal fluctuations with 'mental fatigue' in real-life situations has already been mentioned. However, even in the laboratory fatigue is a problem; in this case it is the 'fatigue' arising from the performance of the task itself. Although this is to a certain extent another aspect of the problem of motivation, it is difficult for even the most constantly motivated subject to keep up his performance for any length of time. The usual solution to this problem is to restrict the length of any test session, and also the number of such sessions to which the subject is exposed. Unfortunately, this in turn imposes constraints on the type of task which can be used, and also the frequency with which performance at it can be assessed; the later constraint places limits on the extent to which the detailed nature of any time of day trend can be described.

Whereas fatigue will be expected to degrade performance at a task, repeated practice will, on the other hand, enhance it. Practice effects of this kind occur with even the most apparently familiar kinds of activity, when these are incorporated into a 'test' situation. Although these effects can (in theory) be removed by 'detrending' the data (see Chapter II), this technique is not a preferred one, since the learning function is itself typically complex, and may well differ in individual subjects. The problem is more usually tackled by taking one or two approaches. The first of these is to administer a sufficient number of tests before the start of the experimental series to ensure that any residual practice effects are small enough to allow them to be ignored. The great advantage of this technique is that the results from each individual in a group can be examined separately, thus enabling intersubject comparisons to be made. The obvious disadvantage is the formidable difficulty of maintaining motivation (or avoiding 'fatigue') over the extended length of the observation period normally required for this approach to be feasible.

The second approach is to 'control' for practice effects by balancing them out in an experimental design of the type frequently used in psychological studies of the effects of a given 'treatment' (see Chapter II). In this kind of design it is, of course, not possible to make intersubject comparisons, and the basic outcome of an experiment is merely a 'mean' rhythm for a group of subjects. Certain assumptions have also to be made concerning the independence of practice effects and treatment order; even when these have been shown to be met, it is still the case that the observed (mean) rhythm represents only that present in the performance of a 'novel' task. This rhythm may not necessarily have the same characteristics as the one that would be seen in a fully practised situation.

The 'between subject' design described in Chapter II is an alternative method of controlling for practice effects. Here each subject is tested only once, separate groups of subjects being assigned to each of the times of day for which an assessment of performance level is sought. However, as pointed out in Chapter II, the problem of 'matching' these groups (e.g. for ability, personality, etc.) is difficult, particularly when the total population from whom subjects can be drawn is limited. Nevertheless, this kind of design is the only one that *can* be used in studies where performance in one session interacts with performance in another, e.g. in certain investigations of memory.

However frequently tests are given during the waking period, approximately one-third of any rhythm being looked for must be absent in any results, since , obviously, 'night' readings are unavailable from sleeping subjects. Performance scores obtained during night hours from subjects who have either been kept continuously awake, or who have been roused at intervals for test sessions, are inevitably confounded by sleep deprivation, or by 'sudden awakening' effects respectively: such scores cannot therefore strictly be considered as 'true' data points in the cycle. But if only 'waking day' performance readings are accepted as true points we are then left with data for which methods for assessing rhythmicity such as cosinor (see Chapter II) are not necessarily appropriate, since such methods make assumptions about the shape of the rhythm over the entire 24 hour period which may not be valid. Thus it is more usual for an investigator working in this area to analyse the test scores he obtains from the point of view of determining the statistical significance of differences in mean level at different times of day (using the more conventional techniques of analysis of variance, or t tests) than to attempt to establish the parameters of the circadian rhythm (such as its amplitude, and phase angle) thought to be responsible for such differences.

Although it can be assumed that many of the authors of the early time of day studies discussed at the beginning of this introduction were well aware of these measurement problems, it is possible that others were not. It is probably fair to say that a greater proportion of the authors of more recent studies have, in designing their experiments, taken account of the complexities necessarily associated with research in this area. To this extent, therefore, the results of these later investigations can be taken as more reliable than those of the pioneers.

RECENT RESEARCH

In this section, the 'post-Kleitman' work will be considered. As was mentioned earlier, much of this more recent work has been influenced by the apparent parallelism between body temperature and performance rhythms, which was itself most clearly described by Kleitman himself.

The data of Blake (1967a) have been taken as providing particularly strong evidence for this parallelism. In a number of what Hockey and Colquhoun (1972) describe as 'immediate information-processing tasks', Blake showed that performance (apart from a 'post-lunch dip') appeared to follow the rise in temperature over the day quite closely, reaching a maximum at 21.00 h (see Figure 1), a time which coincided with the peak of the body temperature rhythm in the population of subjects he employed, namely Naval ratings. However, although Blake's studies represent one of the better examples of recent experimentation in this area, it is possible that the 'late peaking' of performance observed in these studies was due partly to an exceptionally large 'end-spurt' or 'last test of the day' effect, specific to the particular type of subject used, since this late peaking is also seen in other studies with young military subjects (e.g. Colquhoun, Blake, and Edwards, 1969; Adam *et al.*, 1972). On the other hand, Blake's finding that performance at the only truly 'cognitive' test that showed significant variations in his series ('digit-span', a test of short term memory) reached its *lowest* level at 21.00 (see Figure 1) could be argued to militate against this 'subject-specific' interpretation, since the overall trend for performance at this test is in line with that found by some of the earlier observers of 'mental' function mentioned in the introduction (e.g. Gates, 1916a), namely, an initial morning rise, followed by a continuous fall thereafter.

The overall deterioration in short term memory efficiency from morning to afternoon has also been found in other recent studies (Baddeley *et al.*, 1970; Hockey, Davies, and Gray, 1972; Folkard and Monk, 1978), and the prediction that tasks involving both 'immediate information processing' *and* short term memory will show a 'compromise' time of day function has been confirmed by Folkard (1975) for tests of simple logical reasoning. However, in contrast to short term memory, long term retention has been found to be better for material originally presented in the *afternoon* than in the morning (Folkard *et al.*, 1977). This finding has obvious implications for educational time-tabling, which conflict with the conclusions of earlier workers such as Gates.

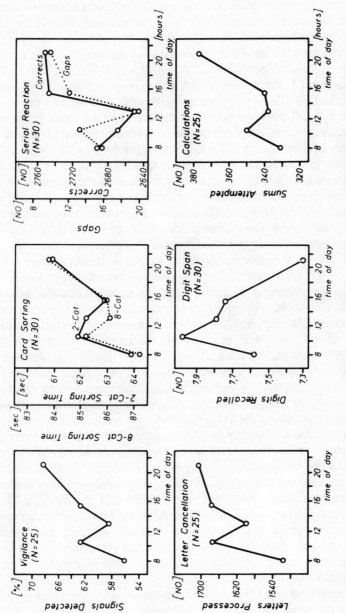

Figure 1   Variation in performance at six different tasks over the waking day. Based on data in Blake (1967a)

There are relatively few recent investigations of tasks which involve 'motor' skills, but those that have been carried out tend to confirm the conclusions of the earlier workers that this type of performance peaks later in the day than the more obviously 'mental' tasks. Of course, the 'purer' the motor task the less performance at its measures psychological processes. It is true that tasks such as the psychomotor 'Kugeltest' (Klein *et al.*, 1977), nut and bolt assembly (Hughes and Folkard, 1976), and rifle aiming (Halberg, 1970), all of which show the later peak, have a clear 'perceptual' component; but the degree to which mentation is involved in such tasks is typically small. In their studies of circadian rhythms in a Zeitgeber-controlled situation, designed to determine whether performance rhythms are truly endogenous, Aschoff *et al.* (1972) used tests of 'grip strength' and 'tapping speed'. But such tests are effectively equivalent to physiological measures, and thus do not measure 'performance' in the sense of the term used in this chapter. Nevertheless, Aschoff *et al.* were also able to show in their studies that, in the obviously mental tasks of simple computation and time estimation, 'time of day' effects, at least *are* endogenous, since they persisted when all Zeitgeber were removed.

All of the studies mentioned so far have been concerned solely with variations in performance during the normal 'waking' day. As was mentioned earlier, any measures of performance taken during 'night' hours must be confounded either by sleep deprivation, or by the effects of 'sudden awakening'. Nevertheless, a number of 'round-the-clock' studies have in fact been carried out, since for practical reasons it is often necessary to know whether or not performance efficiency at a particular type of task is degraded at night, and, if it is, to what extent. Much of the support for these studies has come from military sources, since in defence systems it is clearly of the utmost importance to attempt to ensure a constantly high degree of operational readiness throughout the 24 hour period.

In the process of seeking a work–rest schedule which would achieve this aim, Kleitman and Jackson (1950) and Colquhoun, Blake, and Edwards (1968a) assessed the efficiency of Naval ratings at a range of tasks, some of which simulated the men's actual duties, under the rapidly rotating 'watch-keeping' systems with 4 hour duty spells commonly used in warships. Their results confirmed the prediction from 'normal waking day' studies on enlisted men (such as the series by Blake previously described) that performance levels at those tasks involving 'immediate information processing' would be higher in watches held in the afternoon–evening hours than those held in the morning. In watches held in night hours (either before delayed 'night' sleep, or after a reduced period of such sleep) a degradation in efficiency at such tasks was observed, as was an increase in reaction times. The latter effect, and its relation to the duration of the preceding sleep period, was examined in detail in a similar study by Rutenfranz, Aschoff, and Mann (1972). When the mean watch scores obtained in such studies are plotted on a single 24 hour time scale, the suggestion of a circadian rhythm is very strong (see Figure 2, in which it should be noted that the parallelism with the curve produced by the corresponding mean body temperature readings appears to be quite close).

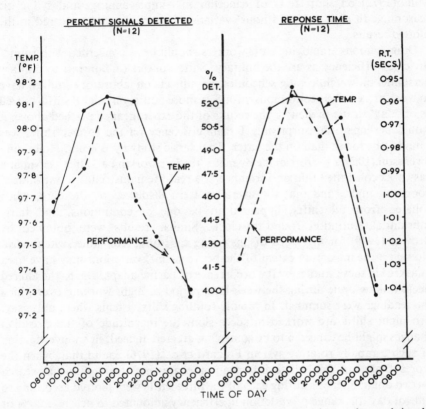

Figure 2   Mean signal detection efficiency, and mean response time to detected signals, in 2 hour sessions at a simulated sonar task, held in the first half of six 4 hour watches commencing at 00, 04, 08, 12, 16, or 20 h, scheduled over a 72 hour period. Average results from four consecutive watch cycles. Overall mean body temperature during each session is also shown. (After Colquhoun, Blake, and Edwards, 1968a)

The results of other (non-watchkeeping) studies, where subjects have either been kept awake, or awakened at intervals, for testing during night hours, provide similarly strong suggestion of the existence of circadian rhythmicity. Thus Klein *et al.* (1977) measured performance on psychomotor, cancellation, and addition tasks, and also on a flight simulator, in various experiments conducted over the complete 24 hour period, and found that the points they obtained in 'night' hours 'fitted' those from daytime testing in such a way as to indicate a pattern of efficiency changes that appeared very clearly as a rhythm (which, again, appeared to parallel that in body temperature). 'Night' tests were also included in the studies by Jansen, Rutenfranz and Singer (1966) on calculation rate and speed at a simultaneously performed tracking task; by Voigt, Engel, and Klein (1968) on auditory reaction time; and by Fort and Mills (1972) on short tests of cancellation, simple aiming, and syllogistic reasoning. In each case, '24 hour' variation in performance appeared in the plotted results.

Organizations employing shift workers should be as concerned with round-the-clock efficiency as are the military. Shift workers (in contrast to military personnel on watchkeeping schedules, or subjects on laboratory studies) have to work more or less continuously for 8 or more hours, on 'night' shifts as well as on 'day' shifts; in view of the results of the experiments described above, it would perhaps be unsurprising if their efficiency on the former shifts was found to be lower than on the latter. The classic study by Bjerner, Holm, and Swensson (1955) of errors made by meter-readers working a 3 shift system at a gasworks confirmed that performance at a real-life industrial task was indeed poorer at night, and that the overall pattern displayed by the data, when collated from all shifts, appeared to be one of continuous, and fairly substantial, variation round-the-clock. Similar results were obtained by Browne (1949) for the speed of answering calls on a telephone switchboard. However, the maximum extent of the between-shift variations may have been 'masked' in these studies by the occurrence of partial adaptation to the altered sleep–waking cycle during the week-long period of night working over which the readings were summed. In rapidly rotating shift systems where only, say, two night shifts are worked in succession, the magnitude of the circadian changes might be expected to be somewhat greater. Indeed, in an investigation of such a rapidly rotating system Folkard *et al.* (1976) found that, when the scores from an 'immediate information processing' task of visual search carried out at intervals during each of the three shifts were plotted according to time of day, the range of variation in efficiency amounted to nearly ±20% of the overall mean (see Figure 3).

In the same study by Folkard *et al.* (1976), it was found that the addition of a considerable memory load to the search task decreased the amplitude of the apparent rhythm, while also altering its phase by about 8 hours (see Figure 3); this differing trend, with high-memory loaded performance being better at night, would, of course, be predicted from the 'waking day' studies of memory tasks reviewed earlier, but it is particularly pleasing to see the prediction confirmed so clearly.*

In sum, the evidence from the recent research that has been conducted in the

---

*Note that the memory involved in this task was of the 'short term' variety. Long term memory would be expected to be worse for material presented at night (see Folkard *et al.*, 1977), and this prediction has been confirmed by Monk and Folkard (1978).

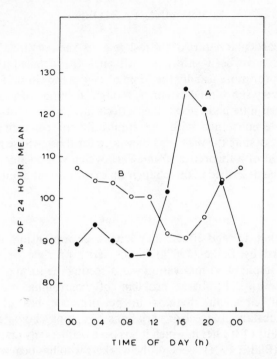

Figure 3 'Round-the-clock' variation in rate of work at a visual search task in a rapidly rotating 3 shift system. A, 'immediate information processing' version; B, 'memory loaded' version. $N = 2$. (Based on data in Folkard *et al.*, 1976)

area adds to that obtained in early studies in providing strong support for the existence of systematic variations in relatively simple performance with time of day that appear to reflect circadian rhythms in 'mental' processes similar to those exhibited by physiological functions. However, much of the research has been concerned only with changes in efficiency during the ordinary waking day. Although the observations that have been made during 'night' hours 'fit' with those from the daytime to give a clear impression of a 24 hour rhythm, these observations have, of necessity, been obtained in conditions such as sleep deprivation, or shift working, which are clearly not normal, and which may themselves be producing the very rhythmicity that is being looked for. Thus there remains the question as to whether or not observed circadian variations in performance represent a truly endogenous periodicity in the underlying process or processes responsible for them. One way to answer this question is to study the ways in which performance 'rhythms' alter in response to changes in the sleep–waking schedule. The effects of such changes are discussed in Chapters V and VII.

MODIFYING FACTORS

Apart from the particular nature of the task (e.g. its 'memory load'), a number of other factors have been shown to influence the detailed form of the circadian rhythm (or more usually the 'time of day' trend) in performance, in some cases to a very substantial extent. Although the mode of action of these factors is at present little understood, their effects are obviously of considerable interest to people concerned with the application of research findings in practical settings, despite the problems they pose for those whose primary aim is the construction of a theoretical framework which will adequately account for the phenomena described in this chapter up to the present point.

Motivation

The suggestion that an 'end-effect' may have been responsible for the 'late peaking' observed by Blake (1967a) in his series of time of day studies described earlier implies that motivation was affecting the form of the diurnal performance curves. The basic problem of controlling motivation in investigations of circadian rhythms in performance has already been discussed. The substantial effect of variations in this psychological 'state' is shown by the results of studies in which it has been deliberately manipulated.

Blake himself (Blake, 1971) is one of the workers who has demonstrated this effect most clearly. In an experiment using the immediate information processing task of letter cancellation, he showed that the variation in performance over the day observed by him in this task under 'normal' conditions was dramatically reduced by introducing an incentive. The latter was provided by announcing each individual's score, immediately after each test session, in the presence of all the members of the group. This supplying of 'knowledge of results' in a social context produced a strong spirit of competition in the subjects, and the resultant heightened state of motivation in the group reduced the extent of the mean time of day variation to a non-significant level (see Figure 4). As might perhaps be expected, the effect of the increased motivation was most marked at times of day when performance was relatively poor (early morning, and after lunch) but barely noticeable at the 'best' time (2100 h).

Chiles, Alluisi, and Adams (1968) have also demonstrated this 'dampening' effect of raised levels of motivation on the amplitude of circadian performance variation. While comparing the effects on performance efficiency of following different work–rest schedules during prolonged confinement to a simulated aerospace vehicle crew compartment, they observed that several of the performance measures taken showed daily variation (which paralleled, at least approximately, the circadian periodicities found in physiological measures such as temperature and pulse rate). However, this variation was not

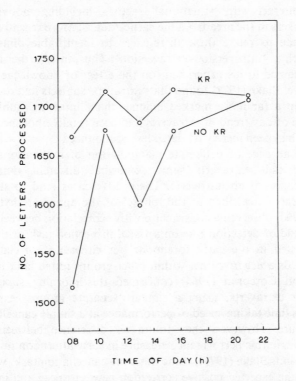

Figure 4   Variation over the waking day in rate of work at a simple letter cancellation task. KR, with 'knowledge of results' incentive (see text); NO KR, without incentive. *N* = 30 and 25 respectively. (Reproduced with permission from M. J. F. Blake (1971). Temperament and time of day. In: *Biological Rhythms and Human Performance*. W. P. Colquhoun (Ed.). London, Academic Press, p.142. Copyright by Academic Press Inc. (London) Ltd.)

significant in a group who were shown the results obtained from earlier groups and were then 'requested to put forth extra effort whenever they sensed any drop in their "sharpness". Thus, they were asked to attempt to prevent the appearance of the low points (or cycling in their performance curves)'. The fact that the subjects were able to do what was asked of them points up the importance of taking the whole 'test situation' into account when considering the results of any particular experiment, and provides a warning of the dangers of generalizing from one subject population to a different one, or even from one individual to another.

Personality Differences

The existence of individual differences in time of day effects, and the way in which these interact with 'situational' factors, including motivation, has concerned workers in the area from the earliest times. More recently, attempts have been made to relate these differences to identifiable dimensions of personality such as 'introversion–extraversion'. Thus, in a further analysis of the results obtained in his experiment on the effect of knowledge of results described above, Blake (1971) found that 'extravert' subjects had responded to the incentive in a far more marked manner than 'introvert' subjects; as a result, the time of day trend in extraverts had been totally abolished, whereas in introverts it had been merely rendered less pronounced.

Even in the absence of deliberate manipulation of motivational state, it would appear that extraverts show somewhat different time of day performance curves from introverts. These differences tend to show up in what is most easily described as the 'phase' of the apparent rhythm. Thus Colquhoun (1960) observed a consistent positive correlation between scores of introversion, and of detection rate on a visual inspection task, within groups of subjects tested in the early forenoon; but either no correlation, or a tendency towards a *negative* one, within other groups tested later in the day. Colquhoun and Corcoran (1964) confirmed this morning superiority of introverts over extraverts, using a similar 'separate groups' experimental design, but this time taking speed of performance at a simple cancellation task as their measure. However, they found no difference between the two personality types in this performance measure in early afternoon test sessions. On the other hand, Blake (1971), using the same cancellation task, was able to show not only the expected positive correlation between speed and introversion in the morning, but also a negative one in the evening; Blake used a 'repeated measures' design with a single group of subjects, tested at various times of day.

In each of the above experiments, individual subjects in a group were tested in complete isolation from each other. Colquhoun and Corcoran (1964) showed that the morning superiority of introverts at the cancellation task completely disappeared when the subjects were seated in company round a table while carrying out the test. This is a striking demonstration of the importance of taking situational factors into account when investigating circadian rhythms in performance. It would appear that the simple fact of being able to see others working at the same task may, at least in an 'experimental' setting, be at least as important in determining the time of day trends observed as the presence or absence of specifically motivating conditions such as knowledge of results.

Effects of physiological rhythms. Apart from the above set of results, more success has been achieved in relating personality factors to observed differences in the rhythm of body temperature (which, as has been shown, tends to parallel that of certain kinds of performance) than to differences in performance rhythms themselves. Thus, Colquhoun and Folkard (1978), in a further analysis of data collected by Blake (1967b), showed that the delayed 'phase' of the temperature rhythm of extraverts demonstrated in the latter report was considerably more marked in 'neurotic' than in 'stable' subjects. Colquhoun and Folkard also showed that these personality factors can determine, to a quite substantial degree, the extent to which the temperature rhythm initially adjusts to a change in the sleep–waking cycle. They analysed data recorded by Adam *et al.* (1972) immediately after such a change induced by a flight across eight time zones, and found that not only was there significantly greater adjustment in extraverts than in introverts, but that the temperature of 'neurotic' extraverts was showing an almost complete phase shift at a time when that of 'neurotic' introverts had hardly altered at all. Again, on the first day of a period of night shifts, night nurses of the neurotic extravert type were shown by Colquhoun and Folkard to exhibit considerably greater rhythm adjustment than those rated as neurotic introverts.

These findings, along with the observation that the temperature readings of extraverts are more variable from day to day than those of introverts, led Colquhoun and Folkard to advance the hypothesis that the rhythmic system of extraverts—particularly, perhaps, 'neurotic' ones—may have an underlying periodicity greater than 24 hours (as has been suggested to be the case for 'evening types', a very possibly related personality grouping). Whether or not this is true, there seems to be little doubt of the importance of personality factors in determining the nature of the temperature rhythm, particularly in abnormal situations. In fact, further evidence of their influence has recently been discovered by the author (Colquhoun and Condon, 1981) in a reanalysis of data originally collected by Colquhoun, Blake and Edwards (1968b) during the course of a study on the rate of adjustment of various rhythms to the altered sleep–waking cycle imposed by 12 days of unbroken night shift working. It was found that the 10 subjects employed in that experiment could be divided into two equally sized groups, one of extraverts and the other of introverts. Despite the small numbers of subjects, and the fact that neither group was a 'neurotic' one, Colquhoun and Condon were able to show that the phase of the temperature rhythm shifted at a significantly faster rate in the extravert group than in the introvert group.

In attempting to account for the various findings described above, an alternative to the hypothesis that extraverts' rhythms have an underlying periodicity greater than 24 hours has been advanced by Colquhoun (1978). He suggested that introverted and/or 'neurotic' people are less 'labile' physiologically (as well as psychologically) speaking, and that, because of this, their rhythms are less likely to respond to changes in the external 'event structure', whether familiar or not. If this is the case, this difference should show up most clearly in physiological measures which are known to be particularly sensitive to exogenous factors. Pulse rate is such a measure, and indeed Colquhoun and Folkard (in an unpublished study from the author's laboratory) have shown, in an analysis of previously unreported data collected by Blake, that a post-prandial rise in this index after a heavy midday meal is significantly smaller in introverts than in extraverts, and apparently virtually absent altogether in 'neurotic' introverts. It has also been oberved (Colquhoun, 1978) that people of the latter type show the least 'post-lunch decrement' in a task of simple calculations; however, owing to the small numbers of subjects so far tested, the reliability of these (apparently associated) physiological and performance differences between 'neurotic' introverts and others cannot yet be taken as established. The same caveat applies to the greater degree of overall post-flight decrement at the calculations task found (Colquhoun, unpublished) to be shown by the neurotic introverts, who, in the reanalysis of the time zone experiment by Adam *et al.* (1972), described earlier, were found to be least adjusted in terms of their temperature rhythm.

Conclusions

Thus, at present, there would appear to be more demonstrations of the effects of personality factors on physiological rhythms, particularly that in temperature, than there are on the performance rhythms that often appear to parallel them in certain respects. Nevertheless, performance rhythms have been shown to be strongly influenced not only by these personality factors, but also by motivation, and by differences in the 'test situation'. In the case of personality, there is a sufficient degree of consistency between the results from physiological and performance studies to warrant the conclusion that there are important links here, which future experimentation will eventually substantiate and, hopefully, explain. In the meantime, the implications of all the findings reviewed in this section for the conduct of experiments in the area of performance rhythms, and for the applicability of the results obtained, clearly cannot be ignored.

AROUSAL, FATIGUE, AND 'EFFICIENCY CHANGES'

The Arousal Hypothesis

The observed parallelism between the rhythm of body temperature and that of performance at a range of immediate information processing tasks has been mentioned several times in preceding sections. The temperature rhythm has been considered by some writers to reflect an underlying circadian variation in 'arousal', or more exactly 'non-sleepiness' (Kleitman, 1963; Colquhoun, 1971). This 'sleepiness' rhythm appears to have been first proposed by Gates (1961a), who based his ideas on the anaemia sleep theory of Howell (1897). Gates hypothesized that the rate of recovery from the anaemic condition through the day is determined by the cumulative effects of diurnal sensory experience and increased brain activity.

Speculative though such a theory may appear to be, it is at least consistent with the observed effects of sleep deprivation. Performance at many tasks has been shown to be depressed by this condition in the morning following a night's loss of sleep (see Chapter V) but to recover later on in the day. Although this recovery is not usually sufficient to restore efficiency to 'normal' levels, the magnitude of the diurnal variation may be increased overall (see, for example, Fiorica *et al.*, 1968). According to Wilkinson (1965), the tasks most affected by sleep deprivation are prolonged, uninteresting, and 'simple' ones, i.e. tasks which, because of their 'unarousing' nature, are least likely to counteract the presumed 'dearoused' (anaemic?) state of the sleep-deprived subject. Blake (1971), in discussing the results of his experiments described earlier in this chapter, argues that those tasks which showed the most clear time of day effects in his series are also tasks of this kind, and that this supports the general notion that changes in arousal underly both sleep deprivation and circadian effects.

There are several difficulties with this theory that improvements in performance during the day reflect increasing arousal (or decreasing sleepiness), and are thus 'complementary' to the detrimental effects of sleep loss. The first is that clear diurnal variation has been shown to exist in tasks which are *not* simple, for example, logical reasoning (Folkard, 1975), complex memory and search (Folkard *et al.*, 1976), and simulated flight (Klein, 1977). Such tasks could hardly be described as 'unarousing'. The second is that tasks which are performed for only as little as a few minutes at a time (see, for example, Fort and Mills, 1972; Folkard, 1975; Folkard *et al.*, 1976) show at least as much variation as the 'long duration' tasks of the Wilkinson type. The third is that, as has been shown earlier in this chapter, efficiency on tasks which test short term memory gets *worse* over the day, rather than better. Finally, it has been demonstrated that *subjectively perceived* arousal, although indeed exhibiting a clear diurnal rhythm, is declining from its peak level at a time when performance at at least some tasks is often reported as still improving (Thayer, 1978).

Attempts have been made to account for at least some of these anomalies by invoking an 'inverted-U' model of the effects of arousal on performance (see Corcoran, 1962). According to this model there is a different optimal level of arousal for any particular task—and perhaps even for any particular set of testing circumstances for a given task. The trouble with this notion, as its critics point out, is that, in the absence of any accepted independent measure of arousal, it is impossible to disprove any assertion made about the presumed effects of variations in its level; the model can, therefore, 'explain' almost anything. Even so, this most flexible of theories has difficulties in accounting for *all* of the complex interactions that have been found between time of day and other presumed arousing conditions such as extraversion, loud noise, or incentives (see Folkard, 1981b, for a discussion of these findings). Thus, if an 'arousal' theory is to account successfully for the totality of the results obtained in studies of circadian variations in performance, it will, as Folkard and Monk (1978) point out, probably have to be a 'multi-factor' theory that recognizes the existence of at least two, if not more, arousing oscillatory systems in the nervous substrate mediating observed behaviour. However, this is not to say that the 'simple' or 'unidimensional' arousal-rhythm hypothesis should be dismissed out of hand; it accommodates the great majority of existing findings, and in any case at present provides the only reasonably adequate conceptual framework in which the results obtained in studies of performance fluctuations over the 24 hour period can be discussed.

Prolonged Performance

Whether or not the finding that performance at prolonged, unarousing tasks such as vigilance does appear to show a fairly pronounced improvement over the day (Blake, 1967a; Colquhoun, 1971) can be accounted for on the 'unidimensional' arousal hypothesis, it has been pointed out by Bonnet and Webb (1978) that, in the experiments where this improvement has been demonstrated, either the test sessions were fairly widely spaced, or the task was alternated with others at frequent intervals. Bonnet and Webb showed that when sessions are 'massed' in such a way that the same test is repeated many times during an extended 'work' period (8 hours in their case) the improvement disappears. This masking of a circadian rhythm by 'fatigue' effects has also been found to occur when the length of *individual* test sessions is itself particularly extended. Colquhoun, Hamilton, and Edwards (1975) tested subjects at an auditory vigilance task for unbroken sessions of 4 hours' duration and found that in this case there was no increase in mean detection rate from a 'morning' to an 'evening' session. Like Bonnet and Webb, Colquhoun and his colleagues observed that, during 'night' hours, such prolonged testing, combined with the sleep deprivation that was a necessary adjunct to the procedure, greatly exaggerated the decline in efficiency that would have been expected from the 'normal' circadian fluctuation. The results of this experiment are shown in Figure 5.

Comparison of the direction and magnitude of the differences between the mean detection rates recorded over the first 2 hours of each 'pair' of watches with the differences obtained for the corresponding times of day in an earlier experiment* that can be considered as a 'control', showed that the prolonged

---

*In this experiment (the results of which are illustrated in Figure 2) the test sessions were of 2 hours' duration only, occurred on different days, and were each preceded by a rest period of at least 8 hours.

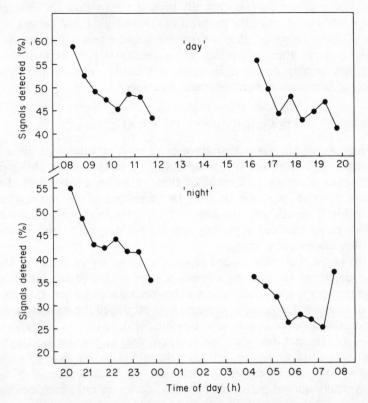

Figure 5   Signal detection efficiency in successive 30 min periods of 4 hour sessions at a vigilance task. Average results from four 'day' trials ($N=11$) and four 'night' trials ($N=12$). (After Colquhoun, Hamilton, and Edwards, 1975)

testing transformed the 'expected' substantial overall rise from 0800–1000 to 1600–1800 to a slight *fall*; and increased the 'expected' overall fall from 2000–2200 to 0400–0600 by a factor which would appear to be no less than about three. Note that, in the case of the 0800–1200 watch, the pronounced 'within session' decrement also masks an improvement that would have been expected *during* this period.

The confounding effects of fatigue on time of day effects in vigilance illustrated by these results (and shown also in the case of multiple task performance, see Coates, 1974) underline the fact that extreme caution should be exercised in generalizing from the typical laboratory experiment in which no attempt is made to simulate 'work' conditions, to real-life situations where, in some cases, fatigue, rather than circadian rhythms, may be the dominant factor in determining actual on-shift performance trends. Of course, as was noted in the introduction, this was clearly recognized by the early workers in this area, and it is not claimed that the present results take us very much further towards a solution of the problem of separating the two factors noted by Gates (1916b). However, they do provide a quantitative estimate of the likely magnitude of their interaction for a particular type of task that is becoming increasingly common in modern industry, namely the human monitoring of automatic or semiautomatic machinery.

MEASUREMENTS OF CHANGE

A large number of the tasks that have been used in studies of circadian rhythms are of a kind where two measures of performance are obtainable, namely speed and accuracy. Typical of these tasks are card-sorting, letter cancellation, and simple calculations. In these tasks, the measure that normally exhibits significant variation is speed; error rates are typically very low, and are rarely reported as varying with time of day, while speed tends to increase from morning to evening.

It will be noted that these 'speed increasing' tasks are examples of those previously described as requiring immediate information processing. Where short term memory is tested, efficiency, as has been shown earlier, exhibits the opposite diurnal trend, tending to *decrease* over the day (but note that *speed* of recall is normally ignored in studies of this function). In the case of efficiency at sensory discriminations such as are involved in the frequently used 'vigilance' type of task, the performance changes observed seem to parallel those seen with the speed measures in immediate information processing tasks; thus the typically quoted performance index, detection rate, increases from morning to evening in line with, say, the rate at which simple computations are performed (see Figure 1).

The fact that the detection rate in vigilance tasks improves over the day would seem to indicate that the efficiency with which sensory discriminations are made increases from morning to evening. However, signal detection theory (Green and Swets, 1966) has clearly demonstrated that a rise in detection rate may not necessarily reflect an increase in the actual ability to discriminate 'signals' from 'non-signals', or noise, but rather a lowering of the decision criterion for making a positive response to 'signal-like' events. Such a shift in criterion results in a rise in both true detection rate and in incorrect detections, i.e. in 'false reports'. Because the false report rate did not, in fact, usually appear to increase in their experiments, it was concluded by Colquhoun, Blake, and Edwards (1968a,b; 1969) that the rise in detection rate over the day consistently found in their studies did indeed indicate, in nearly all cases, a genuine improvement in discrimination efficiency. Although this conclusion may have been correct, it is also true that the false report rates obtained by Colquhoun and his colleagues were (as it typical in vigilance studies) extremely low. Thus the estimates of the signal detection theory 'discriminability' parameter d' which they calculated to support their contention were, of necessity, of low reliability.

In order to gain more reliable estimates of d', Craig (1979) tested subjects at a 'standard' binary discrimination task, with equiprobable signals, at 0800 and 2000, and found no significant change in discriminability between the two times of day. However, both response bias and report confidence did show changes, the latter increasing in the evening. Craig interpreted these results as indicating that time of day influences the decision-making process involved in perceptual judgments, and suggested that a change in this process, rather than an improvement in signal discrimination ability, may be a more probable cause of the increase in detection rates over the day seen with vigilance tasks. Craig further speculated that an analogous shift in the decision 'criterion' may underlie many of the 'speed' changes in immediate information processing tasks referred to above. If this is the case, one might expect to see a change in the 'speed–accuracy trade-off' over the day in the studies which have used such tasks. At first sight, the fact that the error rates have not been reported as increasing over the day would seem to refute this hypothesis. However, as has already been mentioned, overall error rates (where given) are typically very low; they are thus unlikely to have provided sufficiently reliable data for any trends to be detected. The one case where a speed–accuracy trade-off with time of day has been reported for a 'simple' task was step-input pursuit tracking (Buck, 1977). However, since this is clearly a task requiring primarily the execution of gross motor programmes, the question of whether increases in speed over the day in 'typical' immediate information processing tasks indicate changes in strategy, rather than genuine improvements in efficiency, is still an open one, to be answered, perhaps, by further studies with such tasks where the possibility for error is deliberately made much greater.

Despite this somewhat unsatisfactory conclusion, there are, as mentioned above, two types of task in which speed of response is not the normal measure of performance, namely, signal discrimination and memory tasks; is there evidence for strategy change in these cases? Certainly it would seem possible to view the shift in the decision criterion hypothesized by Craig (1979) to be responsible for the changes in performance over the day in signal discrimination tasks as an alteration in the strategy adopted (in this case, in making the required judgments). And in the case of memory, the apparently 'reverse' diurnal changes observed in the efficiency of immediate recall have been interpreted by Folkard and his colleagues (Folkard, 1979a,b; Folkard and Monk, 1979) in a similar light (see below).

Arousal and Strategy Change

Blake (1967a) considered that the finding by Kleinsmith and Kaplan (1963) that induced arousal is detrimental to short term memory was sufficient evidence to enable the observed reverse diurnal trend in efficiency at a digit-span test to accounted for within the unidimensional arousal framework. Additional, more elaboratively supported reasoning for such an account comes from research in the sleep deprivation area, where the presumed lowering of arousal resulting from cumulative partial sleep loss has been shown by Hamilton, Wilkinson, and Edwards (1972) to produce *improved* performance at a (running) digit-span test, whilst simultaneously degrading both speed of computation and efficiency of signal discriminability in a vigilance task. Hamilton and colleagues hypothesized that the improved recall arose from a systematic tendency towards more 'passive' listening as the extent of sleep deprivation, and thus the degree to which arousal was lowered, increased. They proposed a model which accounted for the effects of such passivity by assuming that the latter would delay the decay of traces of recently presented material supposedly held in a 'buffer store'. However, the important part of their argument in the present context was the postulation of a change of strategy accompanying an altered arousal state.

Folkard (1979b) showed that the morning superiority for immediate recall of digit sequences disappears when subjects are specifically instructed to group and rehearse the items during presentation, or to recall the items in a specific order, or both. Folkard and Monk (1979) also demonstrated that the normal morning superiority in short term memory for word lists can be abolished by preventing subvocal rehearsal of the material, thus suggesting that the decline over the day in the performance of tasks involving storage and encoding may be mediated by a strategy change in the use of the articulatory loop. These results were taken as evidence that time of day influences the type of strategy spontaneously adopted; Folkard and Monk (1979) suggested that such a change in processing strategy could itself reflect an increase in attentional selectivity associated with the diurnal increase in arousal level.

As a result of other studies in which he showed that the acoustic similarity effect on short term memory was greater at 1000 than at 1900, and that inter-posing a digit sequence memory task between the presentation of a list of words and its subsequent recall had a greater detrimental effect on list learning at the former time than at the latter, Folkard (1979a) concluded that the suggestion (originally put forward by Folkard and Monk, 1979) that more reliance is placed on maintenance processing in the morning, but more on elaborative processing later in the day, was clearly supported.*

Thus it would appear that time of day fluctuations in the performance of certain tasks, particularly those involving encoding and storage, may indeed reflect underlying changes in the strategies employed in selecting and processing the incoming information, rather than alterations in the actual

---

*The results of all these experiments, and their relation to arousal theory, have been summarized in a review article by Folkard (1981a).

efficiency of such operations; and further, that these changes in strategy may be the mental functions that are most obviously affected by the circadian rhythm (or rhythms) of arousal. This is not to say that the efficiency of the basic systems of information reception and transmission does not also vary in a circadian manner: however, except in the case of the most simple perceptual motor tasks, it may well be that these variations are of relatively minor significance in determining the effective level of performance actually observed at any particular time within the 24 hour cycle.

ENVOI

The conclusion from the evidence presented in this chapter is that performance at a wide range of tasks varies considerably at different times within the waking day; and that measures on such tasks taken at times when the subject would normally have been sleeping 'fit in' with those taken in waking hours in such a way as to strongly suggest the presence of an underlying circadian rhythm in the process or processes underlying the performance. However, it is also clear that the phase, the amplitude, and the detailed 'shape' of these circadian variations can be affected to a greater or less extent by a number of factors, acting either alone or in combination. These factors include the degree of memory load involved in the task, the taking of meals, the level of motivation, the personality type of the individual subject, and the general 'test situation'. It is also apparent that 'fatigue' can influence the nature of the observed trends, though, except in the case of 'vigilance' tasks, systematic attempts to estimate the magnitude of its effects have not as yet been made.

Although in a number of cases variations in performance efficiency round-the-clock appear to closely follow the circadian rhythm of body temperature, it is evident that the notion of a *general* parallelism between performance and temperature rhythms is not really tenable, and that the hypothesis of an actual causal connection between the two may be positively misleading, at least for the great majority of measures of 'performance' in the sense of this term used in this chapter (for fuller discussion see Chapter V). Reservations also apply to the association of performance fluctuations with assumed changes in 'arousal' over the day; nevertheless, at present the arousal-rhythm theory is the only one which can successfully account for a significant proportion of the observed experimental results in the area.

An unanswered question is whether *all* 'time of day' curves represent segments of truly endogenous circadian rhythms, or whether differences in performance at different times of day are caused, in some cases, by the action of exogenous factors which are themselves periodic (see Chapter I). It is true that investigations in isolation chambers have provided fairly strong support for the endogenous nature of at least some performance rhythms, but the observation that the rhythm in a task involving short term memory adjusts to a phase shift of the Zeitgeber at a faster rate than that in one of immediate information processing (Monk *et al.*, 1978) throws some doubt on the generality of the 'endogeneity' hypothesis. Endogenous or not, it cannot really be said that (with the possible exception of immediate recall efficiency) we are significantly nearer to identifying the underlying 'mental' processes responsible for the outwardly observed circadian variations in task performance, nor, indeed, to determining their connection with any particular cyclical physiological state or states. One thing is certain, however: the variations are not ephemeral, since they have been shown in several studies (e.g. Colquhoun, Blake, and Edwards, 1968b) to persist unabated over periods of testing up to as much as 12 days in length, and recently (in unpublished studies by the author and his colleagues) for even longer times, thus confirming the results obtained by the earliest workers, who doggedly tested (only) themselves day after day for months on end.

It is a somewhat depressing fact that, despite a considerable amount of experimentation, little progress in our understanding of the phenomena described in this chapter has been achieved over the last 100 years. Most of the recent findings have simply confirmed (though sometimes on a more reliable basis) those made by the pioneer workers at the turn of the century. One factor which may partly account for this lack of progress is that experimenters are continuing to use 'tasks' or 'tests' which are essentially the same as those which were used in the earliest studies of time of day effects, and that what exactly it is that these tests are measuring is still not understood. Really significant advances are therefore perhaps unlikely to be made until new and more sophisticated methods for assessing cerebral functioning have been developed. However, in the meantime, it would seem that considerable progress could be hoped for if a systematic attempt was made to refine our existing measuring instruments. One way to determine the directions which such refinement should take is to study the manner in which particular manipulations affect the readings given by standard 'tests' at different times of day. Thus, as described in the previous section, Folkard and his colleagues have, by such studies, been able to demonstrate that diurnal variations in performance at accepted tests of short term memory reflect changes in the strategies adopted in processing the information presented for recall, rather than alterations in the basic 'efficiency' of the latter. Not only does this represent a substantial step forward in our understanding of the actual mechanisms underlying the cyclic variations observed in scores of immediate memory, it also gives a clear indication of the nature of the tests which could profitably be used in future studies of circadian rhythms in performance at tasks involving encoding and storage. There is every reason to suppose that a similar approach to existing tests of other types of performance function would yield equally fruitful results.

SUMMARY

This chapter considers performance as it relates to the time period in which it occurs. The early work describing diurnal changes influencing 'mental efficiency' and the relationships between temperature and performance are reviewed. The complex issue of repeated measures and the resultant compounding of 'learning' and 'motivational' effects are noted. A systematic analysis of recent research, emphasizing the task specific nature of the performance/time relationship, provides evidence of clear cut variations linking performance level and time of day. The impact of the modifying factors of motivation and personality are considered. The chapter concludes with a discussion of both conceptual and explanatory issues raised by the data relative to 'arousal' and 'fatigue' and the methodological problems of measuring performance 'efficiency'. The effects of various task dimensions and strategy changes relating to these issues is also explored.

REFERENCES

Adam, J., Brown, T., Colquhoun, P., Hamilton, P., Orsborn, J., Thomas, I. and Worsley, D. (1972). Nychthemeral rhythms and air trooping: some preliminary results from "Exercise Medex". In: *Aspects of Human Efficiency: Diurnal Rhythm and Loss of Sleep.* W. P. Colquhoun (Ed.). London, English Universities Press.

Aschoff, J., Giedke, H., Poppel, E., and Wever, R. (1972). The influence of sleep-interruption and of sleep deprivation on circadian rhythms in human performance. In: *Aspects of Human Efficiency: Diurnal Rhythm and Loss of Sleep.* W. P. Colquhoun (Ed.). London, English Universities Press.

Baade, W. (1907). Experimentelle und kritische Beitrage zur Fragenach den sekundaren Wirkungen des Unterrichts insbesondere auf die Empfanglichkeit des Schulers. *Paedag. Monogr.* Bd. III, Leipzig.

Baddeley, A. D., Hatter, J. E., Scott, D., and Snashall, A. (1970). Memory and time of day. *Quarterly Journal of Experimental Psychology* 22, 605–609.

Bechterew, W. (1893). Uber die Geschwindigkeitsveranderungen der psychischen Processe zu verschiedenen Takeszeiten. *Neurol. Zbl.* 12, 290–292.

Bjerner, B., Holm, A., and Swensson, A. (1955). Diurnal variation in mental performance. A study of three-shift workers. *British Journal of Industrial Medicine* 12, 103–110.

Blake, M. J. F. (1967a). Time of day effects on performance in a range of tasks. *Psychonomic Science* 9, 349–350.

Blake, M. J. F. (1967b). Relationship between circadian rhythm of body temperature and introversion–extraversion. *Nature* 215, 896–897.

Blake, M. J. F. (1971). Temperament and time of day. In: *Biological Rhythms and Human Performance.* W. P. Colquhoun (Ed.). London, Academic Press.

Bonnet, M. H. and Webb, W. B. (1978). The effect of repetition of relevant and irrelevant tasks over day and night work periods. *Ergonomics* 21, 999–1005.

Browne, R. C. (1949). The day and night performance of teleprinter switchboard operators. *Occupational Psychology* 23, 1–6.

Buck, L. (1977). Circadian rhythms in step-input pursuit tracking. *Ergonomics* 20, 19–31.

Chiles, W. D., Alluisi, E. A., and Adams, O. (1968). Work schedules and performance during confinement. *Human Factors* 10, 143–196.

Coates, G. D. (1974). Interaction of continuous work and sleep loss with the effects of the circadian rhythm—II. In: *Sustained Performance and Recovery during Continuous Operations.* B. B. Morgan and G. D. Coates (Eds.). Technical Report ITR-74-2. Norfolk, Virginia USA.

Colquhoun, W. P. (1960). Temperament, inspection efficiency, and time of day. *Ergonomics* 3, 377–378.

Colquhoun, W. P. (1971). Circadian variations in mental efficiency. In: *Biological Rhythms and Human Performance.* W. P. Colquhoun (Ed.). London, Academic Press.

Colquhoun, W. P. (1978). Working efficiency, personality, and body rhythms. *Department of Employment Gazette* 86, 682–685.

Colquhoun, W. P., Blake, M. J. F., and Edwards, R. S. (1968a). Experimental studies of shift work. I: a comparison of 'rotating' and 'stabilized' 4-hour shift systems. *Ergonomics* 11, 437–453.

Colquhoun, W. P., Blake, M. J. F., and Edwards, R. S. (1968b). Experimental studies of shift work. II: stabilized 8-hour shift systems. *Ergonomics* 11, 527–546.

Colquhoun, W. P., Blake, M. J. F., and Edwards, R. S. (1969). Experimental studies of shift work. III: stabilized 12-hour shift systems. *Ergonomics* 12, 865–882.

Colquhoun, W. P. and Condon, R. (1981). Introversion–extraversion and the adjustment of the body-temperature rhythm to night work. In: *Advances in Studies on Night and Shiftwork: Biological and Social Aspect.* A. Reinberg, N. Vieur and P. Andlauer (Eds.). Oxford, Pergamon Press.

Colquhoun, W. P. and Corcoran, D. W. J. (1964). The effects of time of day and social isolation on the relationship between temperament and performance. *British Journal of Social and Clinical Psychology* 3, 226–231.

Colquhoun, W. P. and Folkard, S. (1978). Personality differences in body-temperature rhythm, and their relation to its adjustment to night work. *Ergonomics* 21, 811–817.

Colquhoun, W. P., Hamilton, P., and Edwards, R. S. (1975). Effects of circadian rhythm, sleep deprivation, and fatigue on watchkeeping performance during the night hours. In: *Experimental Studies of Shiftwork.* W. P. Colquhoun *et al.* (Eds.) Opladen, Westdeutscher Verlag.

Corcoran, D. W. J. (1962). Individual Differences in Performance after Loss of Sleep. Unpublished PhD thesis, University of Cambridge, England.

Craig, A. (1979). Discrimination, temperature, and time of day. *Human Factors* 21, 61–68.

Ebbinghaus, H. (1885). *Memory.* Republished in translation, New York, Dover Publications, 1964.

Fiorica, V., Higgins, E. A., Iampietro, P. F., Lategola, M. T., and Davis, A. W. (1968). Physiological responses of men during sleep deprivation. *Journal of Applied Physiology* 24, 167–176.

Folkard, S. (1975). Diurnal variation in logical reasoning. *British Journal of Psychology* 66, 1–8.

Folkard, S. (1979a). Time of day and level of processing. *Memory and Cognition* 7, 247–252.

Folkard, S. (1979b). Changes in immediate memory strategy under induced muscle tension and with time of day. *Quarterly Journal of Experimental Psychology* 31, 621–633.

Folkard, S. (1981a). Circadian rhythms and human memory. In: *Rhythmic Aspects of Behaviour.* F. M. Brown and R. C. Graeber (Eds.). Hillsdown, New Jersey, Lawrence Erlbaum Associations.

Folkard, S. (1981b). Circadian rhythms and shiftwork. In: *Stress and Fatigue in Human Performance*. G. R. J. Hockey (Ed.). New York, John Wiley.

Folkard, S., Knauth, P., Monk, T. H., and Rutenfranz, J. (1976). The effect of memory load on the circadian variation in performance efficiency under a rapidly rotating shift system. *Ergonomics* **19**, 479–488.

Folkard, S. and Monk, T. H. (1978). Time of day effects in immediate and delayed memory. In: *Practical Aspects of Memory*. M. M. Gruneberg, P. E. Morris, and R. N. Sykes (Eds.). London, Academic Press.

Folkard, S. and Monk, T. H. (1979). Time of day and processing strategy in free recall. *Quarterly Journal of experimental Psychology* **31**, 461–475.

Folkard, S., Monk, T. H., Bradbury, R., and Rosenthall, J. (1977). Time of day effects in school children's immediate and delayed recall of meaningful material. *British Journal of Psychology* **68**, 45–50.

Fort, A. and Mills, J. N. (1972). Influence of sleep, lack of sleep, and circadian rhythm on short psychometric tests. In: *Aspects of Human Efficiency: Diurnal Rhythm and Loss of Sleep*. W. P. Colquhoun (Ed.). London, English Universities Press.

Freeman, G. L. and Hovland, C. I. (1934). Diurnal variations in performance and related physiological processes. *Psychological Bulletin* **31**, 777–799.

Gates, A. I. (1916a). Diurnal variations in memory and association. *University of California Publications in Psychology* **1**, 323–344.

Gates, A. I. (1916b). Variations in efficiency during the day, together with practise effects, sex differences, and correlations. *University of California Publications in Psychology* **2**, 1–156.

Green, D. M. and Swets, J. A. (1966). *Signal Detection Theory and Psychophysics*. New York, Wiley.

Halberg, F. (1970). A study of possible variation in rifle markmanship as a function of circadian system phase. *Air Force Contract F29600-69-C-0011: Report No. 1*. University of Minnesota.

Hamilton, P., Wilkinson, R. T., and Edwards, R. S. (1972). A study of four days partial sleep deprivation. In: *Aspects of Human Efficiency: Diurnal Rhythm and Loss of Sleep*. W. P. Colquhoun (Ed.). London, English Universities Press.

Heck, W. H. (1913). A second study of mental fatigue in relation to the daily school program. *Psychological Clinics* **7**, 29–34.

Hockey, G. R. J. and Colquhoun, W. P. (1972). Diurnal variation in human performance: a review. In: *Aspects of Human Efficiency: Diurnal Rhythm and Loss of Sleep*. W. P. Colquhoun (Ed.). London, English Universities Press.

Hockey, G. R. J., Davies, S., and Gray, M. M. (1972). Forgetting as a function of sleep at different times of day. *Quarterly Journal of Experimental Psychology* **24**, 386–393.

Hollingworth, H. L. (1914). Variations in efficiency during the working day. *Psychological Review* **21**, 473–491.

Howell, W. H. (1897). A contribution to the physiology of sleep based upon plethysmographic experiments. *Journal of Experimental Medicine* **2**, 313–345.

Hughes, D. G. and Folkard, S. (1976). Adaptation to an 8-h shift in living routine by members of a socially isolated community. *Nature* **264**, 432–434.

Jansen, G., Rutenfranz, J., and Singer, R. (1966). Uber eine circadiane Rhythmik sensumotorischer Leistungen. *Int. Z. angew. Physiol. einschl. Arbeitsphysiol.* **22**, 65–83.

Klein, K. E., Herrmann, R., Kuklinski, P., and Wegmann, H. M. (1977). Circadian performance rhythms: experimental studies in air operations. In: *Vigilance: Theory, Operational Performance, and Physiological Correlates*. R. R. Mackie (Ed.). New York, Plenum Press.

Kleinsmith, L. J. and Kaplan, S. (1963). Paired associate learning as a function of arousal and interpolated interval. *Journal of Experimental Psychology* **65**, 190–193.

Kleitman, N. (1963). *Sleep and wakefulness.* Chicago, University of Chicago Press.

Kleitman, N. and Jackson, D. P. (1950). Body temperature and performance under different routines. *American Journal of Applied Physiology* **3**, 309–328.

Kraeplin, E. (1893). Uber psychische Disposition. *Arch. Psychiat. Nervenkrkh.* **25**, 593.

Laird, D. A. (1925). Relative performance of college students as conditioned by time of day and day of week. *Journal of Experimental Psychology* **8**, 50–63.

Monk, T. H. and Folkard, S. (1978). Concealed inefficiency of late-night study. *Nature* **273**, 296–297.

Monk, T. H., Knauth, P., Folkard, S., and Rutenfranz, J. (1978). Memory based performance measures in studies of shiftwork. *Ergonomics* **21**, 819–826.

Rutenfranz, J., Aschoff, J., and Mann, H. (1972). The effects of a cumulative sleep deficit, duration of preceding sleep period, and body-temperature on multiple-choice reaction time. In: *Aspects of Human Efficiency: Diurnal Rhythm and Loss of Sleep.* W. P. Colquhoun (Ed.). London, English Universities Press.

Rutenfranz, J. and Hellbrugge, T. (1957). Uber Tagesschwankungen der Rechengeschwindigkeit bei 11-jahrigen Kindern. *Z. Kinderkeilk.* **80**, 65–82.

Thayer, R. E. (1978). Towards a psychological theory of multi dimensional activation (arousal). *Motivation and Emotion* **2**, 1–34.

Voigt, E. D., Engel, P., and Klein, H. (1968). Uber den Tagesgang der Korperlichen Leistungsfahigkeit. *Int. Z. angew. Physiol., einschl. Arbeitsphysiol.* **25**, 1–12.

Wilkinson, R. T. (1965). Sleep deprivation. In: *The Physiology of Human Survival.* O. G. Edholm and A. L. Bacharach (Eds.). New York, Academic Press.

Winch, W. H. (1913). Mental adaptation during the school day, as measured by arithmetical reasoning. *Journal of Educational Psychology* **4**, 17–28; 71–84.

Biological Rhythms, Sleep, and Performance
Edited by Wilse B. Webb
©1982 John Wiley & Sons Ltd.

Chapter 4

Sleep and Biological Rhythms

Wilse B. Webb

The early history of the measurement of variations in physiological functions and the measurement of sleep reveals an extensive and sustained interest in, and interaction between biological system changes and sleep. These will be reviewed first. The literature on biological rhythms shows that sleep has served as a significant experimental variable in that area. A brief review of this is given. The remainder of the chapter outlines the increasing role of chronobiology in sleep research.

PHYSIOLOGICAL VARIATIONS AND SLEEP

Folklore, common sense, and casual observations have recognized major changes of physiological functions in the presence of sleep. Many bodily systems go into a different 'gear' during sleep. The obviousness of these changes associated with sleep led to a long history of speculation and search for their meaning. At least three distinct possibilities have been proposed and explored to account for the simultaneous or near simultaneous occurrence of changes in biological systems and sleep:

(1) the changes are themselves determinants of sleep, e.g. a change in the blood volume results in sleep.
(2) the changes are resultants of or are caused by sleep and/or associated sleep behaviour, e.g. changes in temperature are due to a reclining posture.
(3) the changes *and* sleep are concomitants of some other event or condition, e.g. both sleep and metabolic changes result from 'fatigue' or, perhaps, time cues. The later possibility asserts the potential of a biological rhythm determinant of the change.

Speculations about these relations are found in the writings of the Greeks. Pieron (1913) attributes the earliest to Alcemon writing in the sixth century BC. He attributed sleep to a retreat of the blood into the veins and awakening to an

87

engorgement. Empedocles, some 100 years later, held that sleep was due to the 'cooling' of the blood. The Hippocratic writings, collected some 200 years after Hippocrates' death in about 370 BC, also attributed sleep to a cooling of the blood which resulted in the body becoming 'weak and heavy', the eyes closing, and intelligence waning.

From these writings one cannot forebear recording a remarkably circadian flavoured statement in *The Book of Prognostics* (Adams, 1939).

> 'The patients should wake during the day and sleep during the night. If this rule be otherwise altered it is so far worse, but there will be little harm provided he sleep in the morning for the third part of the day; such sleep as takes place after this time is more unfavorable, but worse of all is to get no sleep . . . .' (page 47)

The explosive growth of life science research in the later half of the 1800s brought a plethora of measurements in the physiological and neurophysiological domains. Relative to sleep, this era was characterized by emerging 'theories' of the causes of sleep centred in various systems. As stated elsewhere (Webb, 1973):

> 'There was a remarkably uniform pattern of the emergence of sleep theories during this period. A new set of findings would be developed about a physiological system and within a few years these findings would serve as an explanatory basis for sleep. For example, as information about the vascular system became available, theories of central anemia or congestion were put forth as likely causes of sleep . . . . Information about nerve cells provoked early inhibition theories of sleep. New data and interest in hematology, and in particular, oxygen and CO_2 characteristics of the blood, led to a plethora of humoral theories of sleep . . . . A new theory seemed to emerge with each new discovery of a bio-chemical process . . . .' (p.3)

But clearly the issue of the mechanisms of sleep was not the primary force behind the discovery and measurement of physiological functions. Sleep, rather, served as a 'condition' for measurement—as a modifier variable.

Kleitman reviews this extensive background in *Sleep and Wakefulness* (1963). His first seven chapters are grouped under the title 'Functional Differences Between Sleep and Wakefulness'. These chapters review the sleep-wakefulness differences of the skeletal musculature, nervous system, blood circulation, respiration, digestion, metabolism, body temperature, and excretion. The focus of the chapters is descriptive. In the three latter chapters he reviews the 'neural' and 'humoral' theories of sleep.

The literature reviewed is remarkable in both its age and its amount. Kleitman finds extensive data prior to this century. Referring to digestion, Kleitman says: 'In general, digestion is not affected in either direction by sleep. This was the considered view of the ancients, and little has been done within recent times to challenge it . . .' (p.53). The respiratory review refers to Aristotle: '(He) is credited with noting that, whereas in the waking state inspiration is active and of short duration and expiration passive and slow, the reverse is often true of sleep.' (p.48). This is followed by consideration in Mosso's work on pulmonary changes in 1878. In reference to reflex excitability, Kleitman notes Pieron's listing in 1907 of eight reports of increased and six reports of decreased reflex excitability (p.14). Studies of oxygen level and CO_2 changes in sleep were reported in an 1866 study (p.51).

With regard to extensity, a few examples will suffice. Kleitman cites 19 studies of electrical–dermal changes in sleep (pp.18–19). There are 55 haematological citations relative to sleep, including pH concentration, blood sugar, potassium, calcium, magnesium, phosphates, corticosteroids, and haemoglobin measures and some 15 studies of blood volume changes (pp.32–33). Reference to circulatory studies of heart rate and blood pressure exceed 100, and respiratory citations (excluding snoring) also exceeded 100.

Kleitman devotes one chapter to performance variations, '24 Hour Variation in Activity and Performance'. This is a remarkable review of the earlier work on performance variations across time and extends from the early work of Lombard (1887) and Dresslar (1892) and extensively reviews his own work in the 1930s relative to the covariations of temperature and performance across the 24 hours.

Throughout this extensive review, while the focus is descriptive, the matter of linkage is a troublesome one—often emerging from incompatible findings. Kleitman comments on Brunton's work as follows:

'Brunton, in a review dealing with the acid output of the kidney and the so-called alkaline tide, listed a number of possible contributory factors which may mask, in one direction or another, the effect of sleep itself, among them variations in food intake, digestive and endocrine tides, posture and muscular relaxation, sweat excretion, quiet and inhibitory influences from higher centers. It is clear that without a control of these factors one may attribute certain changes to sleep when they are only indirectly due to it. It should be emphasized that there are certain 24-hour rhythms—such as that of body temperature, which, even though in the long run are dependent on the alternation of sleep and wakefulness, may persist when one stays awake one or more nights and thus lead to erroneous interpretation of the control test themselves.' (p.64)

Again, he states in his discussion of temperature:

'The effect of sleep on body temperature has long been a topic for debate. It is not that anyone doubts that body temperature falls during the night, but the fall can conceivably be due to rest in the horizontal position and muscular relaxation. In addition, the fact that one's temperature begins to decrease long before bedtime, and follows its usual 24-hour course even if one stays awake the whole night, has been interpreted as showing that sleep is not directly responsible for the low night temperature.' (p.58)

The concerns of Kleitman were by no means new or his alone. The issue of sleep and biological rhythms, in fact, emerged as early as 1875. Fraisse (1963) notes that:

'It has been known for a long time that the pulse, blood pressure, and especially temperature of the body present day–night variations in humans as well as in many animals. There is about 1.8°F difference in the human temperature between the minimum at night and maximum in the afternoon. In 1875, physiologists already attributed this rhythm to the alternation of light and darkness which brought with it the alternation of activity and rest, they therefore thought it possible to reverse this by substituting nocturnal for diurnal activity. The results of their experiments remained very controversial, however, until Toulouse and Pieron found in 1907 that the temperature change was reversed in the case of nurses changing from day to night duty. This reversal was gradual and was not completed until after 30 or 40 days. During the first few weeks the rise in temperature, which usually takes place in the mornings and the early part of the afternoon, grew gradually less marked, until it finally changed to an increasingly rapid drop . . . .' (p.25)

There was a spate of studies in the early 1900s that measured temperature under conditions of displaced sleep and waking schedules. In 1913, Pieron was able to confidently write:

'The fact of reversal proves that the rhythm depends on the conditions of life, on physical and mental activity which normally reaches a peak at a moment determined by cosmic conditions, that is, by the light of the sun. There are, however, modifications of a social nature which explain the fact that this is reached much later in towns than in the country. It is therefore, impossible to speak of one fundamental periodicity. On the other hand the difficulty and slowness of reversal show that the rhythm has been firmly established and tends to maintain its periodicity and oppose the introduction of a new periodicity. Thus, a compromise arises gradually between the past, remembered action, which grows weaker, and the present action, which increases in strength.' (Pieron, 1913)

CHRONOBIOLOGY AND SLEEP

The description of a variation in a system between the state of sleep and waking merely provoked additional questions. The problems raised by the linkages between sleep and system changes form a substantial background of research from which particulars of biological rhythm research emerged. Given a system change and sleep, one can readily vary the sleep condition to explore the interrelations. These fit well the displacement model of biological rhythm research (Chapter I).

Model I: Sleep is replaced by non-sleep and non-sleep behaviour, e.g. the person is kept continuously awake and active for 24 hours.

Model II: the waking period is replaced by sleep behaviour in absence of sleep, e.g. bed rest continued across 24 hours.

Model III: sleep is displaced into an active period and wakefulness replaced the sleep period, e.g. shift work designs.

In these designs, first the variations associated with the sleep period are established. Then if the change did not occur in Model I, did not occur in the presence of sleep behaviour in Model II in the waking subject, or did not 'track' the new sleep period in Model III, sleep would be eliminated as a cause. More critically, if the variation did occur in the absence of sleep (Model I) but in the same time period of sleep, or did not 'track' the sleep behaviour or the displaced sleep period, but did occur in its original time period (Models II and III) notions of an endogenously and temporally ordered system became strong explanatory candidates.

Almost all of the major systems in which variations have been found between sleep or waking have been submitted to one or more of these paradigms. Classical examples extended from Ayles studies in 1866 (cited by Mills, 1966) in which temperature was measured during bed rest across the day to Mills' own renal function comparison of 24 hour wakefulness regime in the early 1950s (Mills, 1951).

Reviews of these experimental variations in systems other than sleep may be found in three chapters in Kleitman (1963, pages 8–61), Mills' 1966 review and in appropriate chapters in Conroy and Mills (1970), Mills (1973), and Saunders (1977).

That Kleitman, the doyen of sleep research, did not more closely link sleep research to biological rhythms, particularly as a circadian rhythm, is puzzling. Kleitman did one of the earliest reviews of the biological rhythm area titled 'Biological rhythms and cycles' (1949). His intensive interest in and comprehension of an endogenous rhythm system is seen in his proposed 'Basic Rest Activity Cycle' which was conceived of as a basic 90 minute ultradian cycle (see Chapter IX). *Sleep and Wakefulness* has one of eight 'parts' entitled 'periodicity' and begins with a chapter, 'the 24 Hour Sleep–Wakefulness and Body-Temperature Rhythms'. As noted above, seven chapters of his book explore the covariation of sleep and other systems. In spite of this, in his 1949 review he concluded that 'The diurnal rhythm is . . . a cycle synchronized with the external periodicity of day and night through the influence of variations in illumination, temperature and other environmental factors . . .'. In 1963, his book distinguished between rhythms which are 'extrinsic' in origin 'likened to a conditioned response' and cycles which are 'intrinsic' in origin. Clearly sleep was considered to be an extrinsically determined rhythm: 'To summarize, the development and maintenance of 24 hour sleep–wakefulness and body-temperature rhythms stems from being born into, and living in, a family and community run according to alternations of light and darkness . . . .' (p.147).

Certainly it would be improper to attribute the slow incorporation of biological rhythm influnces in sleep research to Kleitman. His position is more likely a reflection of the nascent state of both the biological rhythm and sleep areas. There is, however, substantial evidence of an infusion of chronobiology into the sleep domain since the mid-1960s. Since 1958 the UCLA Brain Research Center has published an annual bibliography of the worldwide research literature. These publications are encoded into some 20 categories. In recognition of the perceptible growth of papers which could be so classified, the category of 'biorhythms' was introduced in 1960. Table 1 of Chapter I displays the annual rate of publication of papers within sleep research which could be so designated. Clearly the interaction has been substantial.

Table 1   Biological rhythm aspects of sleep research

Sleep as an independent (phase shift) variable
Identification of temporal aspects of sleep
Variables associated with temporal aspects of sleep
  Species
  Age
  Individual differences
  Extraorganismic variables
  Intraorganismic variables
Time schedules with sleep as the dependent variable
  Time-free environments
  Desynchronous
  Phase shifts

The sleep literature which intersects with the area of chronobiology can be categorized into four areas. These are shown in Table 1.

The first category includes those studies previously referred to in which sleep is eliminated, 'mimicked', or displaced to test the temporal stability of some other biological system. These are the classical biological designs with sleep as the independent phase change variable described in Chapter I and reviewed earlier in this chapter. Within sleep research, the studies of the role of sleep timing relative to endocrine changes such as the growth hormone (LH) is a typical example. Studies in which performance is the primary dependent variable relative to sleep schedule variations are major chapters of this book. Chapter V considers the effects of sleep loss or sleep 'elimination' on performance. Chapter VII reviews the effects of phase shifts of sleep such as shift work designs on performance.

The second category refers to descriptive studies which have identified temporally stable and repetitive aspects of sleep. These are the identification design studies of Chapter I. These have included the measurement and designation of repeated and stable aspects of sleep patterns (sleep onset and termination times) and sleep structure variables such as the REM cycle and are reviewed in this chapter.

The third category are the studies which have defined the variables associated within changes in the defined temporal components of sleep such as species, age, individual differences, and such extraorganismic variables as energy expenditure or sleep surround variables such as noise. The intraorganismic variables are concerned with the effects of modification of the central nervous system by intrusive procedures or by drugs as they modify timing aspects of sleep. The influence of such variables on the temporal aspects of sleep are reviewed in this chapter.

The final category time schedule variations are related to the phase shift design of the first category but differ in that sleep is studied as the dependent variable. In these phase shift designs of this category, sleep may be displaced into the daytime period but rather than studying the continuation of the temperature rhythm or urinary cycle, the effect on sleep during the shift period serves as the primary dependent variable. As reviewed in this chapter, it will also be clear that such phase shift schedules as well as time-free and desynchronous schedules indeed are variables associated with temporal aspects of sleep.

TEMPORAL CHARACTERISTICS OF SLEEP

In Chapter I the primary 'marker' variables of sleep were categorized as pattern measures, structure measures, and subjective measures. Because of the marked variations in these measures due to age and species (see below) these basic measures will be reviewed first for the human adult.

Pattern Measures

Pattern measures, defined by the presence, absence, and placement of sleep, are described within a 24 hour time frame. By observation, objective records, or self-reports, the onset and termination of sleep are recorded. The most frequently reported units are total sleep, number and length of sleep episodes, and placement measures such as onset times or diurnal ratios.

There have been two substantial studies reporting sleep length across a wide age range: a questionnaire study (McGhie and Russell, 1962) and a sleep diary study (Tune, 1960). In addition, a detailed study on college students using questionnaires and sleep diaries simultaneously has been conducted (White, 1975). These studies, and others which have incidentally reported sleep length (e.g. Kripke *et al.*, 1979), are in common accord on sleep length—circa 7½ hours with a standard deviation of approximately one hour.

The more detailed study by White points up some pertinent aspects of this measure.

(1) Questionnaire estimates (either as a direct estimate or derived from estimated bed–waking up times) are correlated 0.80 (circa) with two week diaries.
(2) About 15% of the two estimates varied by more than 1 hour; about 60% by less than 30 minutes.
(3) The population means differ by less than 10 minutes.
(4) The population standard deviation of measures of sleep length is approximately 1 hour.
(5) Within subject standard deviations across two week averages somewhat over 1 hour.
(6) Sleep length on weekends averages one-half hour (plus) longer than on weekdays.

A number of studies have considered the correlates of 'natural' long and short sleepers (see Webb, 1979a) without detecting substantial differences. Several studies have been reported on the chronic reduction of sleep (Johnson and MacLeod, 1973; Webb and Agnew, 1974a).

In the young human adult a 'normative' pattern of sleep is a single nocturnal episode and total sleep time and the length of the sleep period are coterminous. The primary variant is the nap. College students, who are less time bound by regular schedules, show extensive napping. White (1975) reported an average of nearly two naps per week with a mean total time per week of nearly 3 hours from sleep diary data. Evans *et al.* (1977) in a detailed study of naps, reported that only 40% of a student population never or rarely napped. Evans divided naps into replacement naps (making up for lost or soon to be lost sleep) and appetitive naps. The naps of the latter group were significantly 'lighter' than replacement naps. Webb (1978b) has published a speculative paper on napping as a part of the sleep–waking biological rhythm.

Relative to sleep placement, White's data again reveals a range of both between and within subject variability. The population's standard deviation around a mean bedtime during the week of approximately midnight was 1.02 hours; on weekends the standard deviation was 1.34 hours. Wake up time had a standard deviation of 0.89 hour. There was substantial within subject variability, a median standard deviation of 1.12 hours across the two weeks. Johns, Bruce, and Masterton (1974) reported a bedtime between subject standard deviation of 45 minutes using a questionnaire. The extensive presence of shift work which effects sleep placement work is increasingly documented. Bureau of Labour statistics show that, in industrial centres, there is a rise of 6% per decade and in 1978 reported 28% of industrial workers on these schedules. Placement is further confounded by the time zone displacements associated with jet travel. The variations are detailed in Chapter VII.

Several studies have examined the systematic late ('owl') placement of sleep (see Horne and Ostberg, 1977). By an especially devised questionnaire and by temperature measures it is apparent that some individuals systematically place their sleep periods earlier or later than the general population. The determinants of this behaviour — social or biological — is arguable (Webb and Bonnet, 1978).

Structure Measures

The structure of sleep refers to measurements of the ongoing process of sleep. The overall sleep process has been almost exclusively indexed by the EEG. Five reliably discernable EEG patterns appear in sleep (see Chapter I). Figure 1 presents a typical night of sleep in a young human adult using these stages.

The time sharing and placement of these stages have been primarily measurement variables in contemporary sleep research.

By far the most widely used index of these stages has been the proportion of time each stage occupies of total sleep time. Normative figures from the age of 20 through 29 for these data have been extensively reported (Williams, Karacan and Hursch, 1974). These data for young adults are shown in Table 2.

There is differential distribution of the various stages across a full sleep period. This distribution for young adults is shown in Figure 2. A detailed examination of the first half and second half distribution of sleep stages and EEG frequencies across age groups has been reported by Keane, Smith, and Webb (1977).

The most intensively examined temporal component of sleep has been the timing and periodicity of REM sleep. The periodicity of REM was noted in the first paper describing stage 1-REM sleep (Aserinsky and Kleitman, 1953). In their first paper the authors stated that '. . . the first cluster (of eye movements) appeared from 1 to 5 hours after retiring, a second cluster about 2 hours later and additional groups of eye movements at still closer intervals

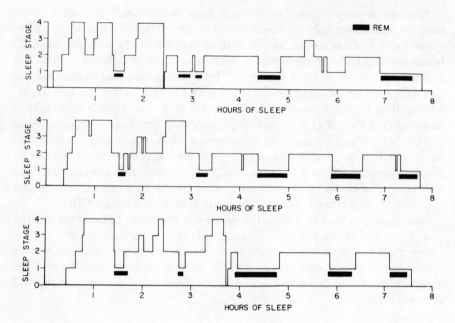

Figure 1   The sleep across three nights of a single subject. The stages of sleep are designated on the vertical axis and hours across the night (11 p.m. to 7 a.m.) on the horizontal axis

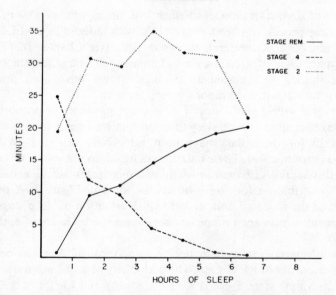

Figure 2   The distribution of stages by hours across the night. Stage 3 essentially parallels stage 4 in distribution and stage 1 is linearly distributed

intervals depending on the length of sleep . . .'. In an early study systematically assessing dream recall Dement and Kleitman (1957) reported that: 'The REM periods occurred at fairly regular intervals throughout the night . . . the average range for the whole group (61 nights) was one REM period ever 92 minutes.'

Table 2   Percentages of sleep stages of 20–29 year old subjects

	Stage 0	Stage 1	Stage 2	Stage 3	Stage 4	Stage REM
M	1	4	49	6	13	14
SD	0.75	2.0	5.0	1.5	5.0	4.0

M, mean; SD, standard deviation.
Adapted from Williams, Karacan, and Hursch (1974).

By 1963, Kleitman was able to state that 'the general character of the cyclical variations in EEG pattern during a night's sleep was confirmed by many investigators who employed the REM–EEG method . . .' (p.98). He follows that statement with 20 reference citations (although none was specifically directed at detailing the cyclicity). He includes this periodicity as a core for his basic rest activity cycle (see Chapter IX).

In 1968, Hartmann published a paper specifically '. . . intended to draw attention to a basic biological cycle . . . the 90 minute "sleep–dream" cycle . . .' (Hartmann, 1968). He reported on the cycle lengths of 15 young adults studied eight or more nights. The defined cycle length was measured from the end of one REM period to the end of the next. The subjects' mean cycle length was 95.8 min. However, the between subject standard deviation was 8.7 min and the average within subject range in cycle length was 63 minutes. Broughton (1975), Globus (1970), Kripke (1974), and Moses *et al.* (1975) have extensively discussed the rhythmic quality of REM episodes.

The large variability in REM cycling was emphasized by Webb (1974b):

'. . . We all know that there is a 90 minute (circa) REM cycle. What we don't all seem to know is that this 90 minute cycle is a mean around an enormous variability of onset times and that each episode is different in length . . . . Let us examine in detail the REM cycling of 22 young adults during 3 nights each. A REM episode was defined as one in which sleep was preceded or succeeded by at least 30 minutes of non-REM and an interval is defined from onset times . . . . Approximately 10% of the first REM episodes occurred before 60 minutes or after 130 minutes, an interval of more than an hour. The mean time of onset was 93 minutes — close enough to 90 minutes to be impressive — but only 17% of the onset times fell within a 20-minute interval around 90 minutes. The time interval between the first episode and the second episode was slightly narrower in range. Although no interval was shorter than 60 minutes, 14% exceeded 120 minutes and 41% of the times fell-within 20 minutes of the 90-minute time period.

In summary, then, although it does appear that there is an approximately 90 minute cycle associated with REM, we must recognize this as a group characteristic which contains a considerable variance . . . .' (p.485)

Recently Feinberg and Floyd (1979) have presented a detailed analysis of REM and non-REM cycling on a large number of subjects across a broad age range. They report systematic changes in the REM cycle interval across the night with differential effects associated with age. Again, it should be noted that while the mean 'cycle' length approximated 90 minutes, the variability was large. For example, the time between the first REM episode and the second in a population of 33 adults was 87.0 min; the standard deviation (presumably of the population) of episodes was 18.5 minutes.

A recent workshop, 'REM sleep: Its Temporal Distribution', published in *Sleep* (Czeiler and Guilleminault, 1980), intensively examined various aspects of this rhythm.

Perhaps because of measurement problems, subjective measures of sleep or sleepiness appear to have been completely neglected in normative temporal studies.

SLEEP RHYTHM MODIFIERS

The previous section describes temporal aspects of typical young adult sleep. While these represent stable temporal characteristics within a range of behaviour and within subject difference they are sharply and systematically modified by four variables: species, age, time schedules, and central nervous system variations. This section will review these in turn.

Species Differences

In regard to sleep structure, all species of mammals and avians tested display an activated phase of sleep similar to REM sleep stage in human adults. This is termed paradoxical sleep (PS) in non-human species. The sleep structure of primates is comprised of the same stages of sleep (1–4, plus 1–REM) as the human. Extensive studies have been reported on the rhesus monkey (Kripke *et al.*, 1979) and the baboon (Bert, 1973). In both species, the proportional distribution of stages were different, with reduced slow wave sleep (stages 3 and 4) and REM sleep amounts. The sleep structure of cats displays essentially a three stage structure with two distinguishable slow wave stages and the PS stage (Ursin, 1971). Ungulated (hoofed) and feline species have significant segments of 'drowsiness' (see Ruckebusch, 1972). The EEG patterns in reptiles and amphibians do not display these characteristic stages and measurement of sleep is disputed (Tauber, 1974). Zepelin and Rechtschaffen (1974) have reviewed the data of a wide range of species and include reports on the total amount of PS and cycle length of PS sleep (onset to onset times) on some 49 mammalia. Total PS % ranges from 34% in the opossum to 6% in the mouse. Birds are reported to have as little as 2–4%. The cycle length extends for approximately 6 min for the chinchilla to 2 hours for the Asian elephant.

Aspects for the patterns of sleep have been less extensively reported. The most extensive data describe the total sleep per 24 hours. The Zepelin-Rechtschaffen review reports on 53 species. Table 3 presents selective data across species for both total sleep and PS drawn from the review.

Table 3

	Total sleep (h)	PS (h)
Opossum	18.0	4.9
Cat	14.5	3.6
Rat	13.6	2.5
Baboon	9.8	0.7
Man	8.0	1.9
Elephant	4.0	1.8
Cow	4.0	0.7
Horse	3.0	0.8

The pattern data on species regarding diurnal placement and such variables as number and length of sleep episodes is sporadic and scattered although relatively extensive data is available on rodents (see Van Twyer, 1969), cattle (see Ruckebusch, 1972), and baboons (see Bert, 1973). Episodes range from very brief bursts and high numbers, typical of small mammalia, to the generally uniphasic patterns of primates. Diurnal placement varies in nocturnal and diurnal animals and in degree of exclusiveness across light/dark periods.

Age and Sleep

Marked changes in both the temporal structure and patterns of human sleep are associated with age.

The structural changes from the age of 3 through the 70s for males and females have been extensively documented in Williams, Karacan, and Hursch (1974). The major change in REM percentages is a decline from about 50% in neonates to about 25% in the early teens. These percentages remain stable until the 70s with some evidence for a small decline in the oldest group. The REM interval (onset to onset times) shows a lengthening across the age groups. Stage 1 percentage increases steadily with age with a consistently larger amount in males across the age range. Stages 3 and 4 show a decline from the late 20s but there is controversy whether this is a decline in 'scored' amounts since these scores utilize an amplitude criterion. There is evidence that while the amplitude of these stages undoubtedly declines, the presence of slow wave sleep, measured by frequency criteria, remains intact (Smith, Karacan, and Yang, 1977).

There can be no doubt about the sharply increased presence of awakenings after the onset of sleep. While percentage of awake time averages about 2% in 30–40 year old males and females, this has doubled in amount by the ages of 50–60 years and continues to rise linearly.

Neonatal sleep structure has been intensively examined. In human neonates two distinct stages of sleep are readily discernable and these are customarily labelled 'Quiet' sleep and 'Active' sleep. Active sleep is characterized by rapid eye movements, grimacing, irregular breathing, and small muscle twitches. The EEG is poorly differentiated. The differentiation of these stages is progressive from prematurity where they are crudely discernible at about 28 weeks (conceptual age). The stages become clearly coordinted with slow waves associated with 'quiet' sleep at about 6 weeks after birth (Parmelee and Stern, 1972). The spindling activity associated with stage 2 adult sleep develops from a very rudimentary form and becomes stabilized during the first year. The 'active' sleep cycle is about 60 minutes in length in the neonate.

Studies of sleep structure relative to age in non-humans have focused on neonatal sleep. These studies have revealed two different developmental formats. Altricial animals show REM sleep changes similar to humans; large amounts of REM (or PS) sleep at birth, reducing in an amount with maturity to a stable level; precocial animals have stable amounts across their life span. Aged rats and mice (Zepelin, Whitehead, and Rechtschaffen, 1972) show limited changes in sleep structure.

The patterns of sleep show dramatic and systematic changes with aging. The human neonate has on the average six sleep episodes distributed across the 24 hour cycle with a mean total sleep of approximately 16 hours. The total length of sleep shows an exponential decline into the late teens where it stabilizes at a mean of about 7.5 hours with a standard deviation of 1 hour. There is some evidence of a slight increase in reported length in the 60s and 70s as well as a significant increase in the standard deviation (Kripke *et al.*, 1979). The primary characteristic of the early change in patterns up to about 5 years results from a decrease in the number of daytime episodes and a consolidation of sleep into a single nocturnal episode. This change, characteristic over the first 16 weeks, is displayed in Figure 3.

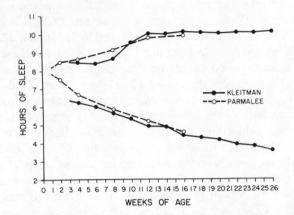

Figure 3   The change in sleep distribution in infants. Sleep from 8 p.m. to 8 a.m. (top line) consolidates in a single episode but changes little in amount; sleep from 8 a.m. to 8 p.m. (bottom line) decreases in two nap periods. (Kleitman, 1963; Parmelee and Stern, 1972)

Modified Temporal Schedules

The classical experimental designs of biological rhythm research (Chapter I), used to determine the endogenous character of a temporal rhythm, have been applied to sleep with impressive evidence of its rhythmic stability. This is to say that sleep has been placed in time-free environments, has been placed in desynchronous or other than circadian schedules, has been eliminated, 'mimicked', and displaced, and measurements have been taken to ascertain the persistence of the sleep tendencies and the time courses of these tendencies. This section reviews these studies relative to sleep. Performance changes are reviewed in Chapter VII.

Human sleep has been recorded in time-free environments in both the laboratory (Webb and Agnew, 1974b) and in the 'natural' environments of the cave (Chouvet *et al.*, 1974). Currently extensive 'free running' studies of sleep and other rhythmic components are being undertaken by Weitzman and his associates (see Weitzman *et al.*, 1980). When thus descheduled, it is clear from these studies that sleep and waking maintain a temporal schedule. However, as typical of most variables (e.g., temperature, urinary flow), the period of the rhythm is extended. In the studies reported by Webb and Agnew the mean displacement of the sleep period was 1.3 hours per 24 hours. Total sleep time increased significantly and the sleep structure shows dynamic changes relative to prior wakefulness, period length, and circadian displacement (see below).

The desynchronous schedules utilize an 'other than 24 hour' design to determine sleep adaptability to alternative time schedules. Resistance to such schedules may be taken as evidence for a circadian endogenous tendency. Studies have utilized 90 min (Carskadon and Dement, 1975), 104 min (Moses *et al.*, 1975), 3 hours (Weitzman *et al.*, 1974), and 9, 12, 18, 20, 30, 36 (Webb and Agnew, 1975a) and 48 hour schedules (Webb, 1978a). In all except the 104 schedule, the waking period (lights on—no sleep permitted) and the sleep period (lights off—sleep permitted) used a 2 to 1 wake/sleep schedule.

In general, total sleep time across experimental sessions is reduced as a function of the distance of the schedules from a 24 hour schedule. Exceptions are found in some subjects in the 48 hour schedule (Chouvet *et al.*, 1974; Webb, 1978a). The effect on sleep stages is complex since each schedule differentially affects prior wakefulness, sleep length, and time of sleep onset and termination. For example, a 12 hour schedule is comprised of two 4 hour sleep periods with 8 hours of prior wakefulness and two different onset and termination times within each 24 hour time period. In general, however, sleep stages respond, as predicted, to these variables with a resultant and remarkable maintenance of stage proportionality across the experimental period (Webb and Agnew, 1977).

Further alternatives to test the rhythmic 'place' of sleep within the 24 hours are to 'displace' sleep from its established place in the 24 hour sequence. As stated previously, this has been accomplished in three ways: eliminate sleep, mimic sleep behaviour, or change its time of occurrence.

The elimination of sleep across the 24 hours and beyond has been persistently studied. The data and findings from these studies relative to their effects on performance are reviewed in Chapter V. The interpretation of these data relative to sleep tendencies as a rhythmic component are complicated. Since sleep is experimentally eliminated the presence of sleep tendencies can only be indirectly measured by decremental performance during the time when sleep has been eliminated. Further, these decrements may not be due to the temporal sleep tendencies but partially or totally attributed to such concepts as 'fatigue' or 'depletion of energy reserves' or 'toxins'. For a discussion of such interaction components see Chapter III.

What can be minimally stated from these designs is that performance is indeed depressed during the 'regular' night period (see Bonnet and Webb, 1978 and Chapter III, *passim*). At least a part of these findings may be inferentially attributable to persistent sleep tendencies. More impressive is the generalized findings of rhythmic 'day'-'night' differential levels of performance in more prolonged deprivations across more than a single 24 hour period. These data are particularly informative since the alternative accounts of 'fatigue' and the like must predict a linear decline of performance.

An alternative procedure used in the biological rhythm designs is to mimic the sleep activity to determine if, say, the temperature decrease occurring during sleep is controlled by the subject being supine. One may also ask whether sleep also is so controlled or is independent of the associated behaviour. In short, if a person is confined to bed will the sleep/waking rhythm persist?

Although this is a commonplace procedure to study the influence of activity and inactivity on a wide range of biological systems (see above) it has not been an active design relative to sleep. The single extensively reported study of sleep and bed rest (Ryback and Lewis, 1971) did not in fact permit sleep to occur during the normal waking period. The time was occupied by varying exercises and tasks. In short, there is no systematic evidence to know to what extent sleep will 'track' inactivity.

The third displacement procedure is that of changing the period of sleep from one time period to another time period. In 'real life' this is the consequence of shift work and jet travel and the complex effects of these schedules on performance are reviewed in Chapter V. A number of laboratory studies have been conducted relative to sleep in such designs. The earlier studies (Weitzman *et al.*, 1970; Webb *et al.*, 1971) found increased wakefulness during daytime sleep and a sharp change in the temporal order of sleep with marked decreases in REM latency. Later studies (Knauth and Rutenfranz, 1972; Foret and Lantin, 1972) have reported and emphasized early awakening from sleep. In these studies and in extensive field surveys it is certain that when sleep is displaced into a new sleep period it is significantly modified and a 're-entrainment' is required for sleep variables.

The problem of measuring the residual sleep tendencies within the original period from which sleep is displaced has most of the complications noted above relative to measuring 'sleep tendencies' during sleep deprivation. The design, however, does have the advantage, at least in laboratory settings, of eliminating sleep deprivation as a variable (albeit the displaced sleep is not precisely that of regular sleep). Unfortunately, with the exception of the series of studies of Taub and Berger (see Chapter VII), reports on performance during the original sleep period have been neglected.

Finally, relative to time schedules and sleep, certain lawful characteristics of sleep as a response to timing variations have begun to emerge. As an independent variable, time may be modified relative to sleep in three major ways: prior wakefulness time can be increased (e.g., sleep deprivation); the sleep period can be shortened, or to some extent, extended; the onset time can be shifted. Relative to performance these changes are discussed in other chapters. Here we note the effects (mostly derived from the designs described above) on sleep *per se*.

Two major effects of prior wakefulness have been established. Latencies have been shown to be exponentially and inversely related to prior wakefulness (Agnew and Webb, 1971). Sleep structure is also systematically affected. Stage 4 sleep in the first 3 hours increases linearly in amount as a function of prior wakefulness to about 30 hours where it becomes asymptotic (Webb and

Agnew, 1973). REM sleep shows a slight decline in amount in the first 3 hours (Agnew and Webb, 1973). This is probably due to the strong presence of stage 4 sleep.

A restriction of the length of the sleep period results in a proportionally greater loss of REM sleep and proportionally less stage 4 sleep due to the differential distribution of these stages across the full sleep period (Figure 3). However, individuals with natural short sleep periods show 'compressed' sleep structures with little or no reduction in the proportion of REM sleep (Webb and Agnew, 1974a). An extension of sleep results in proportionally higher REM sleep in the extended period. A substantial reduction in sleep length results in an extension of total sleep in the subsequent sleep period (Webb and Agnew, 1975b).

As noted above the results relative to sleep period displacement are clear. REM sleep onset latencies are systematically related to the 'time of day' of sleep onset. They are shortest in the morning (8 AM–10 AM) with increasing latencies to a maximum circa 11 PM–1 AM. Latencies show a similar circadian pattern (Webb and Agnew, 1975a). There is also evidence of increased wakefulness within sleep and a modified stage distribution.

In summary, sleep structure response relative to time can be lawfully predicted. Stage 3/4 sleep tendencies increase as a function of prior wakefulness; REM sleep tendencies respond systematically to sleep onset times; sleep latencies show both a prior wakefulness and circadian responsivity; modification of sleep period length differentially affects stage 4 and REM sleep amounts.

Drugs and Central Nervous System Variables

The focus of this series and this volume on performance permits only limited references to the extensive research on the effects of drugs and aspects of the central nervous system and biochemical factors on changes in the temporal aspects of the structure of sleep.

The effects of drugs on sleep have been recently reviewed in the *Pharmacology of Sleep* (Williams and Karacan, 1976). The effect on sleep structure of over 100 substances have been studied with the major concentration in the 'hypnotics'. Most have focused on EEG measures of latency and sleep stage amounts and have used 'insomniac' populations. In very general summary terms, depressants severely reduce the amount of REM sleep, have a limited effect on the timing of REM, and REM amounts show a subsequent rebound on drug withdrawal. On the other hand, other measures of the sleep structure, e.g. stage 2 and slow wave sleep, appear remarkably resistant to change to a broad spectrum of drugs with the exception of stimulants. The latter significantly disturb sleep. There is an increasing salutatory tendency to include post-sleep measures of performance in these studies.

The search for and specifications of the neurophysiological mechanisms of sleep has been contiguous with the advances in the life sciences (Webb, 1973). Since the late 1950s these efforts have dominated sleep research and constituted more than 40% of the research enterprise (Table 1, Chapter I). The research has moved from the earlier lesion studies into highly sophisticated plotting of single cell discharge rates and patterns (see Hobson, McCarley and Wyinski, 1975) and neurochemical studies (see Morgane and Sterne, 1973). By far the greater concentration of these studies has focused on determining the mechanisms underlying the generation of the REM phenomena. A summary of this extensive literature is beyond the bounds of this chapter and the competence of its author.

BIOLOGICAL RHYTHMS AND SLEEP THEORIES

Sleep research has largely been an atheoretical enterprise. As with much of neurophysiology, the search for the mechanisms of sleep has been largely driven by and emergent from empirical findings relative to the central nervous system in general and technical developments in experimentation. 'Miniature' theories, i.e. theories circumscribed to a particular domain of phenomena, have been most prominently developed in two areas: sleep deprivation and REM sleep. The former of these areas generally has been 'arousal' type theories which attempt to account for sleep deprivation in motivational terms (see Kjellberg, 1977). Perhaps because of the profuseness and contradictory nature of the data, the theories about REM sleep have been protean and diverse. The earlier notions, because of the close identification with REM dreams, leaned heavily on Freudian constructs. An alternative was a homoeostatic model which hypothesizes the high presence of REM in infants and its place within sleep to be an endogenous central nervous system 'activation' to offset reduced exogenous stimulation. Later REM 'theories' focused on earlier 'memory' theories or 'drive' theories. In addition, there has been a persistent need to recognize the prime empirical certainty of REM sleep, viz. its ubiquitous rhythmic manifestation across species. As noted, Kleitman incorporated this fact into his earlier concept of a basic rest activity cycle. A current response of the area to this rhythmic characteristic is found in the studies of REM as an ultradian rhythm (Chapter IX). These studies implicitly assume REM to be an ultradian biological rhythm.

Using theory in a broad and loose sense, there have been some attempts to theorize about the function or purpose of sleep. Webb (1979b) reviewed these theories. He divided these into five general categories: restoration, protective, ethological, instinctive, and energy conservation. He noted that most authors tended to combine these categories but that generally one of two distinct positions was held:

(1) sleep was a 'restorative' process in which, during waking, there was a 'loss' or a developed 'noxious' stage which was offset during sleep; or

(2) sleep was an innately elicited, environmentally appropriate behaviour.

Earlier statements about the non-restorative 'determinants' of the sleep response involved an 'instinctive' concept (Moruzzi, 1972; Webb, 1974a; Meddis, 1977). However, a review of the adaptive theories indicates that a biological rhythm model may be considerably more apt than an instinctive model.

An instinctive model focuses on external 'releasor' cues for the occurrence of the response (Tinbergen, 1969). While internal 'causal' factors are incorporated in the model these serve as background or 'motivational components'. Usually the internal factors do not themselves evoke the overt response, 'they merely determine the threshold of the response to sensory stimuli' (p.122). Sleep would then be triggered by such variables as darkness, supineness, etc. The biological rhythm model would reverse this. The primary 'determinant' would be an endogenous, intervening time determined tendency and the 'external' stimuli would serve to modulate or interfere with the response.

Two further differences favour a biological rhythm model. Instinctive behaviour sequences tend to be fully developed systems with 'critical period' age components and with a limited range of individual differences. In contrast, biological rhythm models appear to be more tolerant of developmental sequences and individual differences. It would seem then that the importation of the biological rhythm construct as a 'determinant' of the sleep response may fruitfully enhance the adaptive theories.

It should be noted that such an incorporation will not serve to settle arguments in the restorative–adaptive positions. The restorative theories can be conceptualized as homoeostatic theories. Such models can be developed as temporal models and, importantly, they are intraorganismic in the formulations. Simply, the 'timing' of sleep is a homoeostatic 'depletion' (or 'build up') and sleep length is a function of the rate of 'recovery' within the organism. In stable time sequences both systems may 'explain' sleep behaviours by different assumptions. For example, the short sleeper has either an inherently 'efficient' depletion/recovery ratio or inherent long wake/short sleep rhythm. Arousal from sleep may be hypothesized to be a termination of 'recovery' or a 'phase change'.

These core resemblances, however, do not mean that the approaches are indistinguishable. For the restorative theory a cumulative state change is the independent variable and the timing of sleep is the dependent variable. In contrast, for the biological rhythm theory, time is the independent variable and occurrence or non-occurrence of sleep is the dependent variable. Thus, the research focus of the homoeostatic model is an inwardly directed search for a 'substance' and its change rate. For the biological rhythm model the focus of research is on the stability of occurrences in time.

More critically, while it is true that both theories may be reconciled with data in stable time sequences, their predictions become divergent in altered time schedules. We have noted in Chapter I that time variant research designs from the core of biological rhythm research. In this chapter we have reviewed the responses of sleep in such models. In the three succeeding chapters we shall see the interrelations between sleep and performance in sleep/time varied circumstances (deprivation and varied work–rest schedules). Restoration theories have few or contradictory predictions in such time variations. To the contrary, it is here that biological rhythm concepts, techniques, and theories will be found wanting or will be particularly useful.

In short, of the two distinct positions regarding sleep functions—restorative *vs* non-restorative—it appears likely that the primary testing ground will utilize the methods and constructs of biological rhythm research.

SUMMARY

The chapter reviews the increasing interaction of biological rhythm research and sleep research. In early physiological research, there was a natural confluence of interest in the changes in physiological systems associated with sleep and the question of linkage—sleep as a cause, sleep being caused, or sleep and the system of interest being mutually determined. As sleep schedules could be modified, the independence or stability of systems was tested in such designs. Variation in sleep schedules continues to be a significant technique in biological rhythm research.

In sleep research the temporally organized characteristics of sleep in its patterns and structure have become increasingly apparent as well as systematic modifier variables of these rhythms—species, age, and chronological factors. Since chronological influences involve basic biological rhythm designs—time-free, dis-synchronous, phase displacement—both methodology and findings are of common interest across fields. The chapter concludes with a consideration of sleep conceptualized as a biological rhythm in the context of theories hypothesizing the functional role of sleep.

REFERENCES

Adams, F. (1939). *The Genuine Work of Hippocrates*. Baltimore, Williams and Wilkins.

Agnew, H. W. Jr. and Webb, W. B. (1971). Sleep latencies in human subjects: age, prior wakefulness, and reliability. *Psychonomic Science* 24(6), 253–254.

Agnew, H. W. Jr. and Webb, W. B. (1973). The influence of time course variable on REM sleep. *Bulletin of the Psychonomic Society* 2(3), 131–133.

Aserinsky, E. and Kleitman, N. (1953). Regularly occurring period of eye motility, and concomitant phenomena, during sleep. *Science* 118, 273–274.

Bert, J. (1973). Similitudes et différences du sommeil chez duex Babouins, Papio Handryas and Papio Papio. *Electroencephalography and Neurophysiology* **35**, 209–212.

Bonnet, M. and Webb, W. B. (1978). The effect of repetition of relevant and irrelevant tasks over day and night work periods. *Ergonomics* **21(212)**, 999–1005.

Broughton, R. J. (1975). Biorhythmic variations in consciousness and psychological functions. *Canadian Psychological Review* **16**, 217–239.

Carskadon, M. A. and Dement, W. C. (1975). Sleep studies on a 90-minute day. *Electroencephalography and Clinical Neurophysiology* **39**, 145–155.

Chouvet, G., Mouret, J., Coindet, J., Siffre, M., and Jouvet, M. (1974). Periodicité bicircadienne du cycle veille-sommeil dans des conditions hors du temps. Etude polygraphique. *Electroencephalography and Clinical Neurophysiology* **37**, 367–380.

Conroy, R. T. and Mills, J. N. (1970). *Human Circadian Rhythms.* Baltimore, Williams and Wilkins Co.

Czeiler, C. and Guilleminault, C. (1980). REM sleep: Its temporal distribution. *Sleep.* **198**, 2, 285–346; 377–463.

Dement, W. C. and Kleitman, N. (1957). The relation of eye movements during sleep to dream activity: An objective method for the study of dreaming. *Journal of Experimental Psychology* **53**, 339–346.

Evans, F. J., Cook, M. R., Cohen, H. D., Orne, E. C., and Orne, M. T. (1977). Appetitive and replacement naps: EEG and behavior. *Science* **197**, 687–689.

Feinberg, I. and Floyd, T. C. (1979). Systematic trends across the night in human sleep cycles. *Psychophysiology* **16(3)**, 283–291.

Foret, J. and Lantin, G. (1972). The sleep of transdivets: An example of the effects on irregular work schedules of sleep. In: *Aspects of Human Efficiency.* W. P. Colquhoun (Ed.). London. The English University Press.

Fraisse, P. (1963). *The Psychology of Time.* New York, Harper and Row.

Globus, G. G. (1970). Quantification of the sleep cycle as a rhythm. *Psychophysiology* **7**, 244–253.

Harmann, E. (1968). The ninety-minute sleep dream cycle. *Archives of General Psychiatry* **18**, 280–286.

Hobson, J. A., McCarley, R. W., and Wyinski, P. W. (1975). Sleep cycle oscillation: Reciprocal discharge by two brainstem neuronal groups. *Science* **189**, 55–58.

Horne, J. and Ostberg, O. (1977). Individual differences in human circadian rhythms. *Biological Psychology* **5**, 179–180.

Johns, M. W., Bruce, D. W., and Masterton, J. P. (1974). Psychological correlates of sleep habits reported by healthy young adults. *British Journal of Medical Psychology* **47**, 181–187.

Johnson, L. C. and MacLeod, W. L. (1973). Sleep and awake behavior during gradual sleep reduction. *Perceptual and Motor Skills* **36**, 95.

Keane, B., Smith, J., and Webb, W. B. (1977). Temporal distribution of sleep EEG activity. *Psychophysiology* **14**, 149–157.

Kjellberg, A. (1977). Sleep deprivation and some aspects of performance. *Waking and Sleeping.* **1**, 139–153.

Kleitman, N. (1949). Biological rhythms and cycles. *Physiological Review* **29**, 1–30.

Kleitman, N. (1963). *Sleep and Wakefulness.* Chicago, University of Chicago Press.

Knauth, P. and Rutenfranz, J. (1972). Utersvchungen zum problem des schlafeurhaltens bei experimenteller schichtarbeit. *Internation Archives Arbectsmed.* **30**, 1–22.

Kripke, D., Reitz, M., Pegram, P., Stephens, L., and Lewis, O. (1968). Nocturnal sleep in rhesus monkeys. *Electroencephalography and Clinical Neurophysiology* **24**, 582–586.

Kripke, D. F. (1974). Ultradian rhythms in sleep and wakefulness. In: *Advances in Sleep Research*, Vol. I. E. D. Weitzman (Ed.). New York, Spectrum.

Kripke, D. F., Simons, R. N., Garfinkel, L., and Hammond, E. C. (1979). Short and long sleep and sleeping pills: Is increased mortality associated? *Archives of General Psychiatry* **36**, 103–116.

McGhie, A. and Russell, S. M. (1962). The subjective assessment of normal sleep patterns. *Journal of Mental Science* **107**, 188–202.

Meddis, R. (1977). *The Sleep Instinct*. London, Routledge and Kegan.

Mills, J. N. (1951). Diurnal rhythm in urine flow. *Journal of Physiology* **113**, 528–536.

Mills, J. N. (1966). Human circadian rhythms. *Physiological Review* **46**, 128–171.

Mills, J. N. (Ed.) (1973). *Biological Aspects of Circadian Rhythms*. London, Plenum Press.

Morgane, P. and Stern, W. (1973). Chemical anatomy of brain circuits in relation to sleep and wakefulness. In: *Advances in Sleep Research*, Vol. 1. E. D. Weitzman (Ed.). New York, Halstead Press.

Moses, J. M., Hord, D. J., Lubin, A., Johnson, L., and Naitoh, P. (1975). Dynamics of nap sleep during a 49 hour period. *Electroencephalography and Clinical Neurophysiology* **39**, 627–633.

Moruzzi, G. (1972). The sleep waking cycle. *Ergebnisse du Physiologie* **64**. 1–165.

Parmelee, A. H. and Stern, E. (1972). Development of states in infants. In: *Sleep and the Maturing Nervous System* C. D. Clemente, D. P. Purpura, and F. E. Mayer (Eds.). New York, Academic Press.

Pieron, H. (1913). *Le Problème Physiologique du Sommeil*. Paris, Masson et Cie.

Ruckebusch, Y. (1972). The relevance of drowsiness in the circadian cycle of farm animals. *Animal Behavior* **20**, 637–643.

Ryback, R. and Lewis, O. F. (1971). Effects of prolonged bedrest on EEG sleep patterns in young, healthy volunteers. *Electroencephalography and Clinical neurophysiology* **31**, 529–535.

Saunders, D. S. (1977). *An Introduction To Biological Rhythms*. London, Blackie.

Smith, J., Karacan, I., and Yang, M. (1977). Ontogeny of delta activity during human sleep. *Electroencephalography and Clincial Neurophysiology* **43**, 229–237.

Tauber, E. S. (1974). Phylogeny of sleep. In: *Advances in Sleep Research*, Vol. I. E. D. Weitzman (Ed.). New York, Spectrum.

Tinbergen, N. (1969). *The Study of Instinct*. New York, Oxford Pres.

Tune, G. S. (1960). Sleep and wakefulness in 509 normal human adults. *British Journal of Medical Psychology* **49**, 75–80.

Ursin, R. (1971). Differential effect of sleep deprivation on the two slow wave sleep stages in the cat. *Acta physiologica Scandinavica* **83**, 352–361.

Van Twyer, H. (1969). Sleep patterns of five rodent species. *Physiology and Behavior* **4**, 901–908.

Webb, W. B. (Ed.) (1973). *Sleep: An Active Process*. Glenview, Ill., Foresman.

Webb, W. B. (1974a). Sleep as an adaptive response. *Perceptual and Motor Skills* **38**, 1023–1027.

Webb, W. B. (1974b). The rhythms of sleep and waking. In: *Chronobiology*. L. Scheving and F. Halberg (Eds.). Tokyo, Igakushoin.

Webb, W. B. (1978a). The forty-eight hour day. *Sleep* **1**(2), 191–197.

Webb, W. B. (1978b). Sleep and naps. *Speculations in Science and Technology* **1**(4), 313–318.

Webb, W. B. (1979a). Are short and long sleepers different? *Psychological Reports* **44**, 259–264.

Webb, W. B. (1979b). Theories of sleep functions and some clinical applications, pp.19–35. In: *The Function of Sleep.* R. Drucker-Colin, M. Shkurovich, and M. B. Sterman (Eds.). New York, Academic Press.

Webb, W. B. and Agnew, H. W., Jr. (1973). Stage 4 sleep: influence of time course variables. *Science* **174**, 1354–1356.

Webb, W. B. and Agnew, H. W. Jr. (1974a). The effects of a chronic limitation of sleep length. *Psychophysiology* **11(3)**, 265–274.

Webb, W. B. and Agnew, H. W. Jr. (1974b). Sleep and waking in a time-free environment. *Aerospace Medicine* **45(6)**, 617–622.

Webb, W. B. and Agnew, H. W. Jr. (1975a). Sleep efficiency for sleep-wake cycles of varied length. *Psychophysiology* **12(6)**, 637–641.

Webb, W. B. and Agnew, H. W. Jr. (1975b). The effects of subsequent sleep of an acute restriction of sleep length. *Psychophysiology* **12(4)**, 367–369.

Webb, W. B. and Agnew, H. W. Jr. (1977). Analysis of the sleep stages in sleep-wakefulness regimens of varied length. *Psychophysiology* **14(5)**, 445–450.

Webb, W. B., Agnew, H. W. Jr., and Williams, R. L. (1971). Effects on sleep of a sleep period time displacement. *Aerospace Medicine* **42(2)**, 152–155.

Webb, W. B. and Bonnet, M. H. (1978). The sleep of morning and evening types. *Biological Psychology*, **7**, 29–35.

Weitzman, E., Czeiler, C., Zimmerman, J., and Ronda, J. (1980). Timing of REM and Stage 3 & 4 sleep during temporal isolation in man. *Sleep* **2**, 391–408.

Weitzman, E., Goldmacher, D., Kripke, D., McGregor, P., Kream, J., and Hellman, L. (1970). Reversal of sleep waking cycle: Effect on sleep stage pattern and certain neuroendocrine rhythms. *Transactions of the American Neurological Association* **93**, 153–157.

Weitzman, E., Nogeire, D., Perlow, M., Fukushima, D., Sassin, J., McGregor, P., Gallagher, T. F., and Hellman, L. (1974). Effects of a prolonged 3-hour sleep–wake cycle on sleep states, plasma cortisol, growth hormone and body temperature in man. *Journal of Clinical Endocrinology and Metabolism* **38**, 1018–1030.

White, R. (1975). *Sleep Length and Variability: Measurement and Interrelationships.* Unpublished PhD Thesis, University of Florida, Gainesville, Florida.

Williams, R. and Karacan, I. (1976). *Psychopharmacology of Sleep.* New York, Wiley and Sons.

Williams, R., Karacan, I., and Hursch, C. (1974). *EEG and Human Sleep.* New York, Wiley and Sons.

Zepelin, H. and Rechtschaffen, A. (1974). Mammalian sleep, longevity and energy metabolism. *Brain Behavior Evolution* **7**, 425–470.

Zepelin, H., Whitehead, W., and Rechtschaffen, A. (1972). Aging and sleep in the albino rat. *Behavioral Biology* **7**, 65–74.

Biological Rhythms, Sleep, and Performance
Edited by Wilse B. Webb
©1982 John Wiley & Sons Ltd.

Chapter 5

Sleep Deprivation and Performance

Laverne C. Johnson

BACKGROUND

An accepted technique to determine the functions of a particular organ, system, or behaviour is to remove the organ or system or to prevent the behaviour. This approach has been applied in attempts to understand the function of sleep. Research on sleep deprivation, both total and partial, has a long and active history, but it is only in the past decade or so that serious attention has been given to how sleep loss may affect biological rhythms. Of more importance is the fact that many early studies did not consider the influence of biological rhythms on performance in their evaluation of performance decrement. The importance of time of day in evaluating performance will be discussed later under Behavioural Periodicity.

The first experimental study of sleep loss was reported in 1896 (Patrick and Gilbert). Several review articles have been published summarizing the work since 1896 (Lubin, 1967; Wilkinson, 1969; Naitoh and Townsend, 1970; Johnson and Naitoh, 1974; Johnson, 1975; Naitoh, 1976). Though it has a long history, evaluation of sleep loss effects has not been a major interest of sleep researchers. Webb (1975) has also noted the lack of intensive effort in the area of sleep loss and its effects on human performance. He noted that into 1940, nearly 50 years of research had yielded only 16 human sleep deprivation experiments exceeding one night of sleep loss. Forty-nine subjects were involved in these 16 studies. Between 1940 and 1970, Webb estimates there were about 20 additional studies.

In 1972, the Brain Information Service started its publication of yearly citations in *Sleep Research*. In that first volume, there were 52 citations dealing with total and selective sleep deprivation. In the latest volume, 1979, there are 60 citations, and the number of citations has ranged between 40 and 67 in the intervening years. Only about one-tenth of these studies over the 8 year span were concerned with the effects of sleep deprivation on performance, and some of these performance studies were done using animals. The extensive sleep deprivation studies at the Naval Health Research Center laboratory in San Diego contributed about a quarter of all the performance articles cited in *Sleep Research*. The level of work in this area thus has remained the same even though the number of citations for all areas of sleep research increased from 761 in 1972 to 2066 in 1979.

Webb (1975) speculates that a possible reason for this lack of research effort was that the results were thought to be so obvious and striking that there seemed little need for repetition. The comment is often made that the major consequence of sleep loss is sleepiness. That statement is entirely correct, but measuring the effects of this increased sleepiness on performance is not a simple task. In fact, level of sleepiness *per se* is not linearly related to amount of prior wakefulness and varies with the time of day the question is asked. If I might be permitted a personal observation, a further reason for the dearth of such studies is that prolonged sleep loss studies are extremely demanding on both subjects and researchers and, as one gets older, less energy-demanding areas of sleep research become increasingly intriguing.

Total sleep deprivation obviously implies complete absence of any sleep. There is some conceptual ambiguity as to the completeness of sleep loss and whether total sleep loss even occurs, especially under field conditions. Sleep is a dynamic state, and it is not a 'thing' that can be cleanly excised. Polygraphic analysis has shown that after 72 or more hours of prolonged wakefulness, it is impossible to prevent subjects from obtaining brief 'microsleeps'. Polygraphically, these microsleeps are periods of drowsiness identified in the sleep manual (Rechtschaffen and Kales, 1968) as stage 1. If the subject is not immediately aroused, these microsleeps rapidly progress into sleep stages 2 and 3. As the duration of the vigil increases, microsleeps increase in frequency. Based upon the occurrence of microsleep, Dement (1972) states: 'the notion of total sleep deprivation could be somewhat illusory, and could result merely in a redistribution of activity in sleep and arousal systems in which NREMS stages 1, 2, 3, and 4 would occur in the form of hundreds of microsleeps' (p.337). According to Dement, total sleep deprivation can be likened to a denial of food at usual meal times. Though prohibited from obtaining food at usual meal times, substantial amounts of food can be eaten by numerous quick bites between regularly scheduled meals. Three leisurely meals can, therefore, be replaced with hundreds of 'snacks' if they become necessary to overcome hunger. Similarly, substantial amounts of sleep can be accumulated by redistributing one long sleep period (which is prohibited under total sleep loss conditions) into hundreds of microsleeps to be snatched quickly now and then.

Dement's point is well taken, but there is no evidence to indicate that these brief periods of microsleep serve to mitigate the performance decrement and physiological changes during sustained wakefulness. Subjects exposed to more than 200 hours of wakefulness continued their decline in all areas as sleep loss progressed, in spite of the increasing frequency of microsleep periods (Johnson, Slye, and Dement, 1965; Kollar *et al.*, 1969). The lack of recuperative value from these periods of stage 1 supports those who believe that the drowsy stage 1 periods should not be viewed as physiological sleep but, rather, as a transition period between awake and asleep. Computer analysis (Johnson *et al.*, 1969) of the EEG activity during awake and asleep has indicated that the bursts of 12–14 Hz spindle activity, referred to as sleep spindles (Loomis, Harvey, and Hobart, 1937), first occur during what is classified as stage 2 sleep. Based upon these data, the appearance of the first sleep spindle would be used to define sleep onset, and this criterion has been recommended (Agnew and Webb, 1972; Snyder and Scott, 1972; Johnson, 1973). On the first night of recovery sleep following 264 hours of wakefulness, the physiological indices of the severe loss of sleep were dramatically reversed when the subject entered stage 2 sleep (Johnson, Slye, and Dement, 1965). No physiological changes were seen during stage 1.

It was the recognition of these 'microsleeps', however, that helped to explain some of the discrepancies in the effects of sleep loss on performance. Most of the early total sleep loss studies failed to discover predictable and consistently detrimental effects of total sleep loss on performance. Patrick and Gilbert (1896) did not find a simple monotonic decline in performance as sleep loss progressed. Indeed, the only reliable changes, as a result of total sleep loss, were those in appearance and mood. This lack of total sleep loss effects on performance was surprising, considering how sleepy the subjects were outside the testing room.

HYPOTHESES

The Lapse Hypothesis

Before sleep deprivation studies were able to produce consistent and replicable sets of results, major refinements in the methods of handling performance data were necessary. The *absence* of responses, not the emitted responses, became the major target of research. In contrast to the earlier hypothesis which emphasized accuracy of performance, this new approach stressed that the ever-increasing number of absences or pauses in a subject's responses was the major behavioural symptom of sleep deprivation. Each brief episode of 'no response' constituted performance decrement due to sleep loss. This approach recognized that, even after extended sleep deprivation, there would always be periods during which the sleep deprived subjects would perform accurately, though these periods would become more brief and intermittent as the hours of sleep deprivation accumulated. Broadbent (1955), in his description of this type of behaviour, stated:

'Crudely speaking, a man is not like a child's mechanical toy which goes slower as it runs down. Nor is he like a car engine which continues normally until its fuel is exhausted and then stops dead. He is like a motor which after much use misfires, runs normally for awhile, then falters again and so on' (p.2).

Performance measures (e.g. accuracy) which could not pinpoint these brief periods of 'misfiring' would be less sensitive indicators of the effects of sleep deprivation.

Investigators at Walter Reed Army Institute of Research were instrumental in pointing out the importance of omission of response as a dependent variable (Williams, Lubin, and Goodnow, 1959). Hence, this new approach was labelled 'Walter Reed lapse hypothesis'. The use of 'lapse' as a measure of performance degradation was not, however, originated by this group. Patrick and Gilbert (1896) described the failure of one of their subjects to memorize the digits because of his inability to focus attention. They called such failure a 'kind of mental lapse'. Bills (1958) noted that blocks occurred in mental task performance. Bills also found that the frequency and duration of these blocks increased with fatigue and that errors tended to occur at the time of these blocks. He concluded, after detailed studies of these blocks or lapses, that they were involuntary rest periods which delayed the start of fatigue.

As Lubin (1967) points out, the basic postulate of the lapse hypothesis is that acute sleep loss causes mental and motor lapses. Between lapses, the subject may perform normally. Figure 1 illustrates this point using a 2-choice reaction time test, with 72 trials in each test session (Williams, Lubin, and Goodnow, 1959, p.5). The average of the ten shortest reaction times changes very little, even after 78 hours of total sleep loss. But the average of the ten longest reaction times in each session expands quickly to four times the base line level. Thus, as sleep loss increases, performance becomes more and more uneven, with efficient behaviour alternating with faltering responses or no responses at all. The average or median performance over the entire task is not a sensitive measure of this unevenness. The number of gaps, i.e. periods of no response, has been shown by Wilkinson (1961) to be a good measure.

A supplementary assumption is that task duration will interact with sleep loss to potentiate lapses. That is, on short tasks, the sleep deprived subject can pull himself together, expend more effort, and, for a few minutes, function at a normal level. But, with long tasks, the basic sleep loss deficit will eventually show itself. Figure 2 illustrates the effect of duration on errors of omission in a visual vigilance task (Williams, Kearney, and Lubin, 1965, p.404). Before sleep loss, subjects could perform this vigilance task for 10 minutes with very few errors of omission. After one night of sleep loss, errors start to increase after the seventh minute. After two nights of sleep loss, omissions increase rapidly following 2 or 3 minutes of good performance. Figure 2 gives an

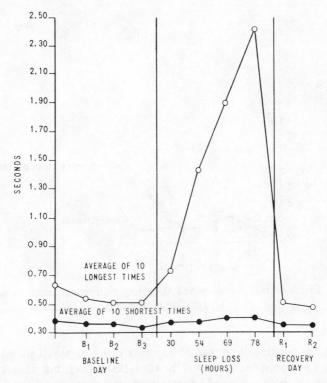

Figure 1   Changes in extreme reaction time with sleep loss. (From Williams, Lubin, and Goodnow, 1959)

exaggerated idea of the smoothness with which the omissions increase. Actually, for each subject, one sees bursts of omission errors, followed by good performance, then another set of omissions, etc. Often, realization that he has missed a signal arouses the subject, so there is a sharp return to good detection following an omitted signal. However, 24 subjects were used in constructing this set of averages, and the waves of uneven performance cancelled each other out.

For the lapse hypothesis, an important aspect of the task is whether it is work-paced or self-paced. Self-paced tasks are those where the subject controls the stimulus display (if any) and can respond at his leisure. In work-paced tasks, the subject cannot control the time when the stimulus appears or its duration and is given a limited time in which to respond. In actual practice, a task may fall somewhere between the ideal self-paced and ideal work-paced conditions. It is easy to change a work-paced task towards a self-paced task simply by extending the permitted response time and allowing the stimulus display to remain unchanged until the subject makes his response.

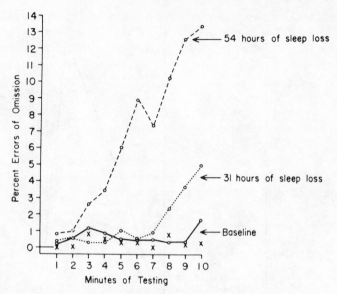

Figure 2   Effect of task duration and sleep loss on performance. (From Williams, Kearney, and Lubin, 1965)

The choice reaction time task of Figure 1 is a typical self-paced task. The subject did not completely control the stimulus display, but almost so. There was a warning click, a 2 second fore-period, and then one of two lights came on. The signal light stayed on until the subject pressed the correct key. What will happen to performance on such a self-paced task? If a lapse hits the subject, then he can recover from the lapse, see which signal light is on, and hit the correct key. This would lead to slowed reaction times, but errors of omission would not usually occur.

The important generalization about self-paced tasks is that the subject, when hit by a lapse, will tend to defer his response until the lapse is over. If the lapse made him forget the stimulus, lose his way in a complex chain of mental operations, or suppress his motor response, then he will most likely start over again. Thus *for self-paced tasks* like adding, problem solving, making judgments, issuing orders, etc., *speed will be impaired but accuracy will remain high.* Our evidence for these statements comes mostly from human subjects, but some anecdotal observations of prolonged periods of operant responding for rats, cats, and monkeys make us suspect that there is some interspecies generalization.

The visual vigilance task of Figure 2 is a typical work-paced task. There was a visual stimulus every second. Sixteen out of every 60 stimuli were signals to press a key. The subject did not control the stimulus display and had to respond to a signal within a second to avoid an error of omission. What will happen to performance on such a work-paced task? If a lapse hits the subject around the time that the signal is displayed, then he will either miss the signal completely, in which case there will be an error of omission, or respond after the lapse is over, in which case there will be a delayed response.

The important generalization about work-paced tasks is that the subject, when hit by a lapse, will generally stop responding. Thus, *work-paced tasks will lead to errors of omission*. Watching a radar screen, monitoring radio communications, or listening to a chain of instructions are all work-paced tasks and will suffer errors of omission under sleep loss.

Another key concept is that of work load. A lapse causes maximum impairment if it hits during a period of information or cognitive processing. Any change in a task which increases the processing time increases the probability of being hit by a lapse.

In general, *as the work load is increased* to the point where the subject can no longer complete the task successfully during base line, *sleep loss will cause errors of omission*. If the work load is held constant and the allowable response time decreased, then the same impairment will result. Conversely, if the allowable response time is increased so that even the slowest worker can ordinarily complete the task, sleep loss of a few nights will cause little impairment.

The Lapse Hypothesis and Memory Impairment

Though there have been many studies on the effects of sleep loss on vigilance, reaction time, and on cognitive tasks such as addition, there have been relatively fewer studies on memory. Memory impairment occurs during sleep loss, but does not fit into the lapse hypothesis quite as easily as impairment of vigilance and cognition. Williams, Lubin, and Goodnow (1959) reported impairment of immediate recall after one night of sleep loss. At the time, they felt that the lapse hypothesis could account for the failure. 'The *S* fails to take in information that is only briefly available' (p.18). They assumed that a lapse occurred during the presentation of the crucial item. But further experiments testing this notion (Williams, Gieseking, and Lubin, 1966) showed that even when sensory registration of every item was verified, practically the same sleep loss deficit for immediate recall was found.

Long term memory was measured by having the subject scrutinize the items on one day and recognize or recall them the next day. In the first study (Williams, Lubin, and Goodnow, 1959), some impairment in this 24 hour delay memory test was found. However, because of an equivocal experimental design and uncontrolled rehearsal by the subject, it was not clear where the impairment occurred. A later study (Williams, Gieseking, and Lubin, 1966) showed that if the items were scrutinized on a base line day and the subject tried to recognize them 24 hours later, then after one night of sleep loss, there was a small non-significant drop. On the other hand, if the items were scrutinized after one night of sleep loss and the subject tried to recognize them

24 hours later, after one night of recovery sleep, there was a significant drop.

These results were interpreted in terms of the usual assumed sequence for the memory process, e.g. sensory registration trace formation, trace storage, retrieval, and playback. Which functions are impaired by sleep loss? Sensory registration was controlled, so we may dismiss this as a factor. During sleep loss, retrieval and playback of a trace acquired 24 hours earlier during base line, was unaffected. Therefore, Williams, Gieseking, and Lubin conclude that one night of sleep loss causes no significant impairment of a trace that has been stored, and causes little difficulty in trace retrieval and playback. (Essentially, this was a self-paced task since the subject was given all the time he needed for recall or recognition.) Both immediate and delayed memory show deficits when the items are presented during sleep loss, so Williams, Gieseking, and Lubin conclude that trace formation and trace storage are impaired during sleep loss.

Two more recent studies (Elkin and Murray, 1974; Polzella, 1975) have attempted to provide more definitive data on the effects of sleep loss on short term recognition memory and the adequacy of the lapse hypothesis. In both studies, a probe recognition memory task was used. Polzella deprived his subjects for 24 hours, while Elkin and Murray's subjects went 55 hours without sleep. In both studies, there was significant memory impairment. However, the explanations for the impairment varied. Polzella concluded that 'the data were consistent with the hypothesis that sleep deprivation increases the occurrence of lapses, periods of lowered reactive capacity, which prevents the encoding of items in short-term memory' (1975, p.194). Elkin and Murray, on the other hands said: 'It is argued that these findings are consistent with the notion that sleep loss causes a deficit in attention leading to misperception and a failure to rehearse adequately material presented for memorization' (1974, p.192). For Elkin and Murray, sleep loss reduces the ability of the subject to attend for extended periods of time.

Buck and Gibbs (1972) have also questioned whether the lapse hypothesis is adequate to explain sleep loss performance decrement in tasks with a high degree of uncertainty as posited by Williams, Kearney, and Lubin (1965). Buck and Gibbs prefer to emphasize change in information processing capability rather than the tendency to take periods of microsleep though they admit the two explanations are not necessarily incompatible.

AN ALTERNATIVE TO THE LAPSE HYPOTHESIS

In a series of three articles, Kjellberg (1977a, b, c) questions the adequacy of the lapse hypothesis and attempts to provide a theoretical framework within which the performance effects of sleep deprivation can be interpreted.

It appears that Kjellberg's objection to the lapse hypothesis, as set forth by the Walter Reed group, was that it dealt with only one dimension of the effects of sleep loss, i.e. dearousal. Lapses were instances of lowered arousal level and lapses are the only major performance manifestations of this dearousal.

After reviewing the empirical findings concerning sleep deprivation and arousal, Kjellberg questions the widely held view that sleep deprivation *per se* leads to dearousal and that 'dearousal is the "pure", uncontaminated effect of SD [sleep deprivation]' (1977a, p.140). Kjellberg maintains that statements about the effects of sleep deprivation on arousal must be formulated in terms of interaction, that is, in terms of how the effects of various situational factors are influenced by sleep deprivation. 'Thus, while it cannot be said that SD leads to dearousal, there is evidence that SD potentiates the influence of sleep-provoking factors in the situation' (1977a, p.142). The work of Bohlin (1971) is cited as an example. Bohlin showed that repetitive stimulus presentation provokes sleep in non-deprived subjects, but also showed that the sleep inducing effects of the repetitive stimulus were more pronounced in sleep deprived subjects. As will be discussed presently, long, monotonous tasks that would lead to lowered involvement and arousal are most affected by sleep loss.

Kjellberg (1977b) also cites evidence suggesting that lapses are not discrete abrupt periods of lowered arousal, but that there is, in most instances, a gradual lowering of arousal which, after reaching a critical level, manifests itself as a performance lapse. Decrements in performance before the occurrences of lapses indicate to Kjellberg that 'if the SD effects are to be regarded as manifestations of lowered arousal this dearousal must lead to other effects beside lapses' (p.147). Attentional deficits are listed as one of the main effects of sleep deprivation and are characterized by weakened attention to external situations as well as a decreased capacity to sustain selective attention to critical aspects of the task or situation.

The main thrust of Kjellberg's argument appears to be his view that lapses are a limited explanation of the effects of sleep loss on performance. When lapses occur, they are the end-point of lowered arousal. Kjellberg does not question the fact that sleep loss influences a subject's response on certain tasks and to certain situational features in a predictable way. In those situations that potentiate lowered arousal, the sleep loss effects are stronger and more predictable. 'The lowered arousal, however, also manifests itself in Ss' subjective state and as a deterioration of the capacity for sustained selective attention' (1977c, p.151). I have no quarrel with Kjellberg's conclusion.

MODIFIER VARIABLES

In overview, one of the most striking features of the variations in performance associated with sleep deprivation are the effects of 'modifier' variables, i.e. variables associated with the ongoing period of deprivation. Those factors for which there is experimental or putative evidence of influence are listed in Table I and briefly discussed in this section. The variables are keyed to this table.

Table 1   Variables effect performance within sleep deprivation

---

Fatigue

Task variables
Duration
Knowledge of results
Difficulty of task
Task pacing
Proficiency level
Task complexity
Memory requirements

Non-task factors
Psychological
(1) high interest
(2) motivation
(3) personality
(4) repeated experiences

Situational factors
(1) exercise
(2) noise
(3) temperature
(4) drugs
(5) breathing atmosphere

Behavioural periodicity

Fatigue

Whether one favours the lapse hypothesis or the interactive concepts of Kjellberg, there is no disagreement that the most common effect of sleep loss is a feeling of fatigue. Fatigue is a concept that appears in studies from all areas and serves as a unifying, though oversimplified, concept. Fatigue is an inevitable consequence of sleep loss. The physical activity necessary to maintain wakefulness during periods of prolonged sleep loss eventually makes it difficult to determine whether failure to respond is due to sleep loss or fatigue. Perhaps when that point is reached, sleep loss and fatigue effects are inseparable and differentiating between the two as causes for performance decrement is not meaningful.

Klein *et al.* (1969), in discussing the importance of fatigue, emphasized that terms like 'work load' and 'stress' should not be used as synonyms for fatigue. For them, stress is part of a work load, and work load is a cause of fatigue; hence, fatigue is the consequence of stress and work load. They emphasize that this discrimination is not only of academic interest but leads to different approaches for measuring effects of long-duration flights. The presence of environmental and situational stressors such as those present in flying, combined with disturbed sleep–wakefulness cycles or disruption in circadian rhythms, undoubtedly will affect both the rate and the ultimate level of fatigue. The rate of recovery of a degraded function will also depend, though probably not in a simple linear fashion, upon the rate of development and final level of fatigue.

Task Variables

Why are some tasks more sensitive to total sleep loss? What factors are responsible for making these tasks sensitive to total sleep loss? Do these factors help explain some of the differences found between laboratory and field studies? Seven factors have been identified. Task duration, whether work-paced or self-paced, and work load have already been mentioned, but they will be listed again and other work will be cited.

Duration of Task. The longer the task, the more sensitive it is to total sleep loss. Total sleep loss of 50 hours causes impairment after only 3 minutes of a visual vigilance task. Seventy hours of total sleep loss cause decrement on a vigilance task after 2 minutes (Williams, Lubin, and Goodnow, 1959). Total sleep loss of one night had no appreciable effect on task performance during the first 5 minutes on a 5-choice test of serial reaction, vigilance, and addition, but clear-cut performance deterioration emerged when performance was evaluated after 15 minute task sessions (Wilkinson, 1961, 1965). Following one night without sleep, the number of additions attempted on the Wilkinson Addition Test decreased significantly from base line level after 10 minutes of testing (Donnell, 1969). Following two nights without sleep, the number of additions attempted was clearly decreased after only 6 minutes. Fifty minutes of testing were required to detect a significant decrease in accuracy after one day of sleep loss, while only 10 minutes were required the second day.

Knowledge of results. By immediately feeding back to the subject information as to how well he had performed each task, total sleep loss of 30 hours did not appear to impair performance on 1 hour 5-choice serial reaction and vigilance tests (Wilkinson, 1961). Immediate feedback of quality of task performance, thus, minimizes the effects of total sleep loss.

Difficulty of task. Performance on difficult tasks is more sensitive to total sleep loss. A simple task, such as addition, can be made very difficult by asking the subject to add quickly. Mental addition at a rate of one addition per 2 seconds did not reveal the effects of 2 nights of sleep loss, but by increasing the speed of addition to one addition every 1.25 seconds, i.e. a 38% speed increase, the effects of sleep loss of 2 nights were detected (Williams and Lubin, 1967).

Task pacing. Self-paced tasks resist sleep loss effects much better than work-paced tasks. In self-paced tasks, even though lapses could prevent the completion of a task by causing the subject to lose his place, as soon as the lapse ends, the task is resumed. The effects of total sleep loss show up in the increased time needed to complete the self-paced tasks, although there are fewer errors of omission and performance accuracy is high.

Proficiency level. Newly acquired skills, such as those involved in driving a car by a person who had just passed his driver's test for the first time, are more affected by loss of total sleep than those skills which have become almost automatic or second nature, like rifle assembly for military personnel.

Task complexity. The more complex the task is, with respect to sequence of mental operations and/or the orderly execution of complex muscular activities, the more likely it is to be sensitive to sleep loss (Wilkinson, 1965; Hockey, 1970). Task complexity, however, may interact with interest. There may be more sleep loss effect on a simple but boring task than on a task that is complex but interesting.

Memory requirements. Any task which requires a short term memory chain will be affected by sleep loss (Williams, Gieseking, and Lubin, 1966; Williams and Williams, 1966).

In summary, the long, work-paced, complex tasks with high attention and vigilance requirements and which do not provide information to the subject on how well he is performing can be expected to show higher sensitivity to total sleep loss.

Non-task Factors

There are three major classes of non-task factors which also influence the outcome of total sleep loss on performance. They are as follows.

Psychological factors. (1) *High interest.* Ax and his colleagues (1967) suggested that interesting tasks resist the effects of loss of total sleep. For example, a battle game used in one study was found to be so interesting that sailors could work on the game for one hour without showing the effects of over 50 hours of total sleep loss (Wilkinson, 1964).

(2) *Motivation.* While tasks of high interest usually have high motivational value, a distinction between high interest and motivation should be made. For example, a serial learning task which may have little interest to the subject can become highly motivating if his performance is monitored by his supervisor. High motivation tasks showed no significant performance decrements after one night of sleep loss, but most of the low motivating tasks resulted in poor performances. In general, high motivation will counteract the effects of total sleep loss, but there is a point beyond which the sheer need for sleep will overwhelm even the subject's willingness to work.

(3) *Personality*. The role that personality factors play in determining sleep loss effects is unclear. No relationship was found between scores on a psychological test of introversion–extraversion and neuroticism and the degree of performance after total sleep loss of one night (Wilkinson, 1959), but, in another study (Corcoran, 1962a), extraverts were affected more than introverts by loss of 60 hours of sleep, as measured by a pursuit tracking task. Following 72 hours of sleep loss, Lester, Knapp, and Roessler (1976) found that subjects who scored high on the Barron Ego Strength Scale and low on the Barratt Impulsiveness Scale detected more signals in a vigilance task.

(4) *Repeated experiences of sleep loss*. Repeated exposures to total sleep loss increased the effects of such sleep loss on task performance (Wilkinson, 1961; Morgan *et al.*, 1973).

Situational factors. (1) *Exercise*. Physical exercises just prior to performing tasks helped reduce performance decrement caused by total sleep loss (Wilkinson, 1965), but, as will be reported later, scheduled exercise periods did not prevent performance decrement over 40 hours of sleep deprivation (Moses *et al.*, 1978).

(2) *Noise*. White noise, 90–100 dB, in an open field lessened the effects of total sleep loss on auditory vigilance performance and on the 5-choice test of serial reaction (Corcoran, 1962b; Wilkinson, 1963).

(3) *Temperature*. A moderate ambient temperature of 30.5 °C does not increase the effects of total sleep loss. There are no conclusive data on the interactions of extreme heat or cold on effects of total sleep deprivation on performances. Occasional cold stresses, e.g. immersing the face in ice-cold water and/or alcohol rubs with an electric fan blowing air onto the subject, help combat spells of extreme sleepiness.

(4) *Drugs*. Though caffeine, in coffee and tea, is frequently used to combat sleepiness, amphetamines appear to be the only drugs which have been studied (Tyler, 1947; Kornetsky *et al.*, 1959; Laties, 1961). Oral intakes of 15 mg dextroamphetamine almost halved the behavioural impairment caused by 68 hours without sleep on a work-paced vigilance task (Kornetsky *et al.*, 1959). Dextroamphetamine was effective in completely eliminating small effects of sleep loss which occurred in self-paced tasks. Depending upon the dosage, alcohol was found to counteract the effect of moderate amounts of total sleep loss (Wilkinson and Colquhoun, 1968).

(5) *Breathing atmosphere*. Hypoxia and inert gas narcosis (especially nitrogen narcosis) produce performance degradations which are similar to the effects of total sleep loss. Hypoxia and inert gas narcosis may potentiate the effects of total sleep loss on performance, although this contention has not yet been studied experimentally.

The above factors, thus, may interact with the effects of sleep loss and may explain why it is difficult to detect sleep loss effects in field studies. In addition to the problem of insuring that total sleep loss actually occurs, the types of tasks, the subjects, motivation and other psychological factors, and the environmental setting all mitigate against marked sleep loss decrements. Sleep loss effects for less than 48 hours of wakefulness will more likely occur on long, repetitive, boring tasks, with no feedback as to accuracy, and preferably work-paced. It is these types of tasks, which are most sensitive to lapses, that have been used by laboratories with positive sleep loss results and which are least likely to be part of operational studies.

Behavioural periodicity. The severity of the effects of total sleep loss depends, in part, on the time of day that measures of performance are obtained (see Chapter III). Sleep deprived subjects may appear quite normal and perform very well in the early afternoon when most have peak behavioural efficiency, but the same subjects will show a marked deterioration in their performance in the early morning when sleep loss effects combine with low behavioural efficiency. Ignorance of behavioural periodicity was a factor in some of the studies reporting no significant effects of total sleep deprivation. Measures of performance taken at different times of the day reflect behavioural periodicity as well as the effects of increasing sleep debt. Klein, Wegmann, and Brüner (1968) have stressed the interaction of sleep loss and circadian rhythms and the need to establish a single time in the 24 hour period as a point of reference. They prefer to use the lowest level in the early morning.

Morgan, Brown, and Alluisi (1970) found, as had Drucker, Cannon, and Ware (1969), that even though performance did not always follow the diurnal cycle during normal work periods, it was likely to do so during periods of continuous operations. With respect to the index of general performance, the subjects were able to maintain their performance near 100% of base line for approximately 18 hours before it dropped to nearly 81% of base line during the last 8 hours of the first 24 hour period of continuous operation. This period happened to be near the end of the first night. Performance improved during the second day of work to above 80% efficiency before falling to a low point of approximately 67% of base line during the night of the second 24 hours of continuous work.

A recent report from our laboratory detailed the circadian variation in performance, subjective sleepiness, sleep, and oral temperature during an altered sleep–wake schedule (Moses *et al.*, 1978). Thirty-eight male students, aged 18–22, participated in the study. Following one base line sleep night, 8 subjects underwent a 60 minute sleep/160 minute wake schedule for 40 hours. Ten subjects pedaled a stationary bicycle (Ex group) and 20 subjects rested in bed (Bdr group) during the same 1 hour interval that the nap subjects were allowed to sleep. Neither the Ex group nor the Bdr group was allowed to sleep during the 40 hour period. There were 10 approximately equally spaced 1 hour treatment sessions during the 40 hours. The Stanford Sleepiness Scale

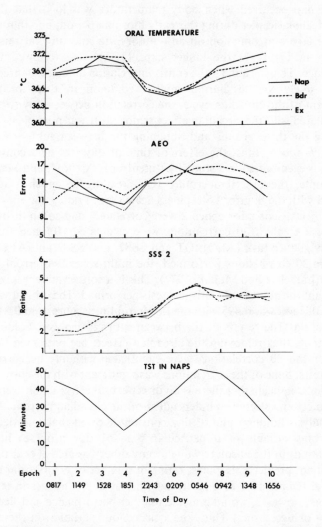

Figure 3   Distribution of oral temperature, performance, self-rated sleepiness, and sleep time in naps during 40 hours. (From Moses *et al.*, 1978)

immediately preceded and followed each session, followed by the Wilkinson Auditory Vigilance Test (40 minutes) and the Wilkinson Addition Test (Wilkinson, 1969) (40 minutes). Oral temperature readings were taken approximately midway between sessions. A more detailed description of the experimental design and the recording techniques has been presented elsewhere (Moses *et al.*, 1975; Lubin *et al.*, 1976).

We were not surprised to find that nap total sleep time (TST) was greater when the nap occurred when body temperature was low, that the subject reported feeling sleepier during this early morning period, and that there were also more errors of omission on an auditory vigilance task at this time. As illustrated in Figure 3, the longer naps (TST) were followed by poorer performance. To determine if the consistent relation among the three variables was due solely to the diurnal rhythm common to them or to effects independent of the circadian cycle, the correlation between any two variables was calculated with the circadian effect removed. It was possible to do this by combining the three groups and obtaining the between subjects correlation *within each epoch*; thus, the effect of time of day was held constant. This approach is exemplified in a study by Rutenfranz, Aschoff, and Mann (1972). For example, the oral temperature (OT) reading at epoch 1 (0817) was correlated with the Stanford Sleepiness Scale (SSS2) rating for epoch 1 across the 38 subjects, scores for epoch 2 were correlated, and so on through epoch 10. Thus, a total of 30 correlations were calculated; 10 each for OT and auditory vigilance task (AEO), OT and SSS2, and SSS2 and AEO. Because there were 30 correlations performed, the multi-stage Bonferroni procedure was used (Larzelere and Mulaik, 1977). This is a conservative test which takes into account the number of statistical tests performed. The critical value of the r at the 0.05 level was 0.495 with the Bonferroni procedure, and 0.313 without the correction. The results of the between subjects analysis, holding time of day constant, thus removing the circadian effect, are presented in Table 2. Only 2 of the 30 correlations were significant without the correction for multiple tests; none of the correlations was significant with the correction.

Our results indicate that there is no direct causal effect among temperature, performance, and sleepiness independent of the circadian rhythm. The results of the analysis holding time of day constant showed that knowledge of the level of one variable at a particular time of day provides little or no information as to the absolute value of any other variable at that time. Thus, one could not predict a sleepiness rating or number of errors from knowledge of the oral temperature at a particular time of day. Changes in temperature across time, however, would indicate whether performance and sleepiness are increasing or decreasing. Thus, the synchronous variation in these variables was due primarily to their common link with time of day. These results support the findings of Rutenfranz, Aschoff, and Mann (1972), who found significant correlations in temperature and reaction time across times of day, but no correlation between the two variables between subjects when time of day was held constant. Rutenfranz and his colleagues (1972) took their analyses a step further by also performing within subject correlations holding time of day constant. They found no significant correlations between temperature and reaction time when time of day was held constant, providing further evidence that temperature and performance were not causally related.

From the analysis of the Nap group alone, it would appear that sleep itself

Table 2 Correlations of oral temperature, sleepiness, and performance holding time of day constant

Measure	E1 (0817)	E2 (1149)	E3 (1528)	E4 (1851)	E5 (2243)	E6 (0209)	E7 (0546)	E8 (0942)	E9 (1348)	E10 (1656)
OT, AEO	0.04	-0.12	-0.01	-0.19	-0.26	-0.04	-0.22	-0.01	-0.20	-0.28
OT, SSS2	-0.18	0.12	-0.13	-0.01	-0.35[a]	0.06	0.17	-0.11	0.18	0.10
SSS2, AEO	0.27	0.26	0.21	0.28	0.34[a]	0.12	0.28	0.21	0.29	0.24

[a]Significant at the 0.05 level without correction for multiple tests (none of the correlations was significant with the correction). (From Moses et al., 1978).

increased sleepiness and was detrimental to performance, since naps on which the most sleep occurred were followed by the highest sleepiness ratings and the poorest performance. The Ex and Bdr groups, however, also reported highest sleepiness and had the worst performance at the same time of day as the Nap subjects, indicating that the circadian variation in these measures was primarily responsible for what appeared to be a detrimental effect of sleep.

The strikingly similar oral temperature curves in the three groups further demonstrate the pervasiveness of the 24 hour rhythm, despite the differences in experimental treatment.

PARTIAL SLEEP LOSS OR REDUCED SLEEP

Relative to total sleep loss, there are fewer performance studies under conditions of partial sleep loss, but partial sleep loss is the most likely type of sleep deprivation to be experienced. The occurrence of fragmented sleep and partial sleep loss in aircrews was clearly documented in our NATO AGARDograph (Johnson and Naitoh, 1974). For effects of partial sleep on sleep *per se* see Chapter IV.

Partial sleep loss is both easy and difficult to define. Decreasing TST by going to bed later or getting up earlier results in a sleep deficit. Partial sleep loss may occur if one sleeps 2 hours, gets up, and then sleeps for 3 hours, gets up, etc.; the fragmented sleep may not equal his/her usual TST. Also, does this fragmented sleep, even when equal to usual TST, have the same recuperative value as uninterrupted sleep? The data are inconclusive. Simply stated, partial sleep loss occurs when there is a reduction of the usual amounts of sleep obtained in 24 hours.

Is a person who sleeps only 4 hours in 24 necessarily suffering from partial sleep loss? Is there a fixed amount of sleep that must be obtained if a sleep debt is to be avoided? The answers appear to be 'no'. There are wide individual differences as to amounts of sleep required. Two men who slept only about 3 hours in each 24 hours reported no sleep loss complaints (Jones and Oswald, 1968). A more extreme example is the report of a 60 year old woman who slept on the average of 1 hour each night with no daytime naps and was reported to be alert, competent, with no need or desire for more sleep (Meddis, Pearson, and Langford, 1973).

Stuss and Broughton (1978) have reported on six additional short sleepers who slept less than 4 hours in 24. Sleep patterns and results on performance tests were studied in one of their subjects who slept only 1.5 hours. A performance battery (calculations, vigilance, sensory motor) was administered after base line, extended, and abbreviated sleep following laboratory adaptation. Stuss and Broughton concluded that the impaired performance found in this subject on most tests following extended sleep (50% extension of base line) indicated that this less than 2 hour sleeper was obtaining his optimum sleep requirement.

Sleep Reduction

While the health and performance of natural short sleepers are of interest to sleep researchers, our interest over the past few years has been on shortened sleep. Those who abruptly shorten their sleep for whatever reason generally return to their usual sleep schedules when allowed to do so. In acute sleep-reduction studies, the data have shown no marked changes in performance, whether this was in subjects allowed only 3 hours for 8 consecutive days (Webb and Agnew, 1965), 5.5 hours for 60 days (Webb and Agnew, 1974), or when sleep was restricted to about 5 hours per day for 3 months (Rutenfranz, Aschoff, and Mann, 1972). The latter study involved 12 young German naval cadets on a training cruise.

In our study of gradual sleep reduction (Friedmann *et al.*, 1977), we found no performance decrement on a battery of cognitive and motor tasks as sleep was reduced from 7.5–8.0 hours to 5.0–4.5 hours in six subjects, and from 6.5 to 5.0 hours in two subjects. In contrast to the acute sleep-reduction studies, the TST of our six 8 hour sleepers was still reduced 1.0–1.5 hours a year later. The two 6.5 hour sleepers returned to 6.5 hours TST when the sleep-reduction period ended, indicating they had already established their minimum sleep lengths.

Although there were no consistent performance decrements in the laboratory or in their graduate studies or work, our subjects began to complain of discomfort between 6.5 and 6.0 hours of sleep. There were complaints of feeling more sleepy, feeling the need for more sleep, and having less vigour and more fatigue (see Figures 4 and 5).

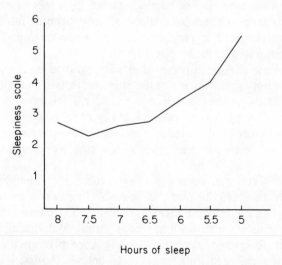

Hours of sleep

Figure 4   Average ratings on Stanford Sleepiness Scale during gradual sleep reduction

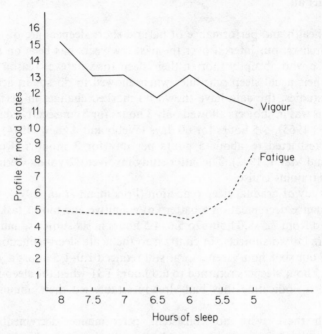

Figure 5   Average ratings on vigour and fatigue scales during gradual sleep reduction

In their interviews, all eight subjects reported difficulty in getting up in the morning as sleep was reduced below 6 hours. This difficulty increased as restriction proceeded to the lowest, 4.5 hour, level. Subjects elected to stop sleep reduction because, as one participant put it, 'I was just too tired' and 'just wanted to sleep'. Others complained of overwhelming fatigue and falling asleep while in class, while playing cards, or while visiting friends, and of difficulty in remaining vigilant while driving.

There was some change in personal efficiency noted by most subjects, but this change did not appear on any of the objective tests or in their school or job performance. As one subject put it when at his lowest sleep level: 'I am noticeably less efficient, less energetic; e.g. I can't seem to study as I used to, I get discouraged more easily, slightly depressed about overcoming difficulties, very much like I feel when I am sick with a cold' (Friedmann *et al.*, 1977, p.248).

Though the Webb and Agnew studies (1965, 1974), that by Rutenfranz, Aschoff, and Mann (1972), and the study by Friedmann *et al.* (1977) have found no significant performance decrement with reduced sleep, in other studies performance impairment has been found. Wilkinson, Edwards, and Haines (1966) observed a decrement in vigilance performance following a single night of sleep reduction from 7.5 to below 3 hours. Performance on both the auditory vigilance and the addition test decreased when sleep was reduced to 5 hours for 2 nights. Hamilton, Wilkinson, and Edwards (1972) found a performance decrement in the number of detections on the auditory vigilance tests and the number of additions completed when sleep was limited to 4 hours. The effect of partial sleep loss was cumulative over a 4 day period.

A study by Hartley (1974) involved the distribution of sleep over the 24 hour period. After a night of normal sleep, 36 subjects were divided into three groups of 12. One group was allowed to continue sleeping normally, one group had 4 hours continuous sleep, and the third group had three 80 minute periods of sleep distributed throughout the 24 hour period, for the next 4 days. Subjects were given a visual vigilance test on each day. Overall performance was better following distributed than following continuous reduced sleep, but worse than following 8 hours of sleep. The main difference between the reduced sleep groups was in their decision criterion. Hartley suggested that this difference mainly reflected the difference in time since the two groups had last slept, and not the amount of sleep *per se*.

Taub and Berger (1976) have also found that changing the phase and duration of sleep affects performance. Because Taub and Berger, as did Hartley, changed the time of day that sleep was obtained as well as the amount of sleep, it is not possible to say that the performance decrement in their subjects was due entirely to the changes in amount of sleep. The importance of circadian influences on performance is well illustrated in this volume.

Fragmented Sleep

It is felt by many sleep researchers in the area of biological rhythms that the fragmentation of sleep and the desynchrony of the physiological rhythms have a greater impact on behaviour. Following changes in both sleep times and sleep–wakefulness cycles, disruption of the circadian cycle was felt to be a more important determiner of performance and of subjective mood changes than the shortened hours of sleep (Taub and Berger, 1973). One of the few studies of sleep during combat conditions documented the effect of fragmented sleep. Sleep of carrier pilots was reported while on duty stations off Vietnam (Brictson, McHugh, and Naitoh, 1974). While TST of the 27 aviators was found to be similar to 28 non-flying personnel, the aviators' sleep–wakefulness cycle was significantly different. The aviators had a far more variable intersleep interval than non-aviators. The more variable a pilot's intersleep interval, the more likely he was to make a landing error.

Laboratory studies of scheduled nap sleep, however, have found little performance decrement. In an extreme variation of the sleep–wake schedule, Carskadon and Dement (1975) placed 5 subjects on a 90 minute day; 30 minutes of sleep, 60 minutes awake, for 5 days. Subjective self-reports of sleepiness and mood revealed initial discomfort on the 90 minute schedule.

However, the sleepiness and mood of the subjects tended to show improvement during the experimental period, approaching base line levels by the fourth or fifth experimental day. Daily 24 hour fluctuations were present on both measures.

In our laboratory, we compared the effects of naps, exercise, and bedrest to sustained performance over a 40 hour period (Lubin *et al.*, 1976). In this study, noted in my discussion of the influence of circadian rhythms, young male naval volunteers were denied normal nocturnal sleep and maintained on a 60 minute treatment/160 minute testing schedule during 40 consecutive hours. Ten subjects bicycled, 20 subjects were allowed to rest in bed but not sleep, and 10 subjects napped. Eight measures of addition, auditory vigilance, mood, and oral temperature were obtained. The Bdr group showed significant impairment on all eight measures and, thus, gave no support to the *forced-rest* theory of sleep function. The Ex group was worse than the Nap and Bdr groups for all measures. Thus, in contrast to Wilkinson's (1965) finding that exercise before a task increased performance levels, scheduled exercise periods were of no benefit to our subjects in overcoming the effects of sleep deprivation. In spite of fragmented, reduced sleep (about 3.7 hours per 24 hours), the Nap group showed no impairment on six of the measures. The results suggest that exercise increases the impairment due to sleep loss, and naps reduce or remove this impairment. Bedrest is not a substitute for sleep.

In summary, while performance decrements do not appear to be a major problem, sleep disruption and sleep deficits appear to raise the 'cost' of maintaining predeficit levels of performance. This cost is sometimes reflected in increased physiological stress-related responses, but, most often, it is reflected in the increased effort to overcome feelings of fatigue. Subjective feelings of fatigue are the major findings whether sleep reduction occurs in the laboratory or in an operational setting.

SUSTAINED PERFORMANCE

The traditional approach to the study of sleep loss effects has been to measure performance on selected tasks or on a battery of tasks at specified time periods during the period of wakefulness. Increasing interest is being directed toward the problem of sustained or continuous, or near continuous, operations. In these situations, the demand to perform is continuous over the total 24 hour period and the demand may persist for days. While the requirement for sustained performance can occur in both military and civilian sectors, most research has been done in military settings. In the civilian sector, sustained operations usually involve emergency situations, but in the military, in this era of possible nuclear warfare, current strategy is based on the probability that a war will be of short duration and relief personnel will not be utilized. The question thus becomes how long can effective performance be maintained without any sleep, and, if sleep is possible, how much sleep is necessary and what are the best times in the 24 hour period to permit sleep.

Diana Haslam and her associates at the Army Personnel Research Establishment in England have conducted studies to answer the question of how long can a person sustain effective performance with no, or only limited, amount of sleep (Haslam, 1981). To obtain information on the performance of 68 soldiers in continuous military operations, field trials of 9 day duration were carried out. The aims were to compare the performance on many tasks of three platoons of infantry scheduled to receive either 0 hour, 1½ hour, or 3 hour blocks of sleep in 24 hours, and to find out for how many days the no-sleep platoon could stay in the field. Assessments indicated that the 0 hour sleep platoon remained effective for physical tasks for 3 days, the 1½ hour group for 6 days, and the 3 hour group for 9 days. Compared with a survival time in the field of 4 days for the no-sleep platoon, 48% of the 1½ hour platoon and 91% of the 3 hour platoon completed the 9 day trial.

Although nearly 50% of the 1½ hour sleep platoon and nearly all of the 3 hour platoon lasted the 9 days, performance over the 9 days deteriorated. On vigilance tasks involving shooting and on cognitive tasks, all three platoons' performance on experiment (no sleep or reduced sleep) days was significantly worse than on control days. For the 0 hour sleep group, performance on day 2 was significantly worse than on day 1 (Figure 6).

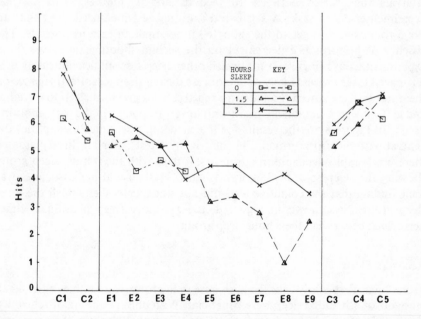

Figure 6 Vigilance shooting. Average number of hits for the three platoons. (From Haslam, 1981)

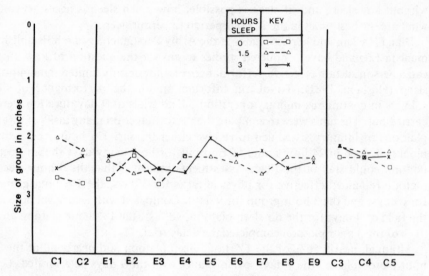

Figure 7   Grouping capacity. Average size of best of three groups for the three
platoons. (From Haslam, 1981)

In the vigilance shooting task, the targets were shown for 5 seconds at time
intervals that varied between 10 seconds and 7 minutes. This was an
experimenter-paced task. A self-paced shooting test measured the ability to
fire 5 rounds at a target so the shots fell in as small an area as possible. The
absence of performance decrement on the second shooting task over the 9
experimental days (Figure 7) confirmed other sleep loss studies indicating that
self-paced tasks are less likely to deteriorate during sleep loss. Performance on
the other tasks followed the pattern expected from previous sleep loss studies
and all followed a circadian pattern with lowest responses in the early morning
hours. In Figure 8 are the results for the encoding task which exemplifies the
general pattern of performance in the cognitive tests. For all three platoons,
there was a rapid decline during the first 4 days with the 0 hour sleep group
showing the steepest drop, but surprising to Haslam and her associates was
their finding that the cognitive tests did not statistically distinguish the three
sleep groups. As shown in Figure 8, the 1½ hour sleep platoon at times
performed better than the 3 hour sleep group.

Recovery Sleep

From their first study, the English research group found that even small
amounts of scheduled sleep were beneficial. With only 1 ½ hours of scheduled
sleep, 48% of the platoon lasted the 9 days. Even though these 48% were still
'in the trenches', their performance on vigilance and cognitive tasks

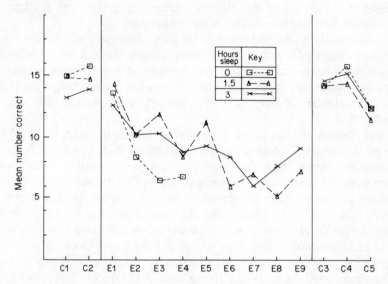

Figure 8   Encoding. Average number correct for the three platoons. (From Haslam, 1981)

deteriorated approximately 50% over the experimental period. These sustained performance studies confirm the earlier sleep loss findings and once again reaffirm the recuperative value of sleep. Since sleep is crucial, the question becomes how much sleep is necessary for recovery, and is there a best time during the 24 hour period to obtain this recovery sleep? Is sleep in the morning as recuperative as sleep in the afternoon?

Paul Naitoh of the Naval Health Research Center has conducted a series of studies addressing the question of circadian cycles and restorative power of brief sleep (Naitoh, 1981 (a)). As a continuation of this group's sleep loss and nap studies, an experiment was conducted on two groups of young sailors to study the recuperative power of a 2 hour nap on task performance and self-ratings of mood, fatigue, sleepiness, and arousal. One group took a 2 hour nap from 0400 to 0600 (the early morning nap) after 45 hours of continuous work. Six hours later, this group took their second 2 hour nap from 1200 to 1400 (the midday nap). For a second group, their only nap was from 1200 to 1400 after 53 hours of continuous work. Circadian rhythm analyses confirmed that the early morning nap was placed near the troughs of many circadian rhythms and the midday nap on the rising limb of the circadian rhythms. On both performance and mood, the early morning nap resulted in severe and prolonged sleep inertia and did not have any recuperative power. In contrast, the midday nap produced a relatively short sleep inertia and had clear recuperative power. Naitoh concluded that the recuperative power of a nap depended not only on its duration but, more importantly, on the hours of prior wakefulness and time of day when it was taken.

A similar study is now under way at the sleep laboratory at the University of Florida. In this study, following 72 hours without sleep, a nap of 2 hours is allowed either before normal sleep times (evening sleep) or during the morning after usual awakening (morning sleep). The goals of the San Diego and Florida studies are similar. If sleep is to be rationed, when should this ration be served?

Diana Haslam and her co-workers, noting that, in Early Call I, the 0 hour sleep group lasted only 4 days, conducted a second study in which 3¾ days of continuous activity were followed by 6 days when there was limited opportunity for sleep. The emphasis in Early Call II was on the recovery process—how much sleep is needed to restore effective performance? Ten soldiers took part in this phase. The aim was to determine if soldiers would remain militarily effective during a period of partial sleep loss following a period of no scheduled sleep. The results indicated that blocks of 4 hours of sleep had a marked beneficial effect upon performance and mood. All 10 subjects completed the study and after a total of 12 hours of sleep over 3 days, performance had recovered to 88% of control values. When testing occurred at 0545 hours, this 88% improvement was not found, reflecting the circadian influence. The 4 hour sleep blocks occurred during the usual night time sleep period. Thus the introduction of 4 hour sleep blocks following 90 hours in which there was no scheduled sleep (and D. Haslam assures me there was little unscheduled sleep) had a marked beneficial effect upon performance.

In a third military study, a team of US Army investigators studied the performance of a 5-man army fire direction control team in a simulated exercise (Francesconi *et al.*, 1978). The study involved a sustained operation component separated by a rest/sleep period of 33 hours followed by a second period of continuous performance. There was some performance decrement during the first 38 hour performance period, but, more importantly, the team performance declined earlier and to a greater extent when they were subjected to the second episode of 38 hours of duty. Analysis of the 33 hour sleep/rest period indicated that some of the team members were unable to sleep effectively even though time for sleep was permitted.

In general, the upper limits of human performance for working intensively and continuously are about 2–3 days when mission tasks are both physical and mental (Francesconi *et al.*, 1978; Haslam, 1981; Naitoh, 1981 (a)). Human effectiveness is eroded during sustained operations in many ways: loss of vigilance, inability to concentrate on the task at hand (wandering mind), slowing down in reading printed instructions and maps, degraded short term memory in retaining commands given, and a tendency to skip routine but critical subsidiary tasks (unwilling to respond). Some of these degradations may occur within the first 12 hours of sustained operations. The adverse effects on human efficiency due to sustained operations are accentuated by an unavoidable daily performance dip between 0300 and 0600.

Sleep loss research has shifted from the effects of acute sleep loss to the minimizing of sleep loss effects over prolonged periods of limited and fragmented sleep. The question is now how much sleep and at what time. Though there are scattered reports of very short sleepers (Jones and Oswald, 1968; Meddis, Pearson, and Langford, 1973), I am impressed with the findings that the minimum sleep time in most surveys is around 4–5 hours. Subjects in our studies of gradual sleep reduction were unwilling to sleep less than 4 hours. But in these studies, none of our subjects maintained a 4 hour sleep schedule after the study ended—most were sleeping between 5 and 7 hours.

More intriguing are the current studies on what are the optimal times for sleep. Most would say at night. Maybe that is only because most of us have done most of our sleeping at night. Can we train ourselves to sleep at other times of the day, or are we trapped by our habits and our circadian rhythms? The latter may be the limiting factor. In an interesting paper, Dr. Naitoh (in press) discusses the chronopsychological approach for optimizing performance. This approach focuses on the diurnal or circadian variations in performance. Naitoh's thesis is that the chronopsychologist should try to improve societal around-the-clock performance by shifting the time of peak performance of some individuals to a different time of day. With this manipulation of individual circadian clocks, Naitoh envisions a society in which there will always be some individuals who are at top efficiency at any given time of the day. Even if such shifting of peak performance is possible, in the era of informed consent and freedom to withdraw, will individuals allow the chronopsychologists to modify their 'clocks'? And, would it work?

SUMMARY

This chapter first reviews the background and major theoretical positions that have evolved in sleep deprivation research. This review emphasizes the paradoxical nature of performance measures in this area—the certainty of decrements and the paradoxes of their ephemeral nature. This is followed by a presentation of the wide range of factors which significantly modify the degree of response decrements under conditions of sleep deprivation: fatigue, task variables, and non-task factors; psychological, situational, and behavioural periodicity. Performance variations associated with partial sleep loss and results of experiments, emphasizing continuous performance, conclude the chapter.

ACKNOWLEDGMENT

This research was supported by the Naval Medical Research and Development Command, Department of the Navy, under Work Unit MF58.524.004-9026.

The views presented in this paper are those of the author. No endorsement by the Department of the Navy has been given or should be inferred.

REFERENCES

Agnew, H. W., Jr. and Webb, W. B. (1972). Measurement of sleep onset by EEG criteria. *American Journal of EEG Technology* 12, 127–134.

Ax, A. F., Fordyce, W., Loovas, I., Meredith, W., Pirojnikoff, L., Shmavonia, B., and Wendahl, R. (1967). *Quantitative Effects of Sleep Deprivation*. US Army Quartermaster Res. Development Res. Rep.

Bills, A. G. (1958). Studying motor functions and efficiency. In: *Methods of Psychology*, pp.459–497. T. G. Andrews (Ed.). New York, Wiley.

Bohlin, G. (1971). Monotonous stimulation, sleep onset and habituation of the orienting reaction. *Electroencephalography and Clinical Neurophysiology* 31, 593–601.

Brictson, C. A., McHugh, M., and Naitoh, P. (1974). *Prediction of pilot performance: Biochemical and sleep-mood correlates under high workload conditions*. Paper presented at the meeting of the AGARD Aerospace Medical Panel Specialists, Oslo, Norway, 29 April – 3 May 1974.

Broadbent, D. E. (1955). Variations in performance arising from continuous work. In: *Conference on Individual Efficiency in Industry*, pp.1–5. Cambridge, England, Medical Research Council.

Buck, L. and Gibbs, C. B. (1972). Sleep loss and information processing. In: *Aspects of Human Efficiency*, pp.47–57. W. P. Colquhoun (Ed.). London, English Universities Press.

Carskadon, M. A. and Dement, W. C. (1975). Sleep studies on a 90-minute day. *Electroencephalography and Clinical Neurophysiology* 39, 145–155.

Corcoran, D. W. J. (1962a). *Individual Differences in Performance after Loss of Sleep*. Unpublished doctoral dissertation, University of Cambridge, Cambridge, England.

Corcoran, D. W. J. (1962b). Noise and loss of sleep. *Quarterly Journal of Experimental Psychology* 14, 178–182.

Dement, W. C. (1972). Sleep deprivation and the organization of the behavioral states. In: *Sleep and the Maturing Nervous System*, pp.319–355. C. D. Clemente, D. P. Purpura, and F. E. Mayer (Eds.). New York, Academic Press.

Donnell, J. M. (1969). Performance decrement as a function of total sleep loss and task duration. *Perceptual and Motor Skills* 29, 711–714.

Drucker, E. H., Cannon, L. D., and Ware, J. R. (1969). *The Effects of Sleep Deprivation on Performance over a 48-hour Period* (HumRRO Tech. Rep. 69-8). Alexandria, Va.: Human Resources Research Office, Div. No. 2 (Armor), May 1969.

Elkin, A. J. and Murray, D. J. (1974). The effects of sleep loss on short-term recognition memory. *Canadian Journal of Psychology/Revue Canadienne de Psychologie* 28, 192–198.

Francesconi, R. P., Stokes, J. W., Banderet, L. E., and Kowal, D. M. (1978). Sustained operations and sleep deprivation: Effects on indices of stress. *Aviation, Space, and Environmental Medicine* 49, 1271–1274.

Friedmann, J., Globus, G., Huntley, A., Mullaney, D., Naitoh, P., and Johnson, L. (1977). Performance and mood during and after gradual sleep reduction. *Psychophysiology* 14, 245–250.

Hamilton, P., Wilkinson, R. T., and Edwards, R. S. (1972). A study of four days partial sleep deprivation. In: *Aspects of Human Efficiency*, pp.101–113. W. P. Colquhoun (Ed.). London, English Universities Press.

Hartley, L. R. (1974). A comparison of continuous and distributed reduced sleep schedules. *Quarterly Journal of Experimental Psychology* **26**, 8–14.

Haslam, D. R. (1981). The military performance of soldiers in continuous operations: Exercises 'Early Call' I and II. In: *Biological Rhythms, Sleep and Shift Work*, pp.435–458. L. C. Johnson, D. I. Tepas, W. P. Colquhoun, and M. J. Colligan (Eds.). New York, Spectrum Publications.

Hockey, G. R. J. (1970). Changes in attention allocation in a multi-component task under loss of sleep. *British Journal of Psychology* **61**, 473–480.

Johnson, L. C. (1973). Are stages of sleep related to waking behavior? *American Scientist* **61**, 326–338.

Johnson, L. C. (1975). The effect of total, partial, and stage sleep deprivation on EEG patterns and performance. In: *Behavior and Brain Electrical Activity*, pp.1–30. N. Burch and H. L. Altshuler (Eds.). New York, Plenum.

Johnson, L., Lubin, A., Naitoh, P., Nute, C., and Austin, M. (1969). Spectral analysis of the EEG of dominant and non-dominant alpha subjects during waking and sleeping. *Electroencephalography and Clinical Neurophysiology* **26**, 361–370.

Johnson, L. C. and Naitoh, P. (1974). *The Operational Consequences of Sleep Deprivation and Sleep Deficit*. NATO AGARDograph No. 193, June 1974.

Johnson, L. C., Slye, E. S., and Dement, W. (1965). Electroencephalographic and autonomic activity during and after prolonged sleep deprivation. *Psychosomatic Medicine* **27**, 415–423.

Jones, H. W. and Oswald, I. (1968). Two cases of healthy insomnia. *Electroencephalography and Clinical Neurophysiology* **24**, 378–380.

Kjellberg, A. (1977a). Sleep deprivation and some aspects of performance. I. Problems of arousal changes. *Waking and Sleeping* **1**, 139–143.

Kjellberg, A. (1977b). Sleep deprivation and some aspects of performance. II. Lapses and other attentional effects. *Waking and Sleeping* **1**, 145–148.

Kjellberg, A. (1977c). Sleep deprivation and some aspects of performance. III. Motivation, comment and conclusions. *Waking and Sleeping* **1**, 149–153.

Klein, K. E., Brüner, H., Ruff, S., and Wegmann, H. M. (1969). *Long duration flight — Long working day fatigue in long distance flights*. Paper presented at AGARD-NATO course on Advanced Operational Aviation Medicine, Institute of Aviation Medicine, GAF. Fürstenfeldbruck, 9–27 June 1969.

Klein, K. E., Wegmann, H. M., and Brüner, H. (1968). Circadian rhythm in indices of human performance, physical fitness and stress resistance. *Aerospace Medicine* **39**, 512–518.

Kollar, E. J., Pasnau, R. E., Rubin, R. T., Naitoh, P., Slater, G. G., and Kales, A. (1969). Psychological, physiological, and biochemical correlates of prolonged sleep deprivation. *American Journal of Psychiatry* **126**, 488–497.

Kornetsky, C., Mirsky, A. F., Kessler, E. K., and Dorff, J. E. (1959). The effects of dextro-amphetamine on behavioral deficits produced by sleep loss in humans. *Journal of Pharmacology and Experimental Therapeutics* **127**, 46–50.

Larzelere, R. E. and Mulaik, S. A. (1977). Single-sample tests for many correlations. *Psychological Bulletin* **84**, 557–569.

Laties, V. G. (1961). Modification of affect, social behavior and performance by sleep deprivation and drugs. *Journal of Psychiatric Research* **1**, 12–25.

Lester, J., Knapp, T. M., and Roessler, R. (1976). Sleep deprivation, personality, and performance on a complex vigilance task. *Waking and Sleeping* **1**, 61–65.

Loomis, A. L., Harvey, E. N., and Hobart, G. A., III. (1937). Cerebral states during sleep, as studied by human brain potentials. *Journal of Experimental Psychology* **21**, 127–144.

Lubin, A. (1967). Performance under sleep loss and fatigue. In: *Sleep and Altered States of Consciousness*, pp.506-513. S. S. Kety, E. V. Evarts, and H. L. Williams (Eds.). Baltimore, Williams and Wilkins.

Lubin, A., Hord, D. J., Tracy, M. L., and Johnson, L. C. (1947). Effects of exercise, bedrest and napping on performance decrement during 40 hours. *Psychophysiology* 13, 334-339.

Meddis, R., Pearson, A. J. D., and Langford, G. (1973). An extreme case of healthy insomnia. *Electroencephalography and Clinical Neurophysiology* 35, 213-214.

Morgan, B. B., Jr., Brown, B. R., and Alluisi, E. A. (1970). *Effects of 48 Hours of Continuous Work and Sleep Loss on Sustained Performance* (Interim Tech. Rep. ITR-70-16). University of Louisville, Performance Research Laboratory, September 1970.

Morgan, B. B., Jr., Coates, G. D., Brown, B. R., and Alluisi, E. A. (1973). *Effects of Continuous Work and Sleep Loss on the Recovery of Sustained Performance* (Tech. Memo. 14-73). US Army Human Engineering Laboratory. University of Louisville, Performance Research Laboratory.

Moses, J. M., Hord, D. J., Lubin, A., Johnson, L. C., and Naitoh, P. (1975). Dynamics of nap sleep during a 40 hour period. *Electroencephalography and Clinical Neurophysiology* 39, 627-633.

Moses, J., Lubin, A., Naitoh, P., and Johnson, L. C. (1978). Circadian variation in performance, subjective sleepiness, sleep, and oral temperature during an altered sleep-wake schedule. *Biological Psychology* 6, 301-308.

Naitoh, P. (1976). Sleep deprivation in human subjects: A reappraisal. *Waking and Sleeping* 1, 53-60.

Naitoh, P. (1981). Circadian cycles and restorative power of naps. In: *Biological Rhythms, Sleep and Shift Work*, pp.553-580. L. C. Johnson, D. I. Tepas, W. P. Colquhoun, and M. J. Colligan (Eds.). New York, Spectrum Publications.

Naitoh, P. (in press, b). Chronopsychological approach for optimizing human performance. In: *Rhythmic Activity of Man*. F. Brown and R. C. Graeber (Eds.). Erlbaum.

Naitoh, P. and Townsend, R. E. (1970). The role of sleep deprivation research in human factors. *Human Factors* 12, 575-585.

Patrick, G. T. and Gilbert, J. A. (1896). On the effects of loss of sleep. *Psychological Review* 3, 469-483.

Polzella, D. J. (1975). Effects of sleep deprivation on short-term recognition memory. *Journal of Experimental Psychology* 104, 194-200.

Rechtschaffen, A. and Kales, A. (Eds.) (1968). *A Manual for Standardized Terminology, Techniques and Scoring System for Sleep Stages of Human Subjects*. Washington, DC, US Government Printing Office.

Rutenfranz, J., Aschoff, J., and Mann, H. (1972). The effects of a cumulative sleep deficit, duration of preceding sleep period and body-temperature on multiple choice reaction time. In: *Aspects of Human Efficiency*, pp.217-229. W. P. Colquhoun (Ed.). London, English Universities Press.

Snyder, F. and Scott, J. (1972). The psychophysiology of sleep. In: *Handbook of Psychophysiology*, pp.645-708. S. Greenfield and R. A. Sternbach (Eds.). New York, Holt, Rinehart and Winston.

Stuss, D. and Broughton, R. (1978). Extreme short sleep: Personality profiles and a case study of sleep requirement. *Waking and Sleeping* 2, 101-105.

Taub, J. M. and Berger, R. J. (1973). Performance and mood following variations in the length and timing of sleep. *Psychophysiology* 10, 559-570.

Taub, J. M. and Berger, R. J. (1976). The effects of changing the phase and duration of sleep. *Journal of Experimental Psychology* 2, 30-41.

Tyler, D. B. (1947). The effect of amphetamine sulfate and some barbiturates on the fatigue produced by prolonged wakefulness. *American Journal of Physiology* **150**, 253–262.

Webb, W. B. (1975). *Sleep, the Gentle Tyrant*. Englewood Cliffs, New Jersey, Prentice-Hall.

Webb, W. B. and Agnew, H. W., Jr. (1965). Sleep: Effects of a restricted regime. *Science* **150**, 1745–1747.

Webb, W. B. and Agnew, H. W., Jr. (1974). The effects of a chronic limitation of sleep length. *Psychophysiology* **11**, 265–274.

Wilkinson, R. T. (1959). Rest pauses in a task affected by lack of sleep. *Ergonomics* **2**, 373–380.

Wilkinson, R. T. (1961). Interaction of lack of sleep with knowledge of results, repeated testing, and individual differences. *Journal of Experimental Psychology* **62**, 263–271.

Wilkinson, R. T. (1963). Interaction of noise with knowledge of results and sleep deprivation. *Journal of Experimental Psychology* **66**, 332–337.

Wilkinson, R. T. (1964). Effects of up to 60 hours' sleep deprivation on different types of work. *Ergonomics* **7**, 175–186.

Wilkinson, R. T. (1965). Sleep deprivation. In: *The Physiology of Human Survival*, pp.399–430. O. G. Edholm and A. Bacharach (Eds.). New York, Academic Press.

Wilkinson, R. T. (1969). Sleep deprivation: Performance tests for partial and selective sleep deprivation. In: *Progress in Clinical Psychology*, Vol. 8, pp.28–43. L. E. Abt and B. F. Riess (Eds.). New York, Grune and Stratton.

Wilkinson, R. T. and Colquhoun, W. P. (1968). Interaction of alcohol with incentive and with sleep deprivation. *Journal of Experimental Psychology* **76**, 623–629.

Wilkinson, R. T., Edwards, R. S., and Haines, E. (1966). Performance following a night of reduced sleep. *Psychonomic Science* **5**, 471–472.

Williams, H. L., Gieseking, C. F., and Lubin, A. (1966). Some effects of sleep loss on memory. *Perceptual and Motor Skills* **23**, 1287–1293.

Williams, H. L., Kearney, O. F., and Lubin, A. (1965). Signal uncertainty and sleep loss. *Journal of Experimental Psychology* **69**, 401–407.

Williams, H. L. and Lubin, A. (1967). Speeded addition and sleep loss. *Journal of Experimental Psychology* **73**, 313–317.

Williams, H. L., Lubin, A., and Goodnow, J. J. (1959). Impaired performance with acute sleep loss. *Psychological Monographs* **73** (14, Whole No. 484).

Williams, H. L. and Williams, C. L. (1966). Nocturnal EEG profiles and performance. *Psychophysiology* **3**, 164–175.

Biological Rhythms, Sleep, and Performance
Edited by Wilse B. Webb
© 1982 John Wiley & Sons Ltd.

Chapter 6

Sleep Structure Variation and Performance

Chester A. Pearlman

From the vantage point of current sleep research, it may be hard to understand the persistent concern of several investigators with the relationship of variations in sleep structure to performance. Two decades of work have produced tantalizing but hardly overpowering results, and fundamental methodological questions remain, such as to what degree it is possible to alter one aspect of sleep structure independently of the whole. Much of this work has been reviewed from somewhat different perspectives by McGrath and Cohen (1978), Ellman *et al.* (1978), and Hoyt and Singer (1978). Many issues, such as methodological concerns, which are treated briefly here, were discussed in greater detail in these reviews. The present chapter also considers studies from 1976 to 1979, which were not covered by these reviews.

In order to appreciate the issues better, it may be helpful to reconstruct the intellectual climate in which these investigations began. The discoveries by Aserinsky, Kleitman, and Dement of the active or REM stage of sleep and the close association between REM sleep and dreaming coincided with the wish of the psychoanalyst, Fisher, to investigate the Freudian theory of dreams outside the analytical treatment situation. Reasoning by analogy with neurotic symptoms which regularly revealed ingenious compromises between repressed infantile wishes and mentation which was acceptable to the conscious mind, Freud (1953) had suggested that dreams involved a similar compromise between repressed infantile wishes and the requirements of the sleeping state. He also quoted with approval the earlier safety-valve notion of Roberts that without the opportunity to go safely mad during dreams, we might go mad during waking. Accordingly, Dement and Fisher wondered if some psychological impairment might result from deprivation of dreaming or REM sleep due to the build up of instinctual drive tension. Although there was no clear indication of how this hypothetical drive tension might affect behaviour, anecdotal reports of hallucinations and other psychotic phenomena following total sleep deprivation (West *et al.*, 1962) seemed consistent with such a possibility. Thus, a natural experimental question was whether effects of total sleep deprivation (see Chapter 5) could be related to selective disruption of various stages of sleep.

EMPIRICAL SEARCH FOR BEHAVIOUR CHANGES

The initial experiments (Dement, 1960, 1964, 1965; Dement and Fisher, 1963) were promising. First, the investigators deprived several subjects of REM sleep by awakening them whenever they showed the characteristic polygraphic patterns of REM sleep. By the end of the first night, many more awakenings were required than would be expected from the normal three to five REM periods per night. Thus, interruption of REM sleep seemed to produce an increased pressure to enter stage REM. This process became even more accentuated on subsequent nights so that after three nights, it became impossible to deprive subjects of REM sleep without preventing sleep altogether. As might be predicted from this evidence of increasing pressure for REM sleep, when the subjects were allowed to sleep undisturbed, most showed a great increase in REM sleep (termed REM rebound) which appeared almost to replenish the amount of REM sleep lost during the deprivation period. Control experiments involving a similar number of awakenings from other stages of sleep did not affect the sleep cycle. Thus, a need for REM sleep appeared to be confirmed. The psychological effects of REM deprivation, however, were less clear. All subjects showed some deleterious effects not noted following control awakenings, such as anxiety, irritability, inability to concentrate, fatigue, and increased appetite with weight gain. Similar effects had been reported following total sleep deprivation, but they are rather non-specific symptoms. The difficulty of defining psychological effects of REM deprivation is understandable because it is not clear what the subject is being deprived of psychologically. What could be so important about the experience of dreaming that one would suffer without it?

Subsequent attempts to clarify the psychological effects of REM deprivation utilized briefer periods of REM deprivation in conjunction with more precise measurement techniques. Most of these studies also evaluated the subjects with the same procedures after a similar number of awakenings from non-REM sleep. These control observations have not yielded significant findings except where specifically noted. The various studies are summarized in Table 1. They will be discussed with reference to the table number.

Study 3 found no specific effects with objective tests. Study 5 noted the non-specific symptoms, but these observations were not confirmed by test findings. Study 6 found no effect of REM deprivation on performance measures, but personality tests indicated that the subjects were less well integrated and less interpersonally effective following REM deprivation.

Clemes and Dement (1967) (study 7) were impressed by observations in animals suggesting that REM deprivation produced increased drive behaviour, such as restlessness, hypersexuality and ravenous appetite (Dement *et al.*, 1967). With tests designed to assess the drive dimension, they found that REM deprived subjects had higher intensity of need and feelings in their TAT story responses and less form appropriateness in their Holtzman protocols. They did not confirm a previous finding (study 4) of increased human movement responses following REM suppression. A more definitive examination of the question of Holtzman human movement responses, however, reported an increase (study 15).

Contrasting findings came from study 10. Despite the fact that each subject's Rorschach and Holtzman protocols following REM deprivation differed from those following base line or control awakenings, the changes were different for each subject so that there was no consistent evidence of altered human movement responses or any other conventional response category. The changes following REM deprivation reflected each subject's base line personality patterns.

This evidence of individual differences in response to REM deprivation was confirmed and expanded in more extensive studies. Cartwright, Monroe, and Palmer (1967) identified three patterns of response to REM deprivation, called disruption, substitution, and compensation. Subjects showing disruption required the most awakenings during the REM deprivation period but showed no REM rebound during recovery nights. Substituters also showed no significant REM rebound, but they regularly reported dreamlike content upon awakening at the onset of REM sleep during the deprivation period. The authors suggested that these subjects might be able to substitute dreamlike experience in other sleep stages for that lost during REM deprivation. The compensators showed the conventional REM rebound during recovery nights.

Study 13 confirmed that subjects showing considerable dreamlike fantasy upon awakening from REM sleep (HOF) showed no REM rebound following REM deprivation and no significant psychological effects. Those low in REM-onset fantasy (LOF) showed the conventional REM rebound and some psychological test changes.

These apparent individual differences need further investigation because of the small number of subjects involved. In a much larger group, Arkin *et al.* (1978) found a significant REM rebound and no evidence of increased dreamlike mentation during stage 2 following REM deprivation, consistent with the LOF reaction pattern. They did not measure REM-onset fantasy, but they did not find another characteristic of the LOF pattern, shorter REM latency (time between sleep onset and the first REM period) on the recovery night following REM deprivation, which presumably results from the increased pressure to engage in REM fantasy. Furthermore, while REM sleep on the recovery night following REM deprivation was increased over base line

Table 1   Studies of REM sleep deprivation

Reference	N	Duration (days)	Measures	Outcome[1]
1. Dement (1960)	8	3–7	Qualitative (see text)	Non-specific disturbances (see text)
2. Dement and Fisher (1963)	21	2–5	Same as above	Same as above
3. Kales *et al.* (1964)	2	6–10	MMPI, Nowlis mood, Clyde mood, Stroop, digit span	0
4. Lerner (1966)	20	2	Holtzman	+ , M responses
5. Sampson (1966)	6	3	MMPI, serial subtraction, digit span	0
6. Agnew, Webb, and Williams (1967)	6	7	(a) Pursuit rotor, reaction time, addition	0
			(b) MMPI, Taylor, Cattell 16PF	+ , irritability and affect lability
7. Clemes and Dement (1967)	6	6	Battery (see text)	0, Nowlis mood −, Holzman form level + , TAT need, feeling
8. Feldman (1969)			Trigrams, number series, pre- and post-deprivation	0
Experiment 1	18	1		
Experiment 2	20	1	Paired associated, post-deprivation; prose passage, post-deprivation	±
9. Empson and Clarke (1970)	10	1	Word list retention; sentence and story retention	0 −
10. Greenberg *et al.* (1970)	4	3	(a) Rorschach, Holtzman	Individually determined; see text
			(b) Digit symbol, paired-associate learning	0
11. Ekstrand *et al.* (1971)	20	1	First list recall, retroactive interference paradigm	0
12. Herman *et al.* (1980)	8	1	Depth perception accuracy	0
13. Cartwright and Ratzel (1972)	10	3	Rorschach, WAIS, (a) LOF, (see text)	+ , Rorschach M, WAIS picture arrangement
			(b) HOF, (see text)	0
14. Chernik (1972)	16	2	Paired associates, pre- and post-deprivation; McNair, Clyde mood scales	0
15. Feldstein (1972)	19	3	Holtzman	+ , M responses

Table 1 (Continued)

Reference	N	Duration (days)	Measures	Outcome[1]
16. Greenberg, Horowitz, and Pearlman (1972)	5	3	Porteus maze while wearing visually inverting prisms	Qualitative (see text)
17. Greenberg, Pillard, and Pearman (1972)	9	1	Habituation to frightening film	–
18. Grieser, Greenberg, and Harrison (1972)	10	1	Recall of anagram solutions	–
19. Koppell et al. (1972)	9	2	Visual evoked potential	+, attend–non-attended difference
20. Muzio et al. (1972)	18	1	Paired-associate retention	–, same as non-REM awakenings
21. Naitoh, Johnson, and Lubin (1973)	14	3	Contingent negative variation	–, same as non-REM deprivation
22. Castaldo, Krynicki, and Goldstein (1974)	8	1	Trigram and paired-associate retention	0
23. Johnson et al. (1974)	7	3	Battery (see text)	0
24. Zarcone, de la Peña, and Dement (1974)	10	2	Inspection time of sexual areas of pictures	+
25. Zarcone et al. (1974)	9	2	Rorschach, primary process: (a) non-psychotics (b) schizophrenics	0 +
26. Allen (1975)	15	1	Sentence retention (a) without tetracycline (b) with tetracycline	0 –
27. Cartwright et al. (1975)	10	1	Recall of self-descriptive adjectives	Qualitative (see text)
28. Lewin and Glaubman (1975)	12	1	Guilford utility test nonsense syllables word list, Guilford word-fluency test	– + 0
29. Moldofsky and Scarisbrick (1976)	7	3	Muscle tenderness	0

Table 1 (Continued)

Reference	N	Duration (days)	Measures	Outcome
30. Puca *et al.* (1976)	10	2	Rosenzweig frustration; Zung depression	+, Extra aggression −
31. Cohen (1977)	25	1	WAIS block design (a) low neuroticism (b) high neuroticism	Impairment 0
32. Lhotsky (1977)	10	1	Erectile response and inspection time with erotic stimuli	0
33. Glaubman *et al.* (1978)	10	1	Guilford consequences test	−
34. Lancey (1978)	16	1	Tourniquet pain tolerance (a) normal MMPI (b) abnormal MMPI	− +
35. Tilley and Empson (1978)	10	1	2 stories, retention	−

+ = Increase; 0 = No Change; − = Decrease

recordings, it did not differ from that observed following non-REM control awakenings, which did not cause any REM suppression. Thus, the nature of the reaction patterns in this group of subjects was somewhat unclear.

Nakazawa *et al.* (1975) and Cohen (1977) investigated the question of individual differences by use of the Maudsley Personality Inventory distinction between high and low neuroticism. They found greater REM pressure (awakenings necessary to produce REM deprivation) and REM rebound in low neuroticism subjects than in high neuroticism subjects, which suggested a connection between low neuroticism and the LOF group of study 13. Cohen, however, found impaired performance on the more difficult WAIS block design items in low neuroticism subjects in contrast to the normal findings of study 13 with LOF subjects. Another study (23) which showed marginal REM rebound following deprivation found no effect on several performance tests or on affect measures.

Study 25 reported no alteration following REM deprivation in Rorschach protocols scored for manifestations of primary process by the schema of Holt and Havel (1960). This procedure assesses such factors as sexual and aggressive drive content, thought deviation, blatency of expression of drive content, reality testing, and the degree to which primary process manifestations are handled adaptively or maladaptively. Alterations in such scores would be expected with any significant change in drive level. Study 30, however, did find increased externally directed aggression on the Rosenzweig picture frustration test. Nevertheless, it became apparent that the notion that

REM sleep provided an opportunity to go safely mad, which was essential to mental health, was untenable. In retrospect, the idea seems like a plausible hypothesis for research, but it deals with only one aspect of psychoanalytical thinking about dreams. The issue is discussed at greater length in Pearlman (in press).

In summary, the initial phase of REM deprivation research revealed a process with a peremptory aspect for many subjects (REM rebound) and some inconclusive personality test changes as well as some evidence of altered drive behaviour in animals. REM deprivation produced no obvious harm, but it did seem to do something. The vacuum left by the demise of the safety valve theory gave rise to several alternative hypotheses to explain the effects of REM deprivation and much additional research to be presented below. Attempts to interpret these findings also had to consider other results of contemporary sleep research. Animal studies had revealed consistent evidence of a REM rebound following deprivation (Jouvet, 1975). Investigation of the phylogenesis of REM sleep showed clear evidence of REM sleep in all mammals studied except the monotreme, *Echidna*. Lesser amounts of REM sleep were found in all birds studied, and suggestive evidence of REM sleep was found in a few reptiles (Rojas-Ramirez and Drucker-Colin, 1977). Slow wave sleep also appeared first in reptiles, but the high voltage slow waves characteristic of stage 4 appeared first in birds. Ontogenetic studies had shown a much higher percentage of REM sleep just before birth and during infancy than in later stages of life in all species studied (Jouvet, 1975).

THEORIES OF REM SLEEP FUNCTION

Some early attempts to account for these data, such as the sentinel hypothesis (that REM sleep originally served to protect sleeping animals from predators by providing periodic arousal in preparation for potential danger), the cortical homoeostasis hypothesis (that REM sleep balances slow wave sleep to keep cortical vigilance within adaptive limits), and the neural growth-promoting hypothesis (that REM sleep provides endogenous stimulation necessary for development of the nervous system in infancy) have proved to be untestable. Since they generated no data, they faded away as contradictory observations were reported (Hennevin and Leconte, 1971; Jouvet, 1975; Pearlman, 1979). Two more recent ideas, the catecholamine-restoration hypothesis (Hartmann, 1973; Stern and Morgane, 1974) and the protein-synthesis hypothesis (Oswald, 1969) have not led to experiments involving human performance. The data supporting these ideas and more extensive data which contradict them are reviewed in Ramm (1979) and Pearlman (1979). Three other ideas about REM sleep, the oculomotor control hypothesis, the drive-facilitation hypothesis and the information-processing hypothesis have yielded supportive findings to be discussed below.

Oculomotor Control

The oculomotor control hypothesis (Berger, 1969) was devised primarily to account for phylogenetic and ontogenetic aspects of REM sleep. Berger suggested that REM sleep provided periodic activation of the neuromuscular pathways involved in binocular depth perception which was necessary in infancy for establishment of these pathways and in adulthood for maintenance, i.e. prevention of loss of function during the quiescence of non-REM sleep. An attractive feature of this hypothesis was the attempt to give some function to the rapid eye movements which spawned the field of modern sleep research. As the likelihood of significant psychophysiological parallelism has waned (i.e. that the eye movements might reflect visual pursuit movements of the dreamer watching the action of the dream) (see Pivik, 1978), the purpose of the intense oculomotor activity during REM sleep is even more obscure. On the other hand, the hypothesis has several severe limitations. The original phylogenetic support, a fair correlation between amount of REM sleep in various species and the degree of partial decussation of the optic tracts, which is a prerequisite for binocular vision, has been diminished by the subsequent findings of significant amounts of REM sleep in moles, which lack oculomotor function (Allison and Van Twyer, 1970), owls, which have immobile eyes, and shrews, which have no conjugate eye movements (Berger, 1972). Similarly, the idea of a need for periodic activation during development is tenuous in view of the severe sensory restriction necessary to produce functional disturbance (Riesen, 1966; Hubel, 1967). Since the arousal accompanying REM deprivation should be an adequate substitute for REM sleep in counteracting deleterious effects of non-REM sleep, the hypothesis also fails to account for the REM rebound following deprivation. Finally, the hypothesis contributes nothing to understanding of the evidence of retention impairment in animals due to post-training REM deprivation (McGrath and Cohen, 1978; Pearlman, 1979).

Despite these theoretical problems, however, studies in humans have found that binocular coordination and accuracy of binocular depth perception are better at the end of REM periods than at the onset, and depth perception is better in the morning than on the preceding evening (Berger and Scott, 1971; Berger and Walker; 1972). Lewis, Sloan, and Jones (1978) confirmed the difference in accuracy of binocular depth perception between beginning and end of REM periods during the second half of the night. They also suggested that the results reported by Berger and Scott were due to the same effect. They did not, however, find improved accuracy from night to morning and concluded that the principal factor was a large decrease in accuracy during non-REM sleep preceding the onset of the REM period. This conclusion is consistent with the transient heterophoria produced by monocular occlusion for 24 hours (Wallach and Karsh, 1963). The recovery to normal function following 20 minutes of binocular experience resembles the mean duration of a REM period. Thus, these findings suggested that binocular coordination and depth perception deteriorate somewhat during non-REM sleep in the latter part of the night and that this impairment is corrected during REM sleep. In contrast, Herman *et al.* (1980) found no difference in accuracy of depth perception between the beginning and the end of REM periods, as well as no effect of REM deprivation. Further understanding of these contradictory findings will depend upon clarification of the role of eye movement in REM sleep.

Drive Facilitation

The drive-facilitation hypothesis is an updated version of the Freudian concept of drive discharge during dreams. It suggests that REM deprivation creates a state of heightened drive tension (Vogel, 1979). This hypothesis is consistent with the previously described anecdotal effects of REM deprivation and the projective test findings. It also fits with the animal observations of hyper-sexuality, increased aggression and hunger, as well as with more recent studies utilizing intracranial self-stimulation which suggested activation of reward mechanisms during REM sleep (Ellman *et al.*, 1978). According to this formulation, REM deprivation lowers the CNS threshold for stimulus bound behaviours with resultant facilitation of sexual, aggressive, or eating behaviours depending upon the context. A limitation of the hypothesis is vagueness of the concept of drive tension. For example, Vogel (1979) directly associated neuronal activity during REM sleep with reduced drive tension during waking with no mediating mechanisms except disinhibition or discharge during REM sleep. Another limitation is failure to account for effects of post-training REM deprivation on animal learning where no change in drive behaviour was observed (Pearlman, 1979). It is also unclear why activation of reward mechanisms during REM sleep should occur, since Freud's idea that preservation of sleep required partial drive discharge during dreaming is no longer tenable (Hobson and McCarley, 1977). Even if such activation were a normal occurrence, it is equally unclear why REM deprivation should intensify the process. Finally, one might expect evidence of increased drive pressure in Rorschach protocols scored for primary process (Holt and Havel, 1960), but as previously mentioned, none was found by Zarcone *et al.* (1974).

Zarcone, de la Pena and Dement (1974) speculated that genetic survival might be favoured by heightened sexual interest during periods of sleep disruption due to stress, presumably by making love not war. They found increased duration of visual fixation on sexual areas of pictures following two nights of REM deprivation. Lhotsky (1977), however, found no increase in erectile response or inspection time with erotic stimuli after one night of REM deprivation.

Another approach to characterizing the inner tension state produced by REM deprivation arose from animal studies showing evidence of increased CNS excitability, such as shortened recovery time for evoked potentials (Dewson *et al.*, 1967) and lowered convulsive threshold (Cohen, Thomas, and Dement, 1970). Kopell *et al.* (1972) studied the effect of REM deprivation on selective attention, as measured by the difference between evoked potentials to flashes recorded while the subject was attending to a stimulus figure and while he was ignoring the stimulus by attending to background changes in his visual field. The amplitude of the principal component of the evoked potential (N_2–P_2), occurring from 190 to 250 msec after the stimulus, was lower during attention to the background after REM deprivation than after non-REM awakenings whereas the amplitude while attending to the figure was similar for both sleep conditions. The authors suggested that this greater difference between the attention and non-attention conditions following REM deprivation was indicative of a narrowing of the attentive field. Narrowing of attention or reduction in the range of cue utilization has been observed in a variety of situations involving increased emotion, arousal, or drive (Easterbrook, 1959). Thus, they concluded that REM deprivation may produce heightened CNS arousal or excitability in humans similar to that in animals. While the difference between REM deprived and control conditions in this experiment seems clear enough, other studies have reported contradictory findings concerning the relationship of amplitude of the N_2–P_2 component of the evoked response to selective attention (see Tueting and Sutton, 1973). The amplitude enhancement with selective attention is more apparent in the late positive component of the evoked response (P_{300}), occurring about 300–400 msec after the stimulus. This component is particularly prominent following meaningful stimuli, i.e. those that require some response in the experimental situation (Karlin and Martz, 1973). Kopell *et al.* (1972) did not report data on the P_{300} component although a similar difference in P_{300} amplitude between attention to figure and background had been found with the same evoked potential procedure by Donchin and Cohen (1967). Those authors noted a much greater difference in the P_{300} component than in the N_2–P_2 component. With this procedure, the P_{300} component has also been found to be linked to another EEG measure of selective attention, the contingent negative variation (CNV) (Donchin and Smith, 1970). The CNV, however, did not show differential change between REM deprivation and stage 4 deprivation (Naitoh, Johnson, and Lubin, 1973). In each condition, the amplitude of the CNV was reduced but to a lesser degree than following total sleep deprivation.

Thus, there is some question about the degree to which the findings of Kopell *et al.* (1972) are related to selective attention. There is also no direct evidence linking a decrease in evoked response to a non-attended stimulus to the narrowing of range of cue utilization described by Easterbrook (1959). Moreover, the emotional state in the situations reviewed by Easterbrook might obliterate differences in amplitude of the N_2-P_2 evoked potential due to the degree of attention to the stimulus. For example, Crighel *et al.* (1976) reported decreased amplitude and wider dispersion pattern of the N_2-P_2 component in anxiety states. Similarly, a standard example of narrowed range of cue utilization, decreased digit memory span in anxiety states, has not been observed with REM deprivation (Kales *et al.*, 1964; Sampson, 1966; Feldman, 1969). Further exploration of the possible relationship between REM deprivation and cue utilization might profitably use other experimental situations, such as size estimation or the receptor–effector span (the amount of perceptual material in a serial array between the point reached by perception and that reached by action, as in copy typing). For details, see Easterbrook (1959). In any event, these considerations suggest that the inner tension state associated with REM deprivation is more complicated than implied by the notion of increased drive. This idea is further discussed below in the section on psychopathology.

Studies of pain perception following REM deprivation have found contradictory evidence concerning an inner tension state. Lancey (1978) noted increased sensitivity to ischaemic pain produced by a tourniquet and decreased duration of tolerance of the pain in normal subjects. An analogous reduction in pain threshold after REM deprivation has been reported in rats (Hicks *et al.*, 1978). Subjects with an abnormal MMPI profile, however, showed greater pain tolerance following REM deprivation. Moldofsky and Scarisbrick (1976) found no consistent change in muscle tenderness with REM deprivation in normal subjects. The direct relation between anxiety and increased pain sensitivity in humans is familiar (see Hill *et al.*, 1952), but studies in rats have suggested decreased fear following REM deprivation (Ogilvie and Broughton, 1976; Hicks and Moore, 1979) despite the increased pain sensitivity.

Given this wide individual variability in spontaneous psychological responses to REM deprivation, a major research strategy has been to focus the experimental situation by measuring performance on specific tasks before and after REM deprivation. Moreover, although the previously discussed suggestion of a relation between hypothetical drive facilitating properties of REM deprivation and reduced range of cue utilization may not be strictly accurate, the intent may be consistent with Easterbrook's (1959) comment that range of cue utilization is equivalent to total information transfer. Accordingly, one might wonder if information transfer were reduced by REM deprivation.

Information Processing

A relationship between sleep and learning has been familiar since Ebbinghaus's observation that sleep retarded forgetting, but subsequent workers always assumed that sleep protected memory traces from interference by waking stimuli, consistent with their view of sleep as a state of cerebral quiescence. The discovery of REM sleep soon suggested the hypothesis of an active role of this stage in information processing. It was based on the coincidence of intense cerebral activity with inhibition of sensory input and motor outflow, which suggested that REM sleep might provide both a memory consolidation mechanism and an efficient time for information processing involving unusual adaptive change, since such reprogramming during waking would probably interfere with ongoing behaviour. For original presentations, see Breger (1967), Dewan (1970), Greenberg (1970), and Pearlman (1970). The clearest support for the information-processing hypothesis has come from animal studies showing increased post-training REM sleep and impaired retention of complex tasks with brief post-training REM deprivation. There is also some evidence that prior REM deprivation impairs learning of aversive tasks (Hennevin and Leconte, 1977; McGrath and Cohen, 1978; Pearlman, 1979). This hypothesis interprets the inner tension state with REM deprivation as a form of impaired adaption. Gross changes in drive behaviour are viewed as release phenomena rather than facilitation. Such effects might result from disruption of inhibitory mechanisms necessary for maintenance of normal behaviour in the stressful experimental situation. In general, the studies showing impaired retention used much briefer periods and less stressful methods of REM deprivation than those showing altered drive behaviour (see Vogel, 1979).

Studies involving information processing in humans have been equivocal although the data to be presented below generally favour the hypothesis as originally formulated. The major problem has been translation of complexity in animal learning to human performance terms. The initial studies by Feldman (1969), Greenberg *et al.* (1970), Muzio *et al.* (1972), Chernik (1972), Castaldo, Krynicki, and Goldstein (1974), and Johnson *et al.* (1974) involved a variety of verbal tasks, such as consonant trigrams, nonsense syllables, number series, and paired associates, tested both before and following REM deprivation. The results consistently showed no effect of REM deprivation on acquisition or retention. Similarly, Ekstrand *et al.* (1971) found no effect of REM deprivation on first list recall in a retroactive interference paradigm learned before sleep disruption.

With total sleep deprivation, retention impairment of somewhat more meaningful material (information items from an almanac, recognition of pictures) had been found. In addition, these tasks involved single exposures rather than learning to criterion (Williams, Lubin, and Goodnow, 1959;

Williams, Gieseking, and Lubin, 1966). Vojtěchovský *et al.* (1971) reported impaired retention of a list of foreign words after one night of total sleep deprivation and impaired story reproduction and paired-associate retention after a second deprivation night. Newman (1939) had also observed that when retention of a story was measured after 8 hours of sleeping or waking, the superior performance of subjects who had slept was most apparent for non-essential information whereas both groups showed equal retention of essential elements of the story. While these results are not inconsistent with the concept of reduced interference during sleep, it seems more likely that sleep, or REM sleep, facilitated retention of a wider range of the material.

Accordingly, the negative results with relatively meaningless stimuli are more understandable, and the finding by Empson and Clarke (1970) of impaired retention of meaningful material (sentences and a prose passage) after one night of REM deprivation seems more significant than an otherwise isolated finding might be. As in the total sleep deprivation studies, the material was presented as a single exposure. Retention of a word list was not impaired in REM deprived subjects, similar to previously discussed studies. Since the REM deprived group had less total sleep than the control group, a possibility remained that the results were due to interference, but this factor was excluded in a replication by Tilley and Empson (1978) which compared the effect of a night of REM or stage 4 deprivation upon retention of two short stories heard once. Stage 4 deprivation resulted in more accurate semantic reproduction (fewer omissions, distortions, and additions; see Horowitz and Berkowitz, 1967) than REM deprivation. On the other hand, with a method similar to that of Empson and Clarke (1970), Levy and Coolidge (1975) found no difference in recall after two hours of primarily REM or primarily Stage 4 sleep, which suggested that the effect of REM deprivation on consolidation is more complex than the conventional retrograde amnesia paradigm.

In a study using two long sentences learned to criterion, Allen (1975) found no effect of REM deprivation upon retention the following day. This finding does not really contradict the results of Empson and Clarke (1970) because of the greater degree of initial learning. Allen, however, did find retention impairment with REM deprivation plus a tetracycline antibiotic although the drug alone had no effect. She suggested that the drug caused protein synthesis inhibition which potentiated the effect of REM deprivation on memory storage. This is unlikely because REM sleep is suppressed by protein synthesis inhibition (Fishbein and Gutwein, 1977), and Allen noted no effect of the drug on REM sleep. Thus, the basis of this combined REM deprivation–drug effect is obscure.

Scrima (1980) provided further evidence of consolidation of memory for meaningful verbal materials during REM sleep in an ingenious study which took advantage of the sleep-onset stage REM frequently found in persons with narcolepsy. After administration of a series of anagrams, subjects took a

20 minute nap. He found better recall after naps consisting of REM sleep than after those consisting of non-REM sleep although recall after non-REM sleep was better than recall after 20 minutes awake. No difference was found with consonant trigrams, similar to the results of REM deprivation studies. Thus, the time course of the possible role of REM sleep is complex. Scrima found an effect of REM sleep at 20 minutes which was not noted by Levy and Coolidge (1975) at 2 hours, but the effect was clear again at 7 hours (Empson and Clarke, 1970; Tilley and Empson, 1978).

In summary, these studies suggest that while most simple verbal tasks are unaffected by REM deprivation, retention impairment may be observed if the task is sufficiently complex or challenging. This distinction is analogous to that of Seligman (1970) between prepared and unprepared learning in animals. Prepared learning is quickly acquired and involves little alteration in the animal's behavioural repertoire (position habits, one-way avoidance, taste aversions). It has a prewired quality. Unprepared learning is slowly acquired and requires unusual adaptive changes in behaviour (difficult discriminations, serial reversals, schedule shifts), analogous to the previously discussed hypothetical reprogramming during REM sleep. Results of REM deprivation studies in animals have generally found no effect upon retention of prepared learning and impaired retention with unprepared types although some discordant findings in mice have been reported (Pearlman, 1979). The remaining studies of REM deprivation in humans have all been derived from this concept.

Greenberg, Pillard, and Pearlman (1972) studied the effect of REM deprivation upon habituation to repeated viewing of a frightening film. Subjects who were REM deprived between the two viewings showed more anxiety on the Profile of Mood States (POMS) after the second viewing than controls. An anxiety-provoking experience is, by definition, something for which the subject is unprepared. As previously discussed, other REM deprivation studies did not show increased anxiety on similar scales, therefore it seems likely that the results reflected defective handling of the anxiety aroused by the film in REM deprived subjects.

In another study of the effect of REM deprivation on reaction to threat, Grieser, Greenberg, and Harrison (1972) used subjects for whom uncompleted items (anagram solutions) on the interrupted task paradigm were threatening while completed items were emotionally neutral. Subjects were selected by Alper's (1957) technique for assessing high ego strength. Such subjects tend to forget uncompleted items. Threat was induced by presenting the anagram procedure as an intelligence test in which the average person should be able to complete more solutions than the subjects were able to do in the time allowed. REM deprivation after the interrupted task procedure impaired recall of the uncompleted items but did not affect recall of completed items. These findings suggested that during REM sleep, the threat associated with uncompleted items was reduced so that recall was similar to that of neutral items. On the other hand, the degree of uncompleted items recalled by REM deprived subjects may have been spuriously low since they had significantly more uncompleted items on original testing than the control-awakening group. Thus, these findings require replication before full acceptance.

In a related study, Cartwright *et al.* (1975) examined immediate and delayed recall of self-descriptive adjectives from the Block Adjective Q-sort test. While all groups showed similar delayed recall, the control-awakening group showed significantly greater improvement over immediate recall than the REM deprived group, a kind of reminiscence. Furthermore, the additional words which the control group recovered on delayed testing were all items implying personal discomfort, which might indicate reduced degree of threat following sleep. The only new words recovered by the REM deprived group were self-affirming items. These results resembled another study by Cartwright (1974) in which solutions to cognitive problems did not differ after periods of REM sleep or waking, but story completions of a TAT picture showed more ability to tolerate and cope with negative possibilities after REM sleep.

The preceding studies interpreted the hypothetical facilitation of unprepared learning by REM sleep as a form of adaptation to threatening aspects of the situations. It is also possible to view the process as a form of creativity. Anecdotal examples of creative dreams are numerous, such as Kekulé's famous dream about the structure of the benzene ring. Lewin and Glaubman (1975) found that REM deprivation impaired performance on the Guilford Utility Test (how many uses can you think of for bricks?), which has been used as a measure of creativity. In contrast to previous reports, they also found significantly better retention of nonsense syllables in REM deprived subjects. The authors concluded that REM deprivation impaired 'divergent' thinking (creativity) but facilitated 'convergent' thinking (rote learning). The facilitation of rote learning was suggested as a possible basis for previous observations of better retention of paired associates after periods consisting principally of non-REM sleep (first half of the night) than after periods consisting mainly of REM sleep (latter half of the night) (Barrett and Ekstrand, 1972; Fowler, Sullivan, and Ekstrand, 1973). Ekstrand *et al.* (1977) reported, however, that these differences disappeared with control for the period of sleep before training of subjects tested after the latter half of the night. In contrast, the impairment of divergent thinking following REM deprivation was confirmed in a study by Glaubman *et al.* (1978) using the Guilford Consequences Test (what would happen, (a) if gravity disappeared?; (b) if all people went blind?). The control-awakening subjects showed more numerous responses, more effective coping responses, and more original ideas than REM deprived subjects.

REM deprivation may also impair some unusual forms of motor learning. A pilot study involving adjustment to wearing visually inverting prisms found some alteration in Porteus maze performance of REM deprived subjects. They showed much more correction of their responses, which resulted in jerky lines, in contrast to control subjects who drew smoother lines (Greenberg, Horowitz, and Pearlman, 1972). This finding suggested deficient visual–motor adaptation to the prisms in REM deprived subjects.

Effects of Performance and Learning on REM Sleep

A corollary of the effect of REM deprivation on information processing is the effect of information processing upon REM sleep. Several animal studies have shown increased REM sleep following training (Pearlman, 1979). Since REM deprivation during the period of increased REM sleep has consistently resulted in impaired retention, these findings were further support for the information-processing hypothesis. Studies in humans, however, have been more equivocal, as with the deprivation effects.

Rechtschaffen and Verdone (1964) reported a small but significant difference in amount of REM sleep between nights when subjects were rewarded for high REM sleep and nights when they were rewarded for little REM sleep. The mechanism remains obscure.

With a stressful film, Baekeland, Koulack, and Lasky (1968) found indications of disturbed REM sleep, such as frequent spontaneous awakenings during and immediately after REM periods. They did not, however, observe increased REM sleep, which is of interest in view of the previously discussed finding of impaired habituation with REM deprivation (Greenberg, Pillard, and Pearlman, 1972). It is possible that this film was too threatening for immediate commencement of normal adaptation processes during REM sleep, as in reactions to traumatic events where sleep is similarly disturbed and interrupted by nightmares involving the traumatic situation.

The first clear evidence relating increased REM sleep to information processing was the report of Zimmerman, Stoyva, and Metcalf (1970) of increased REM sleep during adaptation to wearing visually inverting prisms. Allen *et al.* (1972), however, did not replicate the finding. Recent, more extensive work by Zimmerman, Stoyva, and Reite (1978) has confirmed the absence of any consistent REM augmenting effect of spatially altered vision. These findings were also of interest in view of the previously discussed study of REM deprivation in this situation (Greenberg, Horowitz, and Pearlman, 1972). It is possible that the subject's degree of success at adjusting to the inverted vision may influence his amount of REM sleep. One might expect elevation of REM sleep only in subjects who were successful at mastering the situation, analogous to studies in rats where increased REM sleep occurred in animals which were mastering the task but not in those which failed to learn under the same conditions (see Pearlman, 1979). The work of Zimmerman, Stoyva, and Reite (1978) did not involve sufficient exposure to the distorted vision for thorough adaptation to occur. Accordingly, the effect of inverting prisms on REM sleep needs further study with more careful assessment of the degree of adaptation.

A study of conditioning in infants by Paul and Dittrichova (1975) addressed this issue directly. They found increased REM sleep following sessions in which the babies had been successfully conditioned but no change following training at a task which they failed to acquire.

In a related study, Lewin and Gombosh (1973) found increased REM sleep on a night where the subjects spent the evening engaged in unusual and perplexing activities, compared to a control evening of customary activities. The unusual activities involved running around outside for 5 minutes with instructions to remember everything noticed, followed by administration of parts of the MMPI, Zondi, and Rorschach tests, all given with minimal explanation. Although the only outcome measure for the unusual activity condition was an interview, the authors confirmed that the subjects had been mystified and concluded that this condition created a need for divergent thinking which was reflected in the increased REM time.

Learning of consonant trigrams and paired associates prior to sleep did not alter REM sleep (Castaldo, Krynicki, and Goldstein, 1974), which is consistent with the previously discussed failure of REM deprivation to affect these tasks. On the other hand, results in the more meaningful situation of intensive foreign language learning have been more varied. DeKoninck *et al.* (1975, 1977) found increased REM sleep over base line in four subjects who showed improvement in language test scores and no change in REM sleep in two subjects whose language performance failed to improve. Meienberg (1977), however, found no change in REM sleep in a subject who improved significantly. Somewhat analogous results were observed in a study of two inbred mouse strains which differed in learning ability. While both strains showed some elevation of REM sleep during training, it was more obvious and more closely related to mastery in the better learning strain. Post-training REM deprivation did not affect retention in the poorer learning strain, but it abolished the intersession improvement (reminiscence) characteristic of the better learning strain (see Pearlman, 1979). These findings indicated that learning of the task was possible without involvement of REM sleep but that REM sleep facilitated the performance of some subjects. Similarly, language learning, like paired associates or other rote learning, may not require REM sleep, but REM sleep may affect such factors as fluency or thinking in the new language in some persons. In the analogous situation of recovery from aphasia, Greenberg and Dewan (1969) reported that patients whose speech was improving, had higher amounts of REM sleep than patients whose function had reached a plateau.

A study by Cartwright *et al.* (1977) indicated the limitations of a simplistic concept of information processing in humans which does not consider the meaning of the stimuli to the subjects. They found increased REM time in several subjects who listened to music before going to sleep. A study by Hauri

(1968), which had also involved listening to music before sleep, did not find increased REM sleep, but since only the first half of the night was studied, increased REM sleep during the latter half of the night might have been missed. The results of Cartwright *et al.* cannot be ascribed to the novelty of the presleep procedure since a group which listened to verbal materials did not show increased REM sleep. As there is also no defined information to be processed, it would seem likely that the increased REM sleep was related to unknown factors, such as the previously suggested personal meaning of the stimulus. A similar conclusion was suggested by an earlier report of increased REM sleep in athletes who were forced to suspend temporarily their customary exercise programme (Baekeland, 1970).

The question of personal meaning can be more effectively explored in a clinical setting than with an experimental procedure although the clinical approach suffers from the inherent limitations of observer bias and the small number of subjects that can be thoroughly studied. With these limitations in mind, however, Greenberg and Pearlman (1975) assessed tape-recorded psychoanalytical sessions preceding and following nights which the patient spent in the sleep laboratory for a measure called defensive strain (Knapp *et al.*, 1975). They found that increased REM sleep was associated with fall in strain from evening to morning (analogous to task mastery in animals) and decreased REM latency was correlated with high defensive strain in the evening. This clinical study further supported the idea of responsiveness of the REM system to demands on the nervous system for processing experiences. It also suggested that evidence of demand (shorter REM latency) may differ from evidence of successful mastery or adaptation (increased REM time). On the other hand, if the REM system can be responsive to anything from highly charged psychoanalytical issues to listening to music, measurement of such alterations in sleep structure may serve only as an indication that some kind of information processing is taking place.

Short REM latencies have been observed in a variety of other conditions, such as narcolepsy (Roth, 1978), acute schizophrenia (Feinberg and Hiatt, 1978) and primary depression (depression not clearly related to medical illness or psychogenic maladaptive behaviour) (Kupfer and Foster, 1978), but no study has been made of the relation of REM latency to psychological state in these patients. In addition, Feinberg (1974) noted that short REM latency might result from a primary change in slow wave sleep preceding the first REM period. Thus, further research will be necessary to clarify the relation of these REM parameters to information processing.

ALTERATION OF OTHER SLEEP STAGES

Now, we will consider some effects of varying other aspects of sleep structure. Since it is impossible to deprive a subject of stage 2 sleep without preventing sleep altogether, this research has focused upon those phases of sleep characterized by a predominance of EEG slow waves (stages 3 and 4), which can be altered without awakening the subject. As with the REM deprivation experiments, an early question was whether some effects of total sleep deprivation were related to loss of slow wave sleep. The initial report by Agnew, Webb, and Williams (1964) found a rebound of stage 4 sleep during recovery from two nights in which stage 4 was prevented by use of a tone stimulus which 'moved' the subject to another sleep stage, usually stage 3. This finding suggested that, like REM sleep, there was a requirement for stage 4 sleep. Agnew, Webb, and Williams (1967) replicated this finding. As with their previously discussed study of REM deprivation, they found no effect of stage 4 deprivation upon pursuit rotor performance, discriminative reaction time, or addition. In contrast to REM deprivation, however, the personality tests showed evidence of depression and vague physical complaints suggestive of hypochondriacal concerns which (like REM deprivation) were not behaviourally obvious. Such complaints have been observed during sleep deprivation experiments, but it has been uncertain to what degree they resulted from sleep loss or from musculoskeletal strain involved in staying awake.

Moldofsky and Scarisbrick (1976) investigated this question more carefully. They found increased musculoskeletal tenderness, as measured by a pressure dolorimeter, on mornings following stage 4 deprivation and an increase in musculoskeletal symptoms. A pilot study involving physically fit subjects had not shown these results, which suggested that sedentary life style was a necessary additional factor. The authors concluded that stage 4 sleep disturbance was an important factor in the 'fibrositis' syndrome, which is characterized by similar musculoskeletal complaints without evidence of connective tissue or joint pathology.

Johnson *et al.* (1974) found no significant changes following stage 4 deprivation on the same extensive battery of mood and performance measurements used in their previously discussed REM deprivation study. Some decrement was found in a continuous counting test, which probably measures fatigability, but a similar impairment had been found with REM deprivation. Some decrement in long term verbal retention was also observed, but this did not differ from performance of the REM deprived group. The previously discussed verbal retention test by Ekstrand *et al.* (1971) also found no effect of stage 4 deprivation.

With respect to the question of whether effects of total sleep loss could be related to selective stage disruption, Lubin *et al.* (1974) studied the recuperative effects of REM and stage 4 on performance after two days of complete sleep deprivation. The previously mentioned tests of addition, vigilance, and immediate verbal recall all showed impairment following total sleep loss. On subsequent days, however, recovery of all groups of subjects proceeded at the same rate regardless of whether they were deprived of REM or stage 4 or slept undisturbed. In another experiment, Johnson *et al.* (1974) studied the effects of prior REM or stage 4 deprivation upon the effect of one night of total sleep loss. Once again, the results were negative. Subjects receiving prior REM or stage 4 deprivation actually showed somewhat less impairment than subjects without prior deprivation. These results indicated that for performance on the conventional tests which are sensitive to total sleep loss (see Chapter V for details), the amount of sleep is more important than the kind, and selective sleep cycle disruption appears to make little difference.

Stage 4 and Exercise

Analogous to the idea that learning might increase REM sleep is the common sense notion that fatigue or muscular exercise might increase slow wave sleep (stages 3 and 4), since that aspect of sleep might be involved in restoration (see Baekeland and Lasky, 1966). The restorative aspect has been difficult to define, however (see Horne, 1979). Hobson (1968) reported increased slow wave sleep following a period of exercise in cats, but Hauri (1968) found no effect of 6 hours of strenuous exercise before sleep in humans. With a progressively more demanding midday exercise procedure, however, Shapiro *et al.* (1975) found a progressive increase in stages 3 and 4. Similar patterns were observed in distance runners following a 92 km marathon (Shapiro, 1978). Negative findings with less severe exercise were reported by Zir, Smith, and Parker (1971), Adamson *et al.* (1974) and Horne and Porter (1976). Griffin and Trinder (1978) observed that physically fit subjects had more stage 3 sleep than unfit subjects following moderate exercise although the same difference was noted on base line recordings. Similarly, Zloty, Burdick, and Adamson (1973) found more stages 3 and 4 in experienced distance runners than Baekeland and Lasky (1966) reported for subjects who trained less strenuously. Walker *et al.* (1978), however, noted no difference in slow wave sleep between runners and non-runners.

The increased stages 3 and 4 following the more extreme exercise regimens may resemble that observed in other situations of unusual metabolic demand, such as starvation (MacFayden, Oswald, and Lewis, 1973) and hyperthyroidism (Dunleavy *et al.*, 1974). Increased stages 3 and 4 have also been reported, however, under conditions apparently unrelated to increased metabolic demand, such as prolonged bed rest (Ryback and Lewis, 1971) or a heavy 'visual load' involving 7 hours of monitoring of various scenarios of persons and objects (Horne and Walmsley, 1976). While the sleep effect with bed rest was ascribed to increased metabolic activity involved in maintenance of the muscular system, similar effects were not noted in quadriplegics, who tended to have reduced slow wave sleep (Adey, Bors, and Porter, 1968). Horne (1979) suggested that since the subjects in the study by Ryback and Lewis had television to watch, they may have experienced a heavy visual load similar to the study of Horne and Walmsley. In summary, the range of factors reported to increase slow wave sleep appears to be as broad as that affecting REM sleep. In addition, the amount of stage 4 has been found to be correlated with the duration of previous time awake (Webb and Agnew, 1977) although REM sleep was not significantly affected by this factor. Thus, a possible connection between stage 4 sleep and recovery from exercise seems less clear now than when it was initially proposed. Horne (1979) suggested that slow wave sleep is involved in CNS recovery from fatiguing effects of waking. What the brain might be recovering from remains obscure. Webb has suggested that sleep evolved as an efficient form of immobilization for energy conservation and predator evasion (Webb and Cartwright, 1978). This idea can explain why the only known restorative effect of sleep is restoration of the non-sleepy state, but the hypothesis has some difficulty with the previously discussed fluctuations in sleep structure. Johnson (1973) suggested that because distinction between stage 4 and other stages of non-REM sleep is arbitrarily based on relative prominence of slow waves, it may not be possible to separate hypothetical functions of stage 4 from stages 2 and 3. Since all these stages cannot be suppressed without concomitant REM deprivation, further progress in this area seems uncertain.

PSYCHOPATHOLOGY, PERFORMANCE, AND IMPLICATIONS

The studies discussed above have all involved normal subjects. This section will review studies of sleep structure variation in psychopathological conditions which have assessed some aspect of performance. The initial studies of REM deprivation in schizophrenia were undertaken to determine if such patients might be more likely to show gross psychological impairment than normal subjects. The results were even less impressive than in normals since the previously discussed non-specific symptoms were not apparent despite close observation (Vogel and Traub, 1968).

In depressive states, prolonged REM deprivation has produced significant clinical improvement in several patients. In a double-blind, crossover study comparing three weeks of REM deprivation with control-awakenings in hospitalized depressed patients, Vogel *et al.* (1975) found significant improvement in those with prominent endogenous symptoms, who showed augmented REM pressure (increasing number of awakenings necessary to produce REM deprivation).

Wyatt *et al.* (1971b) found improvement with REM suppression by phenelzine in six atypical depressed patients who showed no endogenous features but who also were not clearly reactive. The connection between REM suppression and improvement was indicated by temporal contiguity, and the presence of increased REM pressure was indicated by large REM rebounds upon drug discontinuation. Subsequent work also found that reactive depressives who responded to a REM-suppressant drug (amitriptyline), showed a REM rebound with drug discontinuation whereas no rebound was found in such patients who failed to improve (Gillin *et al.*, 1978). These results suggested that increased REM pressure in response to REM suppression may be a better predictor of clinical improvement than descriptive diagnostic categories.

Similar benefit from REM suppression by phenelzine has been reported in some patients with narcolepsy (Wyatt *et al.*, 1971a). REM suppression by phenelzine has also been beneficial in patients with neurodermatitis, a skin condition which is frequently influenced by emotional factors (Friedman *et al.*, 1978). Although the performance measures in the studies of depressed, narcoleptic, and neurodermatitis patients were less objective than those of the previously reviewed studies, the results were impressive. The extended periods of clinical observation and the essential exclusion of placebo factors further supported the connection between improvement and REM suppression. Thus, it seems clear that REM deprivation is helpful for some persons.

Since most theories about the function of REM sleep have formulated the effects of REM deprivation in terms of impairment, these findings of improved function have posed a challenge. The oculomotor hypothesis has contributed nothing in this area, but both drive-facilitation and information-processing hypotheses have offered interpretations. Vogel (1979) suggested that drive-enhancing effects of REM deprivation counteracted reduced drive behaviours in endogenous depressed patients, such as anorexia, anhedonia, and reduced sexual interest. He further speculated that this drive facilitation was mediated by the increased CNS excitability produced by REM deprivation and that the periodic neural activity of REM sleep normally reduces such excitability and waking drive behaviour accordingly. Finally, he suggested that symptoms of endogenous depression result from excessive neural activity during REM sleep. The major strength of this hypothesis is the connection between reduced drive behaviour in endogenous depression and the previously discussed evidence of increased drive behaviour with REM deprivation. The major limitation is concretization of the concept of neural activity so that a quantity of discharge during REM sleep is considered to directly affect waking drive tension. Vogel goes further than Freud in suggesting that drive discharge during REM sleep does not merely serve to preserve sleep but tames or modulates drive-oriented behaviour to permit higher organisms greater adaptive behavioural flexibility in the presence of drive motivation. If this were true, one might wonder why the behaviour of endogenous depressed patients is so maladaptive and inflexible. It seems equally plausible to interpret the reduced drive behaviour of endogenous patients as a result of excessive inhibition. Accordingly, improvement with REM deprivation could be due to alteration of the inhibitory processes.

While REM sleep apparently has some modulating influence on drive behaviour, the quantitative relationship suggested by Vogel has similar problems to those of the brain model described in Freud's *Project for a*

Scientific Psychology (see McCarley and Hobson, 1977). Neuroscience research has conclusively shown that nervous activity serves as a transducer of information rather than to discharge quantities of excitation. Pribram and Gill (1976) have indicated how Freud's model can be made more congruent with contemporary thinking by viewing his concept of quantity of excitation as a metaphor for physiological processes underlying higher nervous functions. Vogel's hypothesis, however, requires the literal idea of discharge of excitation to account for the relation of REM sleep to waking drive behaviour. The drive-facilitation hypothesis also has contributed nothing to understanding improvement with REM deprivation in reactive and atypical depressive states, narcolepsy, neurodermatitis, and low back pain (Lancey, 1978), which do not show the evidence of reduced drive behaviour characteristic of endogenous depression.

The information-processing hypothesis interprets impaired function with REM deprivation as deficient adaptation due to absence of the necessary information processing during REM sleep. Accordingly, improved function with REM deprivation suggests that information processing during REM sleep was maladaptive in that situation. This idea deals fairly well with those depressive states in which the patient's usual coping mechanisms, which are facilitated by REM sleep, are more suited to his past life than to the present. REM deprivation may interrupt the maladaptive defensive patterns. Anecdotal evidence of such a phenomenon was noted by Greenberg and Pearlman (1974) in patients receiving REM suppressant, antidepressant drugs who felt well and handled their current life situations efficiently but who seemed out of touch with their inner emotional life. Such a mechanism can also account for the varying duration of improvement following cessation of REM deprivation by the degree to which new ways of coping, which were discovered during the period of REM suppression, become integrated with older maladaptive patterns when normal REM sleep returns. In other cases, REM deprivation may impair the integration of current experience with the fixed pessimistic attitudes characteristic of many depressed persons, with resultant amelioration of mood as long as REM sleep is suppressed.

Some patients with narcolepsy, neurodermatitis, or back pain also have pessimistic attitudes or a tendency to cling to patterns of adaptation more suited to their earlier lives, but the case reports of the patients who improved with REM suppression offer no data on this point. In summary, these studies of sleep structure alteration in psychopathological states have provided exciting leads for future research, but the wider implications for theories of the functions of sleep are not yet clear.

ENVOI

To return to the issues posed at the beginning of this chapter, what can we conclude about the relation of sleep structure variation to performance from a current perspective? A critical problem is the difficulty of conceptualizing the totality of sleep. Most research has dealt either with the active aspects of REM sleep or with the quiescent aspects of slow wave sleep and ignored the inevitable linkage of these states. Research on sleep structure variation will continue to be greatly hampered until progress is made on this point.

An analogous problem exists for theories about individual sleep stages. The restorative and immobilization hypotheses about slow wave sleep are each supported by some data and challenged by other evidence. Similarly, the drive-facilitative aspects of REM deprivation were well known by 1970, but further research has dwindled. In contrast, negative findings on the involvement of REM sleep in information processing were equally well known by 1970, but positive findings in this area have continued to accumulate. Further progress will be enhanced when a way is found to integrate these theories. The reports of beneficial effects of REM deprivation suggest more intensive investigation of psychopathological states with a combination of clinical, psychodynamic, and experimental techniques. Finally, none of the previously discussed research has considered the effect of varying the circadian position of the sleep cycle. Accordingly, future work will have to reassess the reported relations of sleep structure variation to performance from this perspective.

SUMMARY

This chapter reviews the performance effects when the structure of sleep is varied, with particular focus on the extensive studies of REM sleep deprivation. First, presentation of the empirical findings from 35 human subject REM deprivation studies reports on a wide range of performance measures. This is followed by a review of three major theories which have been developed to account for these data (and those of animal studies); the oculomotor theory, the drive-facilitation theories, and the information-processing theories. The more limited data derived from alteration of the other sleep stages are reviewed. In a final section findings emerging from psychopathological conditions, and their associated changes in sleep structure and behaviour changes, are considered.

REFERENCES

Adamson, L., Hunter, W. M., Ogunremi, O. O., Oswald, I., and Percy-Robb, I. W. (1974). Growth hormone increase during sleep after daytime exercise. *Journal of Endocrinology* **62**, 473–478.

Adey, W. R., Bors, E., and Porter, R. W. (1968). EEG sleep patterns after high cervical lesions in man. *Archives of Neurology* **19**, 377–383.

Agnew, H. W. Jr., Webb, W. B., and Williams, R. L. (1964). The effects of stage four sleep deprivation. *Electroencephalography and Clinical Neurophysiology* **17**, 68–70.

Agnew, H. W. Jr., Webb, W. B., and Williams, H. L. (1967). Comparison of stage four and 1-REM sleep deprivation. *Perceptual and Motor Skills* **24**, 851–858.

Allen, S. R. (1974). REM sleep deprivation and protein synthesis inhibition. Effects on human memory. In: *Sleep 1974*. P. Levin and W. P. Koella (Eds.). Basel, S. Karger.

Allen, S. R., Oswald, I., Lewis, S. A., and Tagney, J. (1972). Effects of distorted visual input on sleep. *Psychophysiology* 9, 498-504.

Allison, T. and Van Twyer, H. (1970). Sleep in the moles, scalopus acquaticus and condylura cristata. *Experimental Neurology* 27, 564-578.

Alper, T. G. (1957). Predicting the direction of selective recall. its relation to ego strength and N achievement. *Journal of Abnormal and Social Psychology* 55, 149-165.

Arkin, A. M., Antrobus, J. S., Ellman, S. J., and Farber, J. (1978). Sleep mentation as affected by REMP deprivation. In: *The Mind in Sleep: Psychology and Psychophysiology*. A. M. Arkin, J. S. Antrobus, and S. J. Ellman (Eds.). Hillsdale, Lawrence Erlbaum Associates.

Baekeland, F. (1970). Exercise deprivation: sleep and psychological reactions. *Archives of General Psychiatry* 22, 365-369.

Baekeland, F., Koulack, D., and Lasky, R. (1968). Effects of a stressful presleep experience on electroencephalograph-recorded sleep. *Psychophysiology* 4, 436-443.

Baekeland, F. and Lasky, R. (1966). Exercise and sleep patterns in college athletes. *Perceptual and Motor Skills* 23, 1203-1207.

Barrett, T. R. and Ekstrand, B. R. (1972). Effect of sleep on memory: III. Controlling for time-of-day effects. *Journal of Experimental Psychology* 96, 321-327.

Berger, R. J. (1969). Oculomotor control: a possible function of REM sleep. *Psychological Review* 76, 144-164.

Berger, R. (1972). Evolution of active sleep and coordinated eye movements. In: *The Sleeping Brain*. M. H. Chase (Ed.). Los Angeles, Brain Information Service.

Berger, R. J. and Scott, R. D. (1971). Increased accuracy of binocular depth perception following REM sleep periods. *Psychophysiology* 8, 763-768.

Berger, R. J. and Walker, J. M. (1972). Oculomotor coordination following REM and non-REM sleep periods. *Journal of Experimental Psychology* 94, 216-224.

Breger, L. (1967). Function of dreams. *Journal of Abnormal Psychology* 72, (5, Pt 2).

Cartwright, R. D. (1974). Problem solving: Waking and dreaming. *Journal of Abnormal Psychology* 83, 451-455.

Cartwright, R., Butters, E., Weinstein, M., and Kroeker, L. (1977). The effects of presleep stimuli of different sources and types on REM sleep. *Psychophysiology* 14, 388-392.

Cartwright, R. D., Lloyd, S., Butters, E., Weiner, L., McCarthy, L., and Hancock, J. (1975). Effects of REM time on what is recalled. *Psychophysiology* 12, 561-568.

Cartwright, R. D., Monroe, L. J., and Palmer, C. (1967). Individual differences in response to REM deprivation. *Archives of General Psychiatry* 16, 297-303.

Cartwright, R. D. and Ratzel, R. W. (1972). Effects of dream loss on waking behavior. *Archives of General Psychiatry* 27, 277-280.

Castaldo, V., Krynicki, V., and Goldstein, J. (1974). Sleep stages and verbal memory. *Perceptual and Motor Skills* 39, 1023-1030.

Chernik, D. A. (1972). Effect of REM sleep deprivation on learning and recall by humans. *Perceptual and Motor Skills* 34, 283-294.

Clemes, S. R. and Dement, W. C. (1967). Effect of REM sleep deprivation on psychological functioning. *Journal of Nervous and Mental Disease* 144, 488-491.

Cohen, D. B. (1977). Neuroticism and dreaming sleep: A case for interactionism in personality research. *British Journal of Social and Clinical Psychology* 16, 153-163.

Cohen, H., Thomas, J., and Dement, W. C. (1970). Sleep stages, REM deprivation, and electroconvulsive threshold in the cat. *Brain Research* 19, 317-321.

Crighel, E., Predescu, V., Matei, M., Nica, S., and Prica, A. (1976). Neocortical reactivity to peripheral stimuli in neurotics. *Neuropsychobiology* 2, 258–268.

DeKoninck, J., Proulx, G., Healy, T., Arsenault, R., and Prévost, F. (1975). Intensive language learning and REM sleep. *Sleep Research* 4, 150.

DeKoninck, J., Proulx, G., King, W., and Poitras, L. (1977). Intensive language learning and REM sleep: further results. *Sleep Research* 7, 146.

Dement, W. C. (1960). The effect of dream deprivation. *Science* 131, 1705–1707.

Dement, W. C. (1964). Experimental dream studies. In: *Science and Psychoanalysis*, Vol. VII. J. H. Masserman (Ed.). New York, Grune and Stratton.

Dement, W. C. (1965). Studies on the function of rapid eye movement (paradoxical) sleep in human subjects. In: *Aspects anatomofonctionnels de la physiologie du sommeil*. M. Jouvet (Ed.). Paris, Centre National de la Recherche Scientifique.

Dement, W. C. and Fisher, C. (1963). Experimental interference with the sleep cycle. *Canadian Psychiatric Association Journal* 8, 400–405.

Dement, W. C., Henry, P., Cohen, H., and Ferguson, J. (1967). Studies on the effect of REM deprivation in humans and animals. In: *Sleep and Altered States of Consciousness*. S. Kety, E. Evarts, and H. Williams (Eds.). New York, Grune and Stratton.

Dewan, E. M. (1970). The Programming (P) hypothesis for REM sleep. In: *Sleep and Dreaming*. E. Hartmann (Ed.). Boston, Little, Brown and Co.

Dewson, J. H., Dement, W. C., Wagener, T. E., and Nobel, K. (1967). Rapid eye movement sleep deprivation: A central neural change during wakefulness. *Science* 156, 403–406.

Donchin, E. and Cohen, L. (1967). Averaged evoked potentials and intramodality selective attention. *Electroencephalography and Clinical Neurophysiology* 22, 537–546.

Donchin, E. and Smith, D. B. D. (1970). The contingent negative variation and the late positive wave of the averaged evoked potential. *Electroencephalography and Clinical Neurophysiology* 29, 201–203.

Dunleavy, D. L. F., Oswald, I., Brown, P., and Strong, J. A. (1974). Hyperthyroidism, sleep and growth hormone. *Electroencephalography and Clinical Neurophysiology* 36, 259–263.

Easterbrook, J. A. (1959). The effect of emotion on cue utilization and the organization of behavior. *Psychological Review* 66, 183–201.

Ekstrand, B. R., Barrett, T. R., West, J. N., and Maier, W. G. (1977). The effect of sleep on human long-term memory. In: *Neurobiology of Sleep and Memory*. R. R. Drucker-Colin and J. L. McGaugh (Eds.). New York, Academic Press.

Ekstrand, B. R., Sullivan, M. J., Parker, D. F., and West, J. N. (1971). Spontaneous recovery and sleep. *Journal of Experimental Psychology* 88, 142–144.

Ellman, S. J., Spielman, A. J., Luck, D., Steiner, S. S., and Halperin, R. (1978). REM deprivation: A review. In: *The Mind in Sleep: Psychology and Psychophysiology*. A. M. Arkin, J. S. Antrobus, and S. J. Ellman (Eds.). Hillsdale, Lawrence Erlbaum Associates.

Empson, J. A. C. and Clarke, P. R. F. (1970). Rapid eye movements and remembering. *Nature* 227, 287–288.

Feinberg, I. (1974). Changes in sleep cycle patterns with age. *Journal of Psychiatric Research* 10, 283–306.

Feinberg, I. and Hiatt, J. F. (1978). Sleep patterns in schizophrenia: A selective review. In: *Sleep Disorders: Diagnosis and Treatment*. R. L. Williams and I. Karacan (Eds.). New York, John Wiley & Sons.

Feldman, R. E. (1969). *The Effect of Deprivation of Rapid Eye Movement Sleep on Learning and Retention in Humans.* Doctoral dissertation, Stanford University.

Feldstein, S. (1972). *REM Deprivation: The Effects on Inkblot Perception and Fantasy Processes.* Doctoral dissertation, City University of New York.

Fishbein, W. and Gutwein, B. M. (1977). Paradoxical sleep and memory storage processes. *Behavioral Biology* 19, 425–464.

Fowler, M. J., Sullivan, M. J., and Ekstrand, B. R. (1973). Sleep and memory. *Science* 179, 302–304.

Freud, S. (1953). The interpretation of dreams. *Standard Edition of the Complete Psychological Works of Sigmund Freud.* (J. Strachey, Ed., trans.) Vols. 4, 5. London, Hogarth Press.

Friedman, S., Kantor, I., Sobel, S., and Miller, R. (1978). On the treatment of neuro-dermatitis with a monoamine oxidase inhibitor. The chemotherapy of psychosomatic illness through A-REM suppression. *Journal of Nervous and Mental Disease* 166, 117–125.

Gillin, J. C., Wyatt, R. J., Fram, D., and Snyder, F. (1978). The relationship between changes in REM sleep and clinical improvement in depressed patients treated with amitriptyline. *Psychopharmacology* 59, 267–272.

Glaubman, H., Orbach, I., Aviram, O., Frieder, I., Frieman, M., Pelled, O., and Glaubman, R. (1978). REM deprivation and divergent thinking. *Psychophysiology* 15, 75–79.

Greenberg, R. (1970). Dreaming and memory. In: *Sleep and Dreaming.* E. Hartmann (Ed.). Boston, Little, Brown and Co.

Greenberg, R. and Dewan, E. M. (1969). Aphasia and rapid eye movement sleep. *Nature* 223, 183–184.

Greenberg, R., Horowitz, J., and Pearlman, C. (1972). The relation of dreaming to sensory-motor adaptation. *Psychophysiology* 9, 145.

Greenberg, R. and Pearlman, C. (1974). Cutting the REM nerve: An approach to the adaptive role of REM sleep. *Perspectives in Biology and Medicine* 17, 513–521.

Greenberg, R. and Pearlman, C. (1975). REM sleep and the analytic process: a psychophysiologic bridge. *Psychoanalytic Quarterly* 44, 392–403.

Greenberg, R., Pearlman, C., Fingar, R., Kantrowitz, J., and Kawliche, S. (1970). The effects of dream deprivation: implications for a theory of dreaming. *British Journal of Medical Psychology* 43, 1–11.

Greenberg, R., Pillard, R., and Pearlman, C. (1972). The effect of dream (stage REM) deprivation on adaptation to stress. *Psychosomatic Medicine* 34, 257–262.

Grieser, C., Greenberg, R., and Harrison, R. H. (1972). The adaptive function of sleep: The differential effects of sleep and dreaming on recall. *Journal of Abnormal Psychology* 80, 280–286.

Griffin, S. J. and Trinder, J. (1978). Physical fitness, exercise and human sleep. *Psychophysiology* 15, 447–450.

Hartmann, E. (1973). *The Functions of Sleep.* New Haven, Yale University Press.

Hauri, P. (1968). Effects of evening activity on early night sleep. *Psychophysiology* 4, 267–277.

Hennevin, E. and Leconte, P. (1971). La fonction du sommeil paradoxal: faits et hypothèses. *L'Année Psychologique* 2, 489–519.

Hennevin, E. and Leconte, P. (1977). Étude des relations entre le sommeil paradoxal et les processus d'acquisition. *Physiology and Behavior* 18, 307–319.

Herman, J., Roffwarg, H., Rosenmann, C. J. and Tauber, E. S. (1980). Binocular Depth Perception or Aware State Visual Deprivation, *Psychophysiology*, 17, 236–242.

Hicks, R. A. and Moore, J. D. (1979). REM sleep deprivation diminishes fear in rats. *Physiology and Behavior* 22, 689-692.

Hicks, R. A., Moore, J. D., Findley, P., Hirshfield, C., and Humphrey, V. (1978). REM sleep deprivation and pain thresholds in rats. *Perceptual and Motor Skills* 47, 848-850.

Hill, H. E., Kornetsky, C. H., Flanary, H. G., and Wilder, A. (1952). Effects of anxiety and morphine on the discrimination of intensities of pain. *Journal of Clinical Investigation* 31, 473-480.

Hobson, J. A. (1968). Sleep after exercise. *Science* 162, 1503-1505.

Hobson, J. A. and McCarley, R. M. (1977). The brain as a dream state generator: an activation-synthesis hypothesis of the dream process. *American Journal of Psychiatry* 134, 1335-1348.

Holt, R. R. and Havel, J. (1960). A method for assessing primary and secondary process in the Rorschach. In: *Rorschach Psychology*. M. A. Rickers-Ovsiankina (Ed.). New York, John Wiley and Sons.

Horne, J. A. (1979). Restitution and human sleep: A critical review. *Physiological Psychology* 7, 115-125.

Horne, J. A. and Porter, J. M. (1976). Time of day effects with standardised exercise upon subsequent sleep. *Electroencephalography and Clinical Neurophysiology* 40, 178-184.

Horne, J. A. and Walmsley, B. (1976). Daytime visual load and the effects upon human sleep. *Psychophysiology* 13, 115-120.

Horowitz, M. W. and Berkowitz, A. (1967). Listening and reading, speaking and writing: An experimental investigation of differential acquisition and reproduction of memory. *Perceptual and Motor Skills* 24, 207-215.

Hoyt, M. F. and Singer, J. L. (1978). Psychological effects of REM ('dream') deprivation upon waking mentation. In: *The Mind in Sleep: Psychology and Psychophysiology*. A. M. Arkin, J. S. Antrobus, and S. J. Ellman (Eds.). Hillsdale, Lawrence Erlbaum Associates.

Hubel, D. H. (1967). Effects of distortion of sensory input on the visual system of kittens. *The Physiologist* 10, 17-45.

Johnson, L. C. (1973). Are stages of sleep related to waking behavior? *American Scientist* 61, 326-338.

Johnson, L. C., Naitoh, P., Moses, J. M., and Lubin, A. (1974). Interaction of REM deprivation and stage 4 deprivation with total sleep loss: experiment 2. *Psychophysiology* 11, 147-159.

Jouvet, M. (1975). The function of dreaming: a neurophysiologist's point of view. In: *Handbook of Psychobiology*. M. S. Gazzaniga and C. Blakemore (Eds.). New York, Academic Press.

Kales, A., Hoedemaker, F. S., Jacobson, A., and Lichtenstein, E. L. (1964). Dream deprivation: an experimental reappraisal. *Nature* 204, 1337-1338.

Karlin, L. and Martz, M. J. Jr. (1973). Response probability and sensory-evoked potentials. In: *Attention and Performance IV*. S. Kornblum. New York: Academic Press.

Knapp, P. H., Greenberg, R., Pearlman, C., Cohen, M., Kantrowitz, J., and Sashin, J. (1975). Clinical measurement in psychoanalysis: an approach. *Psychoanalytic Quarterly* 44, 404-430.

Kopell, B. S., Zarcone, V., de la Pena, A., and Dement, W. C. (1972). Changes in selective attention as measured by the visual averaged evoked potential following REM deprivation in man. *Electroencephalography and Clinical Neurophysiology* 32, 322-325.

Kupfer, D. J. and Foster, F. G. (1978). EEG sleep and depression. In: *Sleep Disorders: Diagnosis and Treatment*. R. L. Williams and I. Karacan (Eds.). New York, John Wiley and Sons.

Lancey, S. R. (1978). *The Adaptive Function of the Dreaming Process and the Experience of Chronic Pain*. Doctoral dissertation, University of Notre Dame.

Lerner, B. (1966). Rorschach movement and dreams: A validation study using drug-induced dream deprivation. *Journal of Abnormal Psychology* 71, 75–86.

Levy, C. M. and Coolidge, F. L. (1975). Empson and Clarke re-examined. *Sleep Research* 4, 151.

Lewin, I. and Glaubman, H. (1975). The effects of REM deprivation: Is it detrimental, beneficial, or neutral? *Psychophysiology* 12, 349–353.

Lewin, I. and Gombosh, D. (1973). Increase in REM time as a function of the need for divergent thinking. In: *Sleep*. W. P. Koella and P. Levin (Eds.). Basel, S. Karger.

Lewis, S. A., Sloan, J. P., and Jones, S. K. (1978). Paradoxical sleep and depth perception. *Biological Psychology* 6, 17–25.

Lhotsky, J. (1977). *An Examination of the Effects of Paradoxical Sleep Deprivation on Sexual Behavior in Men*. Doctoral dissertation, Duke University.

Lubin, A., Moses, J. M., Johnson, L. C., and Naitoh, P. (1974). The recuperative effects of REM sleep and stage 4 sleep on human performance after complete sleep loss: experiment 1. *Psychophysiology* 11, 133–146.

MacFayden, U. M., Oswald, I., and Lewis, S. A. (1973). Starvation and human slow wave sleep. *Journal of Applied Physiology* 35, 391–394.

McCarley, R. W. and Hobson, J. A. (1977). The neurobiological origins of psycho-analytic dream theory. *American Journal of Psychiatry* 134, 1211–1221.

McGrath, M. J. and Cohen, D. B. (1978). REM sleep facilitation of adaptive waking behavior: a review of the literature. *Psychological Bulletin* 85, 24–57.

Meienberg, P. (1977). The tonic aspects of human REM sleep during long-term intensive verbal learning. *Physiological Psychology* 5, 250–256.

Moldofsky, H. and Scarisbrick, P. (1976). Induction of neurasthenic musculoskeletal pain syndrome by selective sleep stage deprivation. *Psychosomatic Medicine* 38, 35–44.

Muzio, J. N., Roffwarg, H. P., Anders, C. B., and Muzio, L. G. (1972). Retention of rote-learned meaningful verbal material and alterations in the normal sleep EEG pattern. *Psychophysiology* 9, 108.

Naitoh, P., Johnson, L. C., and Lubin, A. (1973). The effect of selective and total sleep loss on the CNV and its psychological and physiological correlates. *Electro-encephalography and Clinical Neurophysiology* 33 (Supp.), 213–218.

Nakazawa, Y., Kotorii, M., Kotorii, T., Tachibana, H., and Nakano, T. (1975). Individual differences in compensatory rebound of REM sleep with particular reference to their relationship to personality and behavioral characteristics. *Journal of Nervous and Mental Disease* 161, 18–25.

Newman, E. B. (1939). Forgetting of meaningful material during sleep and waking. *American Journal of Psychology* 52, 65–71.

Ogilvie, R. D. and Broughton, R. J. (1976). Sleep deprivation and measures of emotionality in rats. *Psychophysiology* 13, 249–260.

Oswald, I. (1969). Human brain protein, drugs and dreams. *Nature* 223, 893–897.

Paul, K. and Dittrichova, J. (1975). Sleep patterns following learning in infants. In: *Sleep 1974*. P. Levin and W. P. Koella (Eds.). Basel, S. Karger.

Pearlman, C. (1970). The adaptive function of dreaming. In: *Sleep and Dreaming*. E. Hartmann (Ed.). Boston, Little, Brown and Co.

Pearlman, C. (1979). REM sleep and information processing: evidence from animal studies. *Neuroscience and Biobehavioral Reviews* 3, 57–68.

Pearlman, C. (in press). *Medical Psychology of Sleep and Dreams*. New York, Plenum Press.

Pivik, R. T. (1978). Tonic states and phasic events in relation to sleep mentation. In: *The Mind in Sleep: Psychology and Psychophysiology*. A. M. Arkin, J. S. Antrobus, and S. J. Ellman (Eds.). Hillsdale, Lawrence Erlbaum Associates.

Pribram, K. H. and Gill, M. M. (1976). *Freud's 'Project' Re-assessed*. New York, Basic Books.

Puca, F. M., di Reda, L., Livrea, P., Genco, S., Specchio, C. M., Bandiera, L., and Pagano, G. (1976). Modificazioni psicologiche e cataboliti liquorali delle monoamine dopo privazione totale di sonno e dopo privazione selettiva di sonno REM. *Acta Neurologica* 31, 637–646.

Ramm, P. (1979). The locus coeruleus, catecholamines, and REM sleep: A critical review. *Behavioral and Neural Biology* 25, 415–448.

Rechtschaffen, A. and Verdone, P. (1964). Amount of dreaming: effect of incentive, adaptation to laboratory, and individual differences. *Perceptual and Motor Skills* 19, 947–958.

Riesen, A. H. (1966). Sensory deprivation. *Progress in Physiological Psychology* 1, 117–147.

Rojas-Ramirez, J. A. and Drucker-Colin, R. R. (1977). Phylogenetic correlations between sleep and memory. In: *Neurobiology of Sleep and Memory*. R. R. Drucker-Colin and J. L. McGaugh (Eds.). New York; Academic Press.

Roth, B. (1978). Narcolepsy and hypersomnia. In: *Sleep Disorders: Diagnosis and Treatment*. R. L. Williams and I. Karacan (Eds.). New York, John Wiley and Sons.

Ryback, R. W. and Lewis, O. F. (1971). Effects of prolonged bed rest on EEG sleep patterns in young, healthy volunteers. *Electroencephalography and Clinical Neurophysiology* 31, 395–399.

Sampson, H. (1966). Psychological effects of deprivation of dreaming sleep. *Journal of Nervous and Mental Disease* 143, 305–317.

Scrima, L. (1980). The Effect of Isolated PS and Isolated SWS on Recall. *Psychophysiology*, 17, 306.

Seligman, M. E. P. (1970). On the generality of the laws of learning. *Psychological Review* 77, 406–418.

Shapiro, C. H. (1978). Sleepiness of the long-distance runner. *Journal of Physiology* 276, 50 P – 51 P.

Shapiro, C. H., Griesel, R. D., Bartel, P. R., and Jooste, P. L. (1975). Sleep patterns after graded exercise. *Journal of Applied Physiology* 39, 187–190.

Stern, W. C. and Morgane, P. J. (1974). Theoretical view of REM sleep function: Maintenance of catecholamine systems in the central nervous system. *Behavioral Biology* 11, 1–32.

Tilley, A. J. and Empson, J. A. C. (1978). REM sleep and memory consolidation. *Biological Psychology* 6, 293–300.

Tueting, P. and Sutton, S. (1973). The relationship between prestimulus negative shifts and poststimulus components of the averaged evoked potential. In: *Attention and Performance IV*. S. Kornblum (Ed.). New York, Academic Press.

Vogel, G. W. (1979). A motivational function of REM sleep. In: *The Functions of Sleep*. R. Drucker-Colin, M. Shkurovich, and M. B. Sterman (Eds.). New York, Academic Press.

Vogel, G. W., Thurmond, A., Gibbons, P., Sloan, K., Boyd, M., and Walker, M. (1975). REM sleep reduction effects on depression syndromes. *Archives of General Psychiatry* 32, 765–777.

Vogel, G. W. and Traub, A. C. (1968). REM deprivation: I. The effect on schizophrenic patients. *Archives of General Psychiatry* 18, 287–300.

Vojtěchovský, K., Safratová, V., Votava, Z., and Feit, V. (1971). The effect of sleep deprivation on learning and memory in healthy volunteers. *Activitas Nervosa Superior* 13, 143–144.

Walker, J. M., Floyd, T. C., Fein, G., Cavness, C., Lualhati, R., and Feinberg, I. (1978). Effects of exercise on sleep. *Journal of Applied Physiology* 44, 945–951.

Wallach, H. and Karsh, E. B. (1963). Why the modification of stereoscopic depth-perception is so rapid. *American Journal of Psychology* 76, 413–420.

Webb, W. B. and Agnew, H. W. (1977). Analysis of the sleep stages in sleep-wakefulness regimens of varied length. *Psychophysiology* 14, 445–450.

Webb, W. and Cartwright, R. (1978). Sleep and dreams. *Annual Review of Psychology* 29, 223–252.

West, L. J., Janszen, H. H., Boyd, K. L., and Cornelisoon, F. S. Jr. (1962). The psychosis of sleep deprivation. *Annals of the New York Academy of Science* 96, 66–70.

Williams, H. L., Gieseking, C. F., and Lubin, A. (1966). Some effects of sleep loss on memory. *Perceptual and Motor Skills* 23, 1287–1293.

Williams, H. L., Lubin, A., and Goodnow, J. J. (1959). Impaired performance with acute sleep loss. *Psychological Monographs* 73, (14, Whole No. 484).

Wyatt, R. J., Fram, D. H., Buchbinder, R., and Snyder, F. (1971a). Treatment of intractable narcolepsy with a monoamine oxidase inhibitor. *New England Journal of Medicine* 285, 987–991.

Wyatt, R. J., Fram, D. H., Kupfer, D. J., and Snyder, F. (1971b). Total prolonged drug-induced REM sleep suppression in anxious-depressed patients. *Archives of General Psychiatry* 24, 145–155.

Zarcone, V., de la Penna, A., and Dement, W. C. (1974). Heightened sexual interest and sleep disturbance. *Perceptual and Motor Skills* 39, 1135–1141.

Zarcone, V., Zukovsky, E., Gulevich, G., Dement, W., and Hoddes, E. (1974). Rorschach responses subsequent to REM deprivation in schizophrenic and nonschizophrenic patients. *Journal of Clinical Psychology* 30, 248–250.

Zimmerman, J. T., Stoyva, J., and Metcalf, D. (1970). Distorted visual feedback and augmented REM sleep. *Psychophysiology* 7, 298–306.

Zimmerman, J. T., Stoyva, J. M., and Reite, M. L. (1978). Spatially rearranged vision and REM sleep: A lack of effect. *Biological Psychiatry* 13, 301–316.

Zir, L. M., Smith, R. A., and Parker, D. C. (1971). Human growth hormone release in sleep. Effect of daytime exercise. *Journal of Clinical Endocrinology* 32, 662–665.

Zloty, R. B., Burdick, J. A., and Adamson, J. D. (1973). Sleep of long distance runners. *Activitas Nervosa Superior* 15, 217–221.

Biological Rhythms, Sleep, and Performance
Edited by Wilse B. Webb
© 1982 John Wiley & Sons Ltd.

Chapter 7

Work/Sleep Time Schedules and Performance

Donald I. Tepas

INTRODUCTION

Technological development has resulted in significant changes in the way humans relate to and use time. Artificial lighting frees humans from the limits of darkness in a very practical way. Continuous-process manufacturing methods in their present form frequently require round-the-clock operations. Capital equipment costs currently promote the use of equipment for more than 8 hours a day. Rapid forms of transportation make fairly abrupt insertion into different time zones a fairly common event. Societal demand for improved human services and vigilant military operations encourages departures from traditional work schedules. Finally, worker concern with the quality of life has stimulated new interest in non-conventional approaches to work timing.

Overstating the significance of these developments a bit, one might view them as either a romantic challenge to master a new frontier (Melbin, 1978) or a clear threat to human health and happiness (Rutenfranz *et al.*, 1977). In any case, one should not ignore the magnitude and complexity of the variables involved (Tepas, 1976). With around 20% of the work force regularly facing the challenge of what might be termed non-conventional work hours (Maurice, 1975), interest must be directed towards an identification, evaluation, and understanding of the factors operative in the scheduling and use of time.

Rearrangement of existing work schedules along some dimensions is clearly desirable (Carpentier and Cazamian, 1977). Although shift work schemes have frequently been in place for many years, their origins and consequences are, as a rule, quite unknown. Time zone shifts produced by travel seem to be the product of commercial or military goals rather than individual health and happiness factors. In fact, the same variables interact in these divergent approaches to work and rest. However, it is commonly assumed that performance, satisfaction, and healthiness covary in a simple, predictive manner. Keeping in mind the idea that there may be a discrepancy between research findings and popular assumptions, let us examine some of the ways in which human work–rest time schedules can be varied.

THREE MODEL RESEARCH APPROACHES

Through the ages, man has been aware of behavioural and biological performance changes associated with time of day. These changes are not abrupt and discontinuous, but rather rhythmic changes which can be quantified and measured in an objective and continuous manner (Halberg, 1969a). However, the heuristic assignment of these continuous changes to a dichotomy of sleep and waking has considerable explicative value. Such a dichotomous view has been useful as manifest by the classic approach of Kleitman (1963) as well as the more contemporary approach of Johnson *et al.* (1977).

Three basic model research approaches are prominent. In each of these approaches, the temporal location of sleep provides an appropriate anchor for making comparisons. For reasons of simplification and identification, let us label these three approaches as studies of shift worker sleep, time zone shifted sleep, and laboratory shifted sleep. These labels should not be interpreted as overlooking the importance of wakefulness, but rather as an explicative approach to the understanding of what might seem to be quite diverse areas of inquiry.

Shift Worker Sleep

The working hours of people vary within a society and from culture to culture. Nevertheless, the fact is that most people work during daylight hours and that, within a cultural or national group, the working hours of the majority of people cluster around a basic core time period during daylight hours. For example, in America over 73% of the people go to work between 0700 and 0900 (Tasto and Colligan, 1977). Shift workers are those who permanently work outside of this core time period or who rotate or change their work schedule in a manner which results in much of it being outside the basic core time period. This basic core daylight hour work period is usually referred to as the day or morning shift. Work periods immediately following this day shift are usually referred to as afternoon or afternoon/evening shift. Work between the afternoon/evening shift and the day shift, usually with a predomination of non-daylight hours, is said to be night shift work. In America, the starting times for day, afternoon/evening and night shift work centre around 0800, 1600, and 2400 hours, respectively. On a worldwide scale, however, the starting times for these shifts vary over a wide range. It should also be noted that work duration frequently varies from shift type to shift type, from industry to industry, as well as from nation to nation. At best, it is a simplification to speak of day, afternoon/evening and night shift types. However, these terms do appear to translate fairly well across national boundaries, given our current level of sophistication in this area.

Given these three basic types of work shifts, it must also be recognized that one might work the same shift on every work day or one might change shifts following some sort of schedule. Work schedules which call for the same general hours every work day are termed steady or permanent shifts. Work schedules which do *not* call for the same general hours every work day are termed changing or rotating shifts. Rotating shifts vary widely in their form or scheme. Literally thousands of rotating shift schemes are practised with differences in variety of shift types, rate of shift change, and order of shift change (direction) all being factors contributing to this variety. Although the concept of rotating shifts is recognized on a worldwide scale, considerable caution is called for in using this notation since the same term is associated with an extremely broad range of schemes which may emphasize quite different variables. In Europe, for example, it would appear that most forms of rotating shift work involve changes in shift type during a period of less than seven days whereas American forms of rotating shift work mainly involve changes no more frequently than once every seven days (Tepas, Walsh, and Armstrong, 1981).

Conceptually, the notion of permanent shift work may in reality only apply to day shift types. As Van Loon (1963) demonstrated some time ago, those who do not work the day shift may very well 'shift' to the cultural day shift on their days off. In any case, the variety of rotating shift work makes it a simplification to speak simply of permanent and rotating shift schedules. This distinction is a helpful universal concept given our current state of knowledge, but one cannot ignore the obvious heterogeneity possible within this terminology.

Figure 1 provides a schematic representation of the three basic types of shift work. The three time blocks labelled 'work' represent the work times for the day, afternoon/evening and night shifts assuming an 8 hour work duration. The three time blocks labelled 'sleep' indicate the customary rest time of most workers when on these shifts. These sleep/work phases are characteristic of the habits of both permanent and rotating shift workers (Armstrong, Tepas, and Moss, 1980), as well as those observed in laboratory studies of rotating shifts (Webb and Agnew, 1978). Thus, the relationship of work to sleep varies with the three basic shift types. Day workers sleep just prior to work whereas afternoon/evening and night workers sleep immediately after work time. It is also important to note that day and afternoon/evening workers sleep at nearly the same time of day whereas night workers are on the job when others are sleeping but sleep mainly when day workers are on the job.

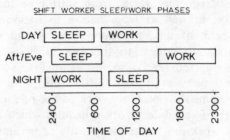

Figure 1   Typical sleep/work phases for three basic types of shift work

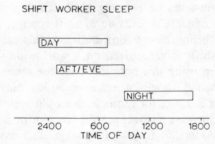

Figure 2   Sleep periods for common shift schedules

A simplification of Figure 1 is presented in Figure 2. In this figure the blocks noting work periods have been eliminated and only the sleep time blocks have been retained. These sleep periods are not rest periods imposed directly by an investigator or an organization. They are the sleep periods of choice selected by experienced shift workers. Individuals working on different shifts sleep at different times of the day. A worker changing from day to afternoon/evening shift, in practice, delays sleep 2 hours or so. Shifting from afternoon/evening work to night work can result in a further delay in sleep of 8 hours. On the other hand, a worker shifting from the afternoon/evening shift to the day shift can be said to advance the time of day at which the sleep period is taken. These are just a few examples of the ways in which changing work shift can advance or delay the time of day at which sleep is taken.

The basic characteristic of shift worker sleep research as defined here is discussed as the behaviours of workers in real life situations. Such research asks how actual field situations influence decisions about sleep as well as influence other behaviours. In most cases we are talking about the chronic effects of shift work schedules on individuals mainly immersed in an existing real world environment. Thus, this approach is more a form of naturalistic observation than it is a version of laboratory experimentation. Variable manipulation and control are potential statistical manoeuvres rather than laboratory manipulations. For the most part the societal time schedules are constant and intended to serve the day shift workers. Those working other shift schedules are faced with an invariant environment and it is their work schedule which is variant and in conflict.

Time Zone Shift Sleep

This model research approach also most frequently involves naturalistic observation. In this case, however, it is the working and resting hours which can be invariant while the societal time schedule is changed. Rapid transportation of an individual from one time zone to another is the origin of the time use problem of interest here. Business, vocational, and recreational factors have all increased the number of individuals experiencing time zone changes in recent years. For example, it is reasonable to estimate that one US airline alone has over 10,000 active employees experiencing time zone changes on a weekly basis. Scheduled airlines transport staggering numbers of individuals from their habitual time zone and abruptly insert them into a new one. Fifty years ago, the number of commercial airline passengers crossing time zones was hardly worth note since much of this industry was less than 10 years old and transcontinental flight was an oddity.

In keeping with the schematic presented in Figure 2, Figure 3 blocks in the projected sleep times of individuals taking a transcontinental US flight crossing four time zones. Assuming that these individuals will fully conform to the time of the new zone in which they arrive, sleep periods for this flight length will be advanced by 3 hours for a west–east flight and delayed 3 hours for an east–west flight. Given the fact that transcontinental flight within the US is commonly more than 3 hours in length and that actual transit time is

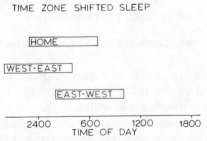

Figure 3 Projected sleep periods for individuals taking a transcontinental US flight crossing four time zones

frequently several hours longer, the time of day at which a flight leaves as well as the personal time demands of the individual traveller can easily modify habitual or home time zone sleep time further. It is important to note that these advances and delays in sleep period may be mandatory products of the time zone shift or they may involve choices made by the traveller or worker.

This is perhaps most evident if we look at the options available when transoceanic flight across more time zones is considered.

Figure 4 provides us with two hypothetical transoceanic flights from the west
to the east. Both flights assume a minimal 16 hours transit time and a 6 hour
change in local time. Given current technology, these are quite reliable times.
Let us assume that the individual involved is habitually a day worker who
usually gets up from sleep at the time point noted by the circled letter A in
Figure 4. Two flights are available, a morning flight with transit time
beginning shortly after getting up or an evening flight with transit time
beginning at 2200 hours. In many cases, the later flight might involve travel
after completion of a normal work day whereas the former schedule starts with
a rested participant.

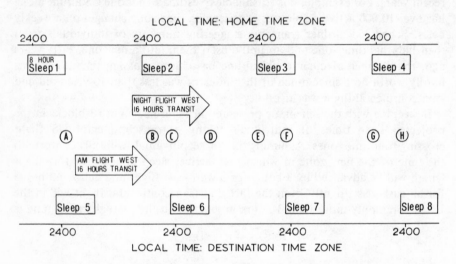

Figure 4   Sleep period options for two hypothetical transoceanic flights

Eight sleep periods are shown on Figure 4. Sleep 1 is, by definition, the
habitual sleep period of the individual when in the home time zone. One
possible option for the traveller is to maintain this sleep schedule independent
of transit and local time options and practices. Should this be practical, sleep
periods 2, 3, and 4 would be selected. Night and morning flights, however,
suggest other sleep period options which the traveller might select. Such a 6
hour shift is indicated by sleep periods 5, 6, 7, and 8. With planning and a
night flight, such a 6 hour shift in habitual sleep period could even be
introduced prior to the flight via an advance, delay, or extension of habitual
sleep time.

Another approach to sleep following transoceanic flight is one in which the
individual would choose to sleep as soon as is practical following transit time.

Napping and other sleep schedule choices are, of course, possible. Thus the combination of flight time, selected sleep, and schedule chosen, can yield a wide variety of possible sleep schemata. Some logical sleep onset time points are shown in Figure 4 by the circled letters B, C, D, E, F, G, and H. This is, of course, a simplification of the actual options available since naps or brief sleep periods may occur at an unscheduled time during transit and other times. In most cases, the options available will result in advanced or delayed sleep periods, with reference to the habitual home time zone sleep period.

Unless an immediate return to the home time zone is made, it would seem some type of shift in the habitual time period must occur if the individual is to participate fully in the society of the flight destination time zone. For the example given in Figure 4 it is important to note that this shift might involve sleep period changes ranging from an immediate 6 hour delay up to 46 hours of wakefulness without sleep, depending upon the strategy chosen. Like shift work schemata, a major issue is how changing time zones advances or delays the time of day at which sleep is taken.

Unlike shift work, where for the most part societal time schedules are constant, the rapid time zone crosser is thrust from one societal time schedule into another which can be quite in conflict with that of the origin time zone. In either case, the individual is faced with adjustment to two competing time schedules. With both shift work sleep research and time zone shifted sleep research one is considering the habits of individuals in real life situations. One must ask how actual field situations influence decisions about sleep as well as influence other behaviours. Social, biological, and performance factors are all relevant and must be considered if improved practices are to be evolved. Both model research approaches take a form more like naturalistic observation than following the strict model of traditional laboratory experimentation.

Laboratory Shifted Sleep

Clearly, many of the timing variables studied by the two model research approaches outlined can also be studied in the laboratory. Whereas field research makes it nearly impossible to control and/or manipulate variables in a way which identifies clearly differential effects, lawful relationships established in the laboratory can serve this role. Although the laboratory can never fully simulate the real world situation, it would be foolish to suggest that most variables identified in the laboratory vanish in the outside world (Webb, 1977). Laboratory research is an essential and primary method for the identification of significant variables and for the refinement of research tools but laboratory defined functional relationships may not take the exact same form in their real world manifestation.

Figure 5 provides us with one example of the manner in which the timing variables under discussion can be studied in the laboratory. In this example,

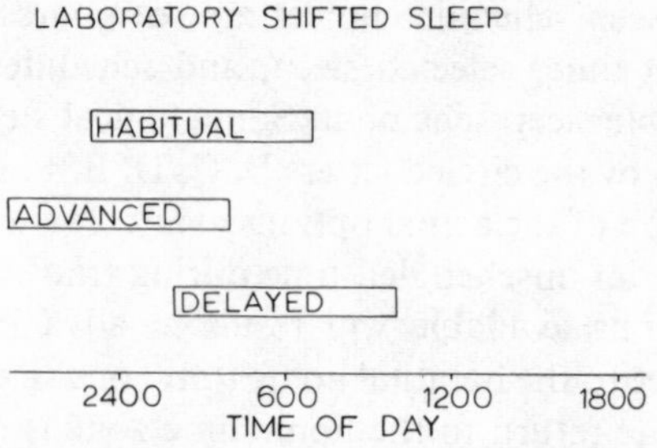

LABORATORY SHIFTED SLEEP

HABITUAL

ADVANCED

DELAYED

2400   600   1200   1800
TIME OF DAY

Figure 5   Sleep periods for laboratory imposed sleep schedules

the habitual time of day at which sleep is taken was advanced or delayed by 3 hours (Taub and Berger, 1976a). It should be noted that this figure has been plotted using the same time scale as was used in Figures 2 and 3. With regard to shifted sleep time, the laboratory sleep schedule imposed as in Figure 5 is identical to what one would expect from a transcontinental US flight crossing four time zones. In a similar manner, the laboratory shifted delayed sleep condition is quite similar to what one would expect from many workers shifting from the day shift to the afternoon/evening shift. This three hour laboratory shifted sleep study imposed a particular sleep treatment on subjects for only one night. Thus, the authors termed this a study of acute shifts in the sleep–wakefulness cycle, and the study is akin to observations on the effects of a single time zone shift exposure or the effects of a shift work schedule which calls for daily shift changes.

Although the chronic effects of years of shift work cannot be duplicated in the laboratory, some approximation can be obtained by repeated cycles of an imposed work–rest schedule. For example, one can place subjects on unusual work schedules for extended time periods as members of confined crews (Chiles, Alluisi, and Adams, 1968), attempt to establish stabilized shifts in the laboratory (Colquhoun, Blake, and Edwards, 1969), or place individuals on sleep–wake schedules whose cycle is shorter or longer than 24 hours (Webb, 1978). In most cases, the participants are college students or military personnel and the imposed schedules may be applied for days, weeks, and even months. In some cases, a clear effort is made to use 'synthetic work' to simulate real world conditions rather than use more traditional laboratory tasks (Morgan, 1974).

Since laboratory shifted sleep research approaches generally use workers who are not representative of the civilian working class, one must approach these studies with a modest degree of caution. If nothing else, one might argue that the laboratory-studied population is healthier and therefore more resistant than the general working population. One can argue, however, that variable effects in such a health population may in fact be even more virile in a population of older or more representative industrial workers. So long as one does not insist on a direct translation and/or application of laboratory functional relationships to the field, the main danger associated with laboratory shifted sleep research approaches appears to be one of assuming that all or the most significant variables will be evident. Laboratory research is good at establishing the clear legitimacy of variables, but it cannot be expected to identify the entire universe or relative weight of operative variables in the field situation.

THE FINDINGS

Background

In the US, research using some form of the laboratory shifted sleep model approach appears to have been the preferred strategy of choice. The impressive study of Mott *et al.* (1965) is perhaps the lone significant exception prior to 1970 and extensive investigations using the other model research approaches are not yet common in the US. European investigators, on the other hand, have established a broader approach and have widely used the shift worker in their research designs. Given differences in social customs and working conditions, one is faced with the perplexing question of the degree to which European findings can be extrapolated to other field conditions (Tepas, 1979). As already noted, rotation schedules and shift starting times vary greatly from one country to another.

Early US laboratory sleep research, on the other hand, has played an important role in structuring variable selection for all three model research approaches. Early research by Kleitman (1933) firmly demonstrated that diurnal changes in body temperature are associated with changes in performance. Kleitman's first book (1939) and the work of Halberg (1969a) starting in the 1940s provide important benchmarks for the scientific community. Although these two investigators demonstrate a clear interest in how time-of-day changes in *performance* relate to time schedules, their research in practice emphasizes biological dependent variables. Kleitman and Jackson (1950), in fact, proposed quite directly that there is a firm parallelism between body temperature and performance. They then argue in favour of the use of body temperature as a valid indirect estimate of alertness and efficiency. See Chapter III for a further discussion of this matter.

The position that body temperature and other physiological variables are a valid indirect estimate of performance, although historically dated at this point in theoretical development, plagues much of the research in this area. Performance measurement has been viewed by many as being obtrusive, time-consuming, and insensitive. As a result, many key studies do not include any form of performance measurement. One is led to infer from these omissions that the authors assume a simple and direct relationship between the physiological measurements and performance. A second form of omission is also frequently evident in the literature. Key studies indicate in their methods sections that performance was measured but fail either to report details of the performance task used or any of the behavioural data.

In addition, it must be noted that views of performance and biological clock have significantly evolved and become more significant in the last 20 years. Performance is not a simple concept and different tasks do tap different mechanisms. This is discussed in Chapter III. Developing a task to measure sleep loss, for example, requires consideration of a number of fairly specific factors if impairment is to be detected (Wilkinson, 1968). In a similar sense, it is now reasonable to speak in the plural of biological clocks. Although models for the biological clock(s) vary, the ability to desynchronize the phase relationships of one or more rhythms within an individual by various means is well established. Edmunds (1976) provides a number of examples of this. One wonders how often investigators have failed to report performance data simply because it did not fit in with earlier stated views of performance as a unitary concept.

In reviewing the research findings flowing from our three model research approaches, much of this historically conceptual naïveté becomes evident. Physiological variables are presented as indirect measures of performance. Performance measures when presented may appear to be quite insensitive measures as used or interpreted. Details concerning performance measurement technique or relations to physiological data may not be evident or of obvious concern. Few, if any, studies provide a good match between sophisticated performance measurement, biological rhythm study method, and/or theory use. In a very real sense, this is also a time schedule problem. Most active researchers in the area are well aware of the naïveté of their past efforts and the practical limits of their current efforts. As a new and developing problem area, it is clear that research only now approaches some of the issues. For the present time, however, one must wrestle with the bias of the past, making unsupported assumptions and arbitrary deletions when they seem to fit with a current perception of the field.

Shift Worker Sleep

Several excellent reviews of the effects of shift work are available (Carpentier and Cazamian, 1977; Rutenfranz *et al.*, 1977; Rutenfranz and Colquhoun, 1979; Rutenfranz, Knauth, and Angerbach, 1981). It is quite clear from these reviews that shift work effects are complex and require consideration of physiological, social, and performance variables if one is to assess the benefits and hazards of various forms of shift work. Although the findings to date with regard to many variables are conflicting or controversial, sleep variables are consistently found to be related to shift work dimension. Night work results in sleep problems. Whether these problems should be labelled 'disturbances' akin to clinical problems, a fairly simple problem of chronic sleep deprivation, or some combination of these two diagnoses, is not yet clear.

The laboratory shifted sleep research studies using polysomnographic recordings (Weitzman *et al.*, 1970; Kripke, Cook, and Lewis, 1971; Webb, Agnew, and Williams, 1971) found that acute shifts result in sleep disturbances. More recent studies in the laboratory of chronic shift workers (Knauth and Rutenfranz, 1972; Foret and Lantin, 1972; Wedderburn, 1975; Walsh, Tepas, and Moss, 1981) can be viewed as emphasizing the problem of chronic sleep deprivation. The most consistent polysomnographic finding of these later studies is that day sleep by people working at night results in a decrease in total sleep time. This is in keeping with survey data showing that night work shows concomitant decreased sleep length.

Figure 6 shows the results of three independent survey studies of permanent shift workers. All three studies show similar findings, although not all of the differences are significant in the data from Mott *et al.* (1965). Afternoon/ evening shift work is accompanied by the longest sleep length whereas night work is accompanied by the shortest sleep. Figure 7 shows the results of three independent survey studies of rotating shift workers. All three studies show similar and significant differences which mirror the data from the permanent shift workers. Visual comparison of Figures 6 and 7 also suggests that the sleep of rotating shift workers on night work is shorter than that of permanent night shift workers.

As noted earlier, the timing of sleep periods with respect to work periods varies with shift type, but varies in the same manner for most permanent and rotating shift workers. Since sleep length also varies with shift type in a similar manner for both permanent and rotating shift work, one can conclude that most rotating shift workers change their behaviours as they change shift in a manner predictable from permanent shift worker data. With regard to sleep, it appears that rotating shift workers have not developed any unique way to handle shift work. This is especially interesting since the Ostberg (1973) data is from European workers on a rotating shift system.

The finding that afternoon/evening shift workers sleep the longest is worthy of special note even though the difference is small. It suggests that afternoon/ evening workers sleep longer because their sleep onset and waking times are less subject to social and job demands. Given their usual time of day for sleeping, there is little available to tempt them to delay sleep onset and few social obligations to interfere should they choose to sleep in. As Webb and Agnew (1975) have pointed out, social factors can lead day shift workers to delay the onset of the sleep period, but they must still get up at a specific time to keep their job. In any case, it is difficult to account for the difference

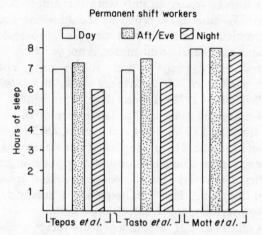

Figure 6   Mean sleep length in hours from three independent surveys of permanent shift workers. Data from Mott *et al.* (1965), Tasto *et al.* (1978), and Tepas, Walsh, and Armstrong (1981). The Tasto *et al.* data include a correction of an error from the original report

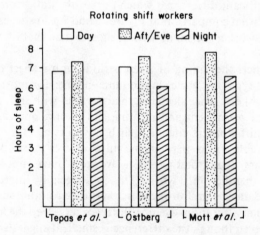

Figure 7   Mean sleep length in hours from three independent surveys of rotating shift workers. Data from Mott *et al.* (1965), Ostberg (1973), and Tepas, Walsh, and Armstrong (1981)

between day shift and afternoon/evening shift sleep times simply on the basis of time of day circadian physiological differences or on the basis of differential fatigue effects.

Given the conclusion that night shift work results in sleep deprivation, one would predict that performance sensitive to sleep deficits would yield significant differences if the performance of day shift and night shift workers were compared. This is the case. Figure 8 shows the performance of matched groups of permanent day shift and night shift workers on the Williams–Lubin experimenter-paced addition task before and after sleep in the laboratory during the usual work week (Tepas *et al.*, 1981). These workers slept in the laboratory at their usual sleep period but went to their job every work day as normally employed. The differences between groups on polysomnographic total sleep time, presleep performance, and post-sleep performance are all statistically significant. Between groups, post-sleep performance is different from presleep performance. Within groups, pre- and post-sleep performance is not significantly different. Given the times these workers were tested, the performance deficit of the permanent night shift workers in this study cannot be mainly produced by the time of day at which testing was conducted.

The finding that within groups there was no significant difference between pre- and post-sleep performance is not surprising if one takes the traditional approach that there is a firm parallelism between body temperature and performance. Kleitman and Jackson (1950) noted many years ago that performance prior to going to bed is usually about the same as that immediately after getting up. To take this position one must assume that the diurnal temperature rhythm of the permanent night shift workers has changed from that of day workers, conforming to their work–sleep schedule. Lobban and Tredre (1966) have gathered physiological rhythm data from chronic shift workers which suggests that gross rhythm adaptation of this sort may not occur. If one takes the opposite approach and assumes firm parallelism

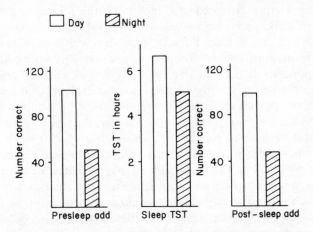

Figure 8   Pre- and post-sleep performance on the Williams–Lubin addition task, and EEG total sleep time as a function of work shift for permanent shift workers. Data from Tepas *et al.* (1981)

between physiological rhythms and performance with no changes in rhythm associated with night shift work, one cannot explain the large difference between day shift post-sleep performance and night shift presleep performance since the time of day for testing is nearly the same for both cases.

Clearly, the above data suggest that factors other than physiological rhythms effect performance. It is also very clear that the performance of real night shift workers can be significantly poorer than that of day shift workers. The unfortunate fact is that studies of the performance of night shift workers are rare and studies of industrial performance at night are unclear as to situational factors which probably obscure the results (Rutenfranz and Colquhoun, 1979). As will be noted in discussing laboratory shifted sleep research, it is quite possible that there are several performance rhythms which correlate in different ways with various physiological rhythms. One possibility is that for some behaviours night shift performance might even be better than day shift performance. Monk and Embrey (1981) have recently confirmed this variation in the first study to explore this possibility in chronic shift workers. In this study of the performance of six computer operators, the relationship between temperature and performance was varied by manipulating the memory load of the task used.

It is important that the existence of significant deficits in worker performance at night not be overlooked. Early field studies by Browne (1949), Bjerner, Holm, and Swensson (1955) and others found worker performance on the job to be the poorest in the early morning hours. More recently, Patkai, Akerstedt, and Pettersson (1977) have shown similar time of day performance changes using laboratory-grade choice reaction time performance measurements made at the job site. Given the research control problems noted above and the factors discussed in Chapter III, the robust nature of these effects in shift worker populations cannot be denied. It is the expectations to these effects which may be more difficult to confirm with additional research.

In sum, the literature shows without question that shift work effects sleep. Of most importance is the fact that night shift work reduces sleep length. Clearly these time-of-work/time-of-sleep interactions are complex and the product of physiological, social, and job factors. Without a doubt, night shift work can seriously impair performance. Shift work is not villainous in all respects. It is reasonable to suggest that some forms of shift work may have positive physiological or social effects which outweigh the anticipated performance deficits. It is also reasonable to suggest that some forms or types of performance might in fact be better at night. Two obvious dangers exist. Research which depends solely upon physiological variables to identify shift work hazards could be quite misleading. Research which depends upon a single performance measure to identify shift work effects can also be quite misleading. More research on real shift workers using performance measures is needed to fill in a dire gap.

Time Zone Shifted Sleep

As we noted in our discussion of Figure 4, individuals travelling rapidly through time zones have many options available to them. It is interesting to note that Strughold (1952) stressed the significance of sleep as a variable as well as the relationship of sleep to time zone shifts in his pioneering paper on global flights. Unfortunately, the literature published following this paper does not provide us with an extensive systematic survey of any notable size which might give us an accurate insight as to the options available for travellers to choose from. Obviously, time zone shifted sleep research deals with what is colloquially referred to as 'jet lag' or 'jet fatigue'. This terminology is of questionable or practical value. There is little in the literature to support the notion that all time zone crossing jet travel mandates deficits. When deficits occur, there is nothing to clearly suggest that the deficits are strictly the unique product of the variables associated with jet travel. It is surprising that so-called jet lag has been accepted as a popular concept yet the voluntary practical choice behaviour of travellers has never been systematically studied in a satisfactory manner.

To date the literature includes only a small number of field studies and only a few of these include satisfactory subject samples. These data do suggest that individual differences in time zone shift effects are significant and cannot be ignored (Reinberg, 1970). Thus, sample size is an issue of concern. In most studies, traveller choice with regard to sleeping and waking behaviour appears to have been eliminated as a variable for major study due to the experimenter's demand for regular measurement schedules, the use of regular civil airline flight schedules which do not yield ideal designs, or job schedule requirements when the subjects are aircrew members. Similar to the shift work area research, sleep variables are frequently reported as being related to time zone shift experiences. Once again, the question is whether these sleep problems should be labelled 'disturbances' akin to clinical problems, a fairly direct problem of total sleep deprivation, or some combination of these two diagnoses.

Logs and observations of aircrew members can be viewed as supporting the idea that both sleep disruption and cumulative sleep loss are problems (Nicholson, 1970; Preston and Bateman, 1970). A major problem in deciphering this question is the fact that aircrew members are pushed through demanding schedules by their airlines (Nicholson, 1972; Preston, 1974). Preston *et al.* (1973) studied stewardesses in the laboratory and were able to demonstrate significant decrements in performance associated with a laboratory simulated time zone shift. Sleep logs collected from the eight women in this laboratory study indicate a decrease in sleep period length in the four women administered the time zone change condition. Obviously, in-flight on the job aircrew performance and physiological measurement is an attractive approach which is difficult to conduct but does merit future research (Preston, 1978).

Time zone shift sleep polysomnographic recordings have been made from only a small number of individuals. In addition to suffering from study design errors of the sort inherent in many field studies, these observations fail to report a standard complement of sleep measures. The data suggest that time zone shifted sleep results in a decrease in sleep latency, an increase in the percentage of slow wave sleep (stages 3 and 4), and perhaps a decrease in absolute REM (rapid eye movement sleep) time. Total sleep time is not reported and we are not informed as to the specifics of the sleep period imposition in these studies. These time zone shifted sleep effects appear to be remarkably similar to those of the night shift worker (Walsh, Tepas, and Moss, 1981). This view emphasizes the problem of chronic sleep deprivation. Evans *et al.* (1972) comment that the results obtained in their sleep and time zone change study are more in keeping with the effects associated with total sleep deprivation than they are with the laboratory studies of acute time shifts. Endo, Yamamoto, and Sasaki (1978) conclude that time zone shifted sleep is a complicated summation of '. . . sleep deprivation, sleep reversal, nap, shift in sleep onset time and change in circadian rhythm'.

Studies of time zone shifts provide us with some of the most interesting findings if we consider their findings with regard to the issue of whether there is a parallelism between physiological measures and performance. Studies by Hauty and Adams (1966a,b,c) and Klein and his associates (Klein *et al.*, 1970; Klein, Wegmann and Hunt, 1972) do not report sleep data but they do relate rectal temperature and other physiological measures to various performance tasks. The results of these two groups of studies do not agree in many respects. These differences in findings may be related to differences in flight schedules, traveller home of origin, traveller demographics, or several other experimental design issues. It is unfortunate that many have concentrated on the differential findings of these studies when the similarities in their findings seem more relevant at this point. For both groups of studies, the results indicate quite clearly that physiological variables do not adjust to time zone shifts as fast as some performance variables. In each study there is evidence that not all performance variables adjust at the same rate and therefore it is implied that the rate of adjustment can be changed by performance task selection or manipulation. The data also agree in that they demonstrate that not all physiological variables adjust at the same rate.

The data of Endo, Yamamoto, and Sasaki (1978) play a very important role in spanning some gaps in the literature. In their field study they have shown that the pulse rate adaptation to time zone shifts can be slower and different from that of sleep. It also appears that in at least one of their studies the participants were aircrew members performing their usual duties. This does not appear to have been true in the Hauty and Adams studies or in the Klein studies which involved actual air flights. Although two of the polysomnographic subjects in the Evans study were experienced aircrew members, the significance of this cannot be clearly assessed from this study. Given the fact that there is little data published from field studies of experienced aircrew members while performing their usual duties, there is a clear need for additional research. As was true with studies of shift worker sleep, Monk and his colleagues have provided us with some interesting preliminary data which may indicate not all time zone shift effects need be clear decrements. A study of one subject suggests that when memory load is manipulated traveller rate of adaptation may be more rapid and adaptation time quite minimal (Monk *et al.*, 1978). As the authors note, this finding must be approached with caution and does call for further research.

In sum, the literature shows without question that time zone shifts do effect sleep. There is some data to suggest that the major effect on sleep is one of reducing sleep length and perhaps fragmenting sleep in a variety of ways. Clearly, there are time-of-flight/time-of-sleep interactions which are complex and the product of physiological, social, and job factors. Most would agree that time zone shifts can impair performance. However, there is reason to believe that effects can be manipulated or minimized. Unfortunately, there is a significant need for additional research since most of the studies reported to date involve very small samples and incomplete variable measurement. As with the shift work research, there is clear evidence that there need not be a firm parallelism between physiological measures and performance measures. Thus, research which depends upon a single performance measure or a single physiological measure to identify time zone shift hazards can be quite misleading.

Laboratory Shifted Sleep

In their study of three groups of college students, Taub and Berger (1973a,b; 1974a,b; 1976a,b,c) provide an excellent example of the sort of refinement possible with laboratory shifted sleep research. They also provide an excellent example of the limitations of laboratory shifted sleep research. In this study, the habitual sleep period of highly selected subjects was advanced, delayed, extended, shortened, or studied under habitual time conditions. Performance, mood, and polysomnographic measures were made. Advancing or delaying sleep had no effect on total sleep time and for the most part simply increased or decreased measures of sleep latency in a predictable direction. Extending or reducing the sleep period resulted in increases or decreases in total sleep time in the anticipated directions and also produced quite predictable sleep stage changes. Two, three, and four hour changes in sleep time period were used with treatment combinations administered only once in repeated measures designs.

Performance deficits were reported by Taub and Berger for the advanced and delayed sleep period conditions as well as those for extending and shortening sleep. They also interpret their data as showing that these effects are most evident in short sleepers. These findings are quite important for at least three reasons. First, they demonstrate that relatively small changes in habitual sleep period can result in sleep and performance deficits. Second, they demonstrate that performance measures can be more sensitive than the sleep measures in that performance decrements were frequently evident with no significant changes in total sleep time. Third, these results clearly demonstrate the importance of knowing the usual habits of participants in studies. Imposition of absolute timing schedules on individuals without knowledge of their usual choice with regard to such matters does not appear to be in order unless sample sizes are large enough to control for this. Since this study used highly selected male college students who were only administered a given treatment combination once, the results must be approached with caution and the findings may be strictly limited to acute exposure. Repeated exposure to such conditions with other populations might yield quite different results. It should also be noted that napping and drug use were prohibited in this study, something not characteristic of the real world, but a common limitation characteristic of laboratory shifted sleep model research studies.

Acute studies of this sort are helpful in elucidating probable variables for future consideration. They may apply directly to those situations in which inexperienced travellers make time zone shifts, or new workers experience rapidly changing shift work schemes for the first time. However, another approach to the laboratory shifted sleep research model is to study the performance of crews and individuals exposed to a specific work-rest cycle for days or months. A review of factors relevant to this approach will be found in Chapter III. These studies frequently use multiple performance tasks which have been arranged into a standard battery which can be repeatedly and automatically administered. Since some effort has been made to model these batteries in keeping with the demands of modern man-machine systems, they have been termed 'synthetic work' (Morgan, 1974).

A current review of synthetic work research findings (Alluisi, Coates, and Morgan, 1977) yields conclusions quite similar to those written by Ray, Martin, and Alluisi (1961) over 15 years earlier: 'Within broad limits, performance does not appear to vary significantly as a function of the work-rest cycle, provided the work-rest and sleep-wakefulness ratios are held constant and the period does not exceed one week.' Studies of continuous synthetic work with total sleep loss for periods as long as 48 hours in length demonstrate that the deficits produced are more pronounced in some tasks than in others. While this provides another example of the notion that performance and performance decrement are not unitary concepts, it is difficult to extrapolate these findings in a very specific way to other studies due to the fact that the tasks included in these test batteries are fairly unique and apparatus-bound. Perhaps the most significant contribution of these studies is their demonstration that time-of-day effects can interact with or be masked by on-going performance when a variety of stressors are introduced (Alluisi, 1972). The fault of this approach lies in its strength: it is difficult to evaluate the degree to which synthetic work is a valid substitute for real work. The fact that these studies most frequently use students as subjects makes this consideration even more important.

Laboratory studies of shift work have been pioneered by Colquhoun and his associates (Chapter III). Colquhoun (Colquhoun, Blake, and Edwards, 1968a,b; 1969) and Blake (1967) have made noble efforts to insure that laboratory results do not reflect the transient effects of being a guest in the laboratory, but rather the stabilized effects of a particular rotating or 'permanent' shift. These efforts have gradually evolved to the sophisticated and more current research of Folkard, Monk, and their colleagues (Folkard *et al.*, 1976; Monk *et al.*, 1978; Monk and Embrey, 1981; Folkard and Monk, 1981) which dramatically challenges many earlier research assumptions. Given the Kleitman suggestion that body temperature is a reasonable estimate of performance, many investigators have been willing to substitute temperature measurement for performance measurement. When temperature was measured, the expectation was that performance would vary with time of day so that maximum performance would occur in the middle of the waking period with minimal performance coming during the night and early morning hours. At best, this now appears to be an idealistic conception.

Folkard *et al.* (1976) had two students live in the laboratory. During this time they were placed on a rapidly rotating shift system having the following sequence: 2 days of rest, followed by 2 days on day shift, followed by 2 days on afternoon/evening shift, followed by 2 days on the night shift. This sequence was repeated until 18 days had passed and the study ended. This is the laboratory version of the so-called 'continental shift system'. On work days in the laboratory, the subjects did an industrial assembly task. A visual memory and search task (MAST) was used as the performance measure. This paper and pencil task varied memory load by varying the size of the target letter subset for which the subjects searched. Low MAST targets resulted in performance which paralleled the rectal temperature recordings in the traditionally expected manner. High MAST targets, however, resulted in performance in the opposite direction: performance was best around midnight and worst in the afternoon.

This clear evidence that performance is not a single rhythm has been confirmed by Monk and Embrey (1981) in a study of six computer operators on a rapidly rotating shift system. Froberg (1979) using a different performance task has also collected supportive information in a total sleep deprivation study. In this case, the high memory load task was a digit span test and the lower memory task was a simple coding test. Interestingly, the difference between the two tasks decreased as sleep deprivation increased with the high memory load task conforming more and more with the low memory load task and the temperature curve. Monk et al. (1978) have reported data from two subjects working 21 consecutive night shifts in the laboratory. High and low MAST targets were again used and this study provides additional evidence confirming their earlier studies as well as the notion that the various performance rhythms have different adaptation rates.

Laboratory shifted sleep research discussion would not be complete without reference to a series of studies examining the effects of non-24 hour days on sleep. Even when talking about night shift work or time zone shifted sleep, the initial unstated bias one exercises is one which anticipates that all sleep should fit a stereotype which assumes that the normal regimens of things is one whereby about 8 hours out of every 24 hours is dedicated to sleep. This also seems to carry with it the further assumption that is is normal for sleep to be linked with time of day just as it is true for other physiological and behavioural variables. Sleep researchers have examined this with the studies of sleep-wakefulness schedules other than 24 hours in length.

Webb (1978) provides an excellent review of studies in which the sleep–wake schedule has been longer or shorter than 24 hours. If one examines the percentage of the assigned sleep periods marked by polysomnographic signs of sleep, the data indicate that the percentage of sleep time decreases as the wake-sleep schedule gets longer or shorter than the traditional schedule of 8 hours of sleep and 16 hours of wakefulness. One should consider these findings in several ways. First, they are a clear demonstration that sleep is bound by time-of-day factors, just like most other physiological and performance measures. Second, they suggest that the time required to adapt or adjust to a new non-24 hour schedule may be a good way to separate different sleep variables. Third, perhaps we can think of different kinds of 'sleeps' just as we can think of different kinds of performance. Thus, we can contemplate correlation of various sleep type time-of-day functions with various performance time-of-day functions.

A final word of caution is in order. One must not forget that research following the laboratory shifted sleep model research approach can be quite misleading if directly accepted at face value. A study by Webb and Agnew (1978) provides one with a good example of this. This laboratory study placed six young adults on a rapidly rotating shift work schedule in the laboratory. The total sleep times for these subjects during base line recording and for each of the three shifts is shown in Figure 9. The data in this figure should be compared with data collected using the shift worker sleep model research approach. This was presented in Figure 7. The two sets of data agree in that sleep time was greatest for the afternoon/evening shift. However, the reduced sleep length characteristic of night shift worker sleep is not evident in the

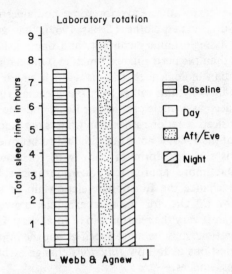

Figure 9   Mean sleep length in hours for subjects on a laboratory rapidly rotating shift schedule. Data from Webb and Agnew (1978)

laboratory rotation study. The laboratory study does an excellent job in demonstrating that sleep behaviours vary with shift, but fails to demonstrate the significant sleep reduction characteristic of night shift work. It also results in a general overestimation of the sleep length of actual shift workers. In this case, direct extrapolation from the laboratory to the field situation would be misleading. This is not a case of a laboratory study producing poor quality data, but rather a fine demonstration of a critical difference between many laboratory studies and the field situation. As Webb and Agnew note, the subjects in their study were unaffected by the general social environment and pressures characteristic of most shift work. Thus, this study provides indirect evidence of the degree to which social factors probably influence the real-world shift work situation.

DISCUSSION

As new scientific fields develop, the sorts of questions which are asked change. As Johnson *et al.* (1977) noted, sleep research started out asking if a person can function effectively without sleep. In the 1960s this question changed to asking if one type of sleep is more important than another. In the 1970s the question seemed to evolve around how much sleep do we need. This change in questions asked was part of a normal evolutionary developmental process whereby the naïveté of our initial question became apparent with the collection of additional knowledge and we moved on to a more sophisticated, yet equally naïve question. We are now ready for some new questions, and these are perhaps old questions in new clothes (Tepas, 1969). One can no longer think of performance as a single unitary concept, and one must study performance functions rather than *the* performance function. One can no longer think of a diurnal or circadian biological rhythm as a single unitary concept, and one must study circadian rhythms rather than *the* circadian function. One can no longer think of sleep as a single problem or issue, and one must think how the various forms of sleep function rather than what is *the* function of sleep.

The question of the 1980s is not *a* question but rather questions. It is not, for example, what is the best form of shift work or how does sleep effect performance. One more appropriate question might be: how does the continental shift change the functional relationship of sleep REM time to MAST performance? Or, for another example, how does duration on permanent night shift vary the relationship of total sleep time to vigilance task hit rate? The questions may be more specific, but the important thing is that we are asking questions as to how *functions* change or how the relationship between functions changes.

This new sophistication may be a timely development. The electronic revolution may increase the monotony of many industrial jobs. Should this be the case, our existing literature will serve us well as we attempt to solve night work problems associated with the performance of relatively simple tasks. However, it is quite reasonable to suggest that many of these simple tasks will be performed in the future by robots and automated devices. This leaves man available to perform the more complex problem-solving tasks. As has been pointed out in this chapter and in Chapter III, there are many reasons to suggest that different time-of-day functions fit these tasks. Should this be the case, there will be a pressing need for additional research. Dated approaches which assume that performance varies with time of day in a simple way could yield some quite disastrous applications efforts.

Shift work research, time zone shift studies, and laboratory shifted sleep studies have all demonstrated that shift work, sleep, and performance are not simple variables influenced in a fairly direct and identical manner by time of day. Although synchrony of physiological and performance variables may be common, desynchrony of these variables may be more the rule than the exception under real world conditions. In a similar vein, the current love affair with the sine wave should not lead us astray (see Chapter II). Reinberg *et al.* (1978), for example, have made a noble effort to calculate acrophase data from more than one shift work study in an effort to determine if the amplitude of the circadian rhythm is related to the ability of shift workers to adjust rapidly to shift changes. This may be a productive approach for some problems, but we should never assume that all time-of-day functional relationships will fit the same mathematical model. One wonders how often in the past investigators have discarded data simply because it did not fit the sine wave temperature model. Let us hope that there is a growing willingness to explore apparent functional relationships taking other forms.

What we are proposing is that there is an evolution in our thought about time schedules and performance which has and is developing as we refine our methods and improve our data base. As Williams, Lubin, and Goodnow (1959) pointed out in their classic study of total sleep deprivation, the initial problem is one of finding sensitive performance measures. As we develop sophistication in our performance measurement, parallel changes in our constructs must be developed and used. Lacy (1967) pointed out over 10 years ago that the term 'arousal' does not refer to a simple single process, but rather to several complexes of arousal process which need not occur simultaneously. Workers in the timing/performance areas of research commonly continue to treat terms like activation and arousal as if they were simple non-actuarial entities. Most of the conceptions used by workers in the time/performance area beg for more sophisticated conceptual development. It is, for example, not enough to simply develop a sensitive performance task said to be a memory and search task. The concept of memory load must be more fully developed to make it less task specific in the sense that the concept can easily be allocated to other task and data banks.

Two of our model research approaches are oriented towards real-world field research observation whereas the remaining model research approach fits more with the traditional notion of isolated, more basic perhaps, laboratory research. In practice, however, the research reviewed provides an outstanding example of how the distinction between applied and basic research has become quite fuzzy. Investigators, methods, and subject populations are moving in and out of the laboratory with ease as dictated by practical or philosophical matters. This is a fine example for investigators in other areas of research who have not as yet been as liberated from the traditions of their training. However, it is important to note this liberty has also frequently been characterized by an inferior regard for traditional concerns with issues of sample size, subject selection, and data selection. The need for improvement along these lines is obvious to almost any reader of the literature, and more concern for these matters is in order if the exciting findings in these areas of research are to have more widespread scientific acceptance and public use.

Data gathered by all three model research approaches manifests the importance of social factors in effecting many of the findings. Indeed, as was pointed out earlier, it is also noted that the findings of this research are relevant to the everyday activity of a large percentage of the population. Although technological developments may be pressing humans to use time in more different ways, the issues of choice and flexibility also appear to be growing concerns. The Glickman and Brown (1974) report on changing schedules of work makes this quite clear. Webb and Agnew (1975) have suggested that much of our working population is 'job-bound' in that they can go to sleep when they wish but must get up at a specific time to go to work. The result, they suggest, is sleep deprivation. Inflexible working hours result in sleep deprivation, since people appear to choose to stay up later. Some work shifts do not result in people getting up to go to work. These shifts, as well as various forms of flexi-time work, are not as job-bound with regard to sleep. Since various forms of shift work and flexi-time may both be on the increase, it is reasonable to sugest that a growing percentage of the working population will in fact have additional choices available to them with regard to when they work and when they sleep. Although in absolute time this increased flexibility may be quite small, it probably does represent a significant social intervention which deserves scientific examination. One should not forget that perhaps the majority of US workers do not have to report when they are in and on the job (Feinsilber and Mead, 1980).

The introduction of one additional variable, flexibility *vs* inflexibility of working hours, provides a good example of the wide range of problems still left for exploration. Figure 10 is a preliminary effort to provide a systematic classification of the many work schedule phenomena which probably exist in our society. Under both flexible and inflexible hours categories, one has both permanent and rotating shifts. The terms 'chronic' and 'acute' refer to how long a person has worked on a particular shift system and allows us to include both laboratory and field studies within one figure. Clearly, this scheme does not allow the classification of all possible work schedules. For example, it does not take note of the direction in which changes are made or whether changes are made in a voluntary manner. It ignores many social and physiological variables which one knows deserve consideration. It does, however, provide a convenient way to visualize some of the shift variables which are or will require study. Above all, this chart makes our current ignorance of time and performance relationships quite clear.

Intervention and extrapolation to new subject populations and problems is an important and testy issue. For example, little research data has been gathered from women. Akerstedt and Froberg (1977) have reported what may be the first study of the effects of sleep deprivation on normal women. Many years ago, Mellette *et al.* (1951) reported that the time-of-day variations in body temperature are different for men and women. They report differences in time of temperature minimum and maximum as well as differences in level and rate of change. The Akerstedt and Froberg (1977) modest suggestion that women may respond to sleep deprivation differently from men, together with this study of temperature change differences, suggest that sex is an important variable for future consideration given the fact that more and more women are joining the working population.

The origin of the shift schemes practised in most industrial plants is not known, but it seems reasonable to suggest that they were based on factors other than scientific fact. In the future, we can expect the scientist to play a

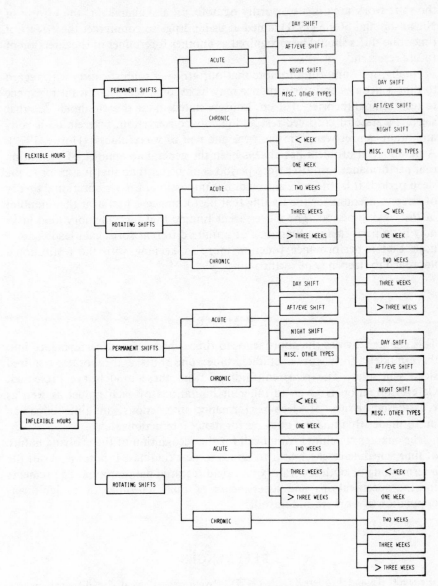

Figure 10   Proposed classification of work schedule phenomena

more active role as new shift work schemes are contemplated. This has already occurred in the time zone shifted research area where Graeber, Sing, and Cuthbert (1981) have made a pioneering effort to counteract the effects of transmeridian flight. The efforts of Ehret (1981) to extrapolate animal data to the shift work area is also worthy of note. In a similar light, the efforts of Nicholson and Stone (1981) aimed at using drugs to counteract the effects of time zone shifts should be recognized as another forerunner of the direction of future research.

Finally, it is important to note that our growing sophistication with regard to time schedules and performance may have some very significant relevance to restitutional theories of sleep. Loosely stated, these theories hold '. . . that sleep is a state of enforced rest and energy conservation, wherein both body and brain can recover from the wear and tear of wakefulness' (Horne, 1979). A paradoxical problem has always been the general acceptance of the notion that performance just after sleep period is no better than that just prior to the sleep period. It is difficult, although not impossible, for a restitutional theory of sleep to account for the finding that performance is best near the midpoint of the waking period. The more recent finding that high memory load tasks may have performance functions of a quite different sort again leads one to hope that a performance function more in keeping with the restitutional approach to sleep may be forthcoming.

SUMMARY

This chapter divides the approaches to time schedules and performance into three models: shift worker studies, time zone shifts and laboratory shifted sleep schedules. The research findings from these models are presented. Careful attention is given to inherent limitations of each model as well as cross-design issues of sleep–performance interactions, multiple circadian performance rhythms and time–performance interactions.

The chapter concludes with a call for the recognition of the evolving nature of time schedule research as it responds to new findings. It notes issues of the intermeshing of both laboratory and field research data into the requirements for the specifications and assessments of time schedules of a significant population of workers and travellers.

REFERENCES

Akerstedt, T. and Froberg, J. E. (1977). Psychophysiological circadian rhythms in women during 72 h of sleep deprivation. *Waking and Sleeping* 1, 387–394.

Alluisi, E. A. (1972). Influence of work–rest scheduling and sleep loss on sustained performance. In: *Aspects of Human Efficiency*. W. P. Colquhoun (Ed.). London, English Universities Press.

Alluisi, E. A., Coates, G. D., and Morgan, B. B. Jr. (1977). Effects of temporal stressors on vigilance and information processing. In: *Vigilance: Theory, Operational Performance, and Physiological Correlates*. R. R. Mackie (Ed.). New York, Plenum.

Armstrong, D., Tepas, D. I., and Moss, P. D. (1980). Sleep reports from two samples of rotating shift workers. *Sleep Research* 9, 267.

Blake, M. J. F. (1967). Time of day effects on performance in a range of tasks. *Psychonomic Science* 9, 349-350.

Bjerner, B., Holm, A., and Swensson, A. (1955). Diurnal variation in mental performance; a study of three-shift workers. *British Journal of Industrial Medicine* 12, 103-110.

Browne, R. C. (1949). The day and night performance of teleprinter switchboard operators. *Occupational Psychology* 23, 121-126.

Carpentier, J. and Cazamian, P. (1977). *Night Work*. Geneva, International Labour Office.

Chiles, W. D., Alluisi, E. A., and Adams, O. S. (1968). Work schedules and performance during confinement. *Human Factors* 10, 143-196.

Colquhoun, W. P., Blake, M. J. F., and Edwards, R. S. (1968a). Experimental studies of shift-work I: A comparison of 'rotating' and 'stabilized' 4-hour shift systems. *Ergonomics* 11, 437-453.

Colquhoun, W. P., Blake, M. J. F., and Edwards, R. S. (1968b). Experimental studies of shift-work II: Stabilized 8-hour shift systems. *Ergonomics* 11, 527-546.

Colquhoun, W. P., Blake, M. J. F., and Edwards, R. S. (1969). Experimental studies of shift-work III: Stabilized 12-hour shift systems. *Ergonomics* 12, 865-882.

Edmunds, L. N. Jr. (1976). Models and mechanisms for endogenous timekeeping. In: *An Introduction to Biological Rhythms*. J. D. Palmer (Ed.). New York, Academic.

Ehret, C. F. (1981). New approaches to chronohygiene for the shift-worker in the nuclear power industry. In: *Night and Shift Work: Biological and Social Aspects*. A. Reinberg, N. Vieux, and P. Andlauer (Eds.). Oxford, Pergamon.

Endo, S., Yamamoto, T., and Sasaki, M. (1978). Effects of time zone changes on sleep: West-East flight and East-West flight. *Jikeikai Medical Journal* 25, 249-268.

Evans, J. I., Christie, G. A., Lewis, S. A., Daly, J., and Moore-Robinson, M. (1972). Sleep and time zone changes. *Archives of Neurology* 26, 36-48.

Feinsilber, M. and Mead, W. B. (1980). *American Averages*. New York, Doubleday.

Folkard, S., Knauth, P., Monk, T. H., and Rutenfranz, J. (1976). The effect of memory load on the circadian variation in performance efficiency under a rapidly rotating shift system. *Ergonomics* 19, 479-488.

Folkard, S. and Monk, T. H. (1981). Individual differences in the circadian response to a weekly rotating shift system. In: *Night and Shift Work: Biological and Social Aspects*. A. Reinberg, N. Vieux, and P. Andlauer (Eds.). Oxford, Pergamon.

Foret, J. and Lantin, G. (1972). The sleep of train drivers: An example of the effects of irregular work schedules on sleep. In: *Aspects of Human Efficiency*. W. P. Colquhoun (Ed.). London, English Universities Press.

Froberg, J. E. (1979). *Performance in Tasks differing in Memory Load and its Relationship with Habitual Activity Phase and Body Temperature*. Stockholm, Forsvarets Forskningsanstalt FOA rapport C 52002-H6.

Glickman, A. S. and Brown, Z. H. (1974). *Changing Schedules of Work*. Kalamazoo, W. E. Upjohn Institute for Employment Research.

Graeber, R. C., Sing, H. C., and Cuthbert, B. N. (1981). The impact of transmeridian flight on deploying soldiers. In: *The Twenty-Four Hour Workday: Proceedings of a Symposium on Variations in Work–Sleep Schedules*. L. C. Johnson, D. I. Tepas, W. P. Colquhoun, and M. J. Colligan (Eds.). Cincinnati, DHHS (NIOSH), 81-127.

Halberg, F. (1969a). Chronobiology. *Annual Review of Physiology* 31, 675-725.

Halberg, F. (1969b). Circadian system of nonhuman primates. In: *Circadian Rhythms in Nonhuman Primates*. F. H. Rohles (Ed.). Basel/New York, S. Karger.

Hauty, G. T. and Adams, T. (1966a). Phase shifts of the human circadian system and performance deficit during the periods of transition: I. East-West flight. *Aerospace Medicine* 37, 668–674.

Hauty, G. T. and Adams, T. (1966b). Phase shifts of the human circadian system and performance deficit during the periods of transition: II. West-East flight. *Aerospace Medicine* 37, 1027–1033.

Hauty, G. T. and Adams, T. (1966c). Phase shifts of the human circadian system and performance deficit during the periods of transition: III. North-South flight. *Aerospace Medicine* 37, 1257–1262.

Horne, J. A. (1979). Restitution and human sleep: A critical review. *Physiological Psychology* 7, 115–125.

Johnson, L. C., Naitoh, J. M., Moses, J. M., and Lubin, A. (1977). Variations in sleep schedules. *Waking and Sleeping* 1, 133–137.

Klein, K. E., Bruner, H., Holtman, H., Rehme, H., Stolze, J., Steinhoff, W. D., and Wegmann, H. M. (1970). Circadian rhythms of pilots' efficiency and effects of multiple time zone travel. *Aerospace Medicine* 41, 125–132.

Klein, K. E., Wegmann, H. M., and Hunt, B. I. (1972). Desynchronization of body temperature and performance circadian rhythm as a result of outgoing and home-going transmeridian flights. *Aerospace Medicine* 43, 119–132.

Kleitman, N. (1933). Studies on the physiology of sleep VIII. Diurnal variation in performance. *American Journal of Physiology* 104, 449–456.

Kleitman, N. (1939). *Sleep and Wakefulness.* Chicago, University of Chicago Press.

Kleitman, N. (1963). *Sleep and Wakefulness* (2nd edn) Chicago, University of Chicago Press.

Kleitman, N. and Jackson, D. P. (1950). Body temperature and performance under different routines. *Journal of Applied Physiology* 3, 309–328.

Knauth, P. and Rutenfranz, J. (1972). Untersuchungen zum problem des schlafver-haltens bei experimenteller schichtarbeit. *International Archives Arbeitsmed* 30, 1–22.

Kripke, D. F., Cook, B., and Lewis, O. F. (1971). Sleep of night workers: EEG recordings. *Psychophysiology* 7, 377–384.

Lacy, J. I. (1967). Somatic response patterning and stress: Some revisions of activation theory. In: *Psychological Stress.* M. H. Appley and R. Trumbull (Eds.). New York, Appleton-Century-Crofts.

Lobban, M. C. and Tredre, B. E. (1966). Daily rhythms of renal excretion in human subjects with irregular hours of work. *Journal of Physiology* 185, 139–140.

Maurice, M. (1975). *Shift Work.* Geneva, International Labour Office.

Melbin, M. (1978). Night as frontier. *American Sociological Review* 43, 3–22.

Mellette, H. C., Hutt, B. K., Askovitz, S. E., and Horvath, S. M. (1951). Diurnal variation in body temperatures. *Journal of Applied Physiology* 3, 665–675.

Monk, T. H. and Embrey, D. E. (1981). A field study of circadian rhythms in actual and interpolated task performance. In: *Night and Shift Work: Biological and Social Aspects.* A. Reinberg, N. Vieux, and P. Andlauer (Eds.). Oxford, Pergamon.

Monk, T. H., Knauth, P., Folkard, S., and Rutenfranz, J. (1978). Memory based performance measures in studies of shiftwork. *Ergonomics* 21, 819–826.

Morgan, B. B. Jr. (1974). Effects of continuous work and sleep loss in the reduction and recovery of work efficiency. *American Industrial Hygiene Association Journal* 35, 13–20.

Mott, P. E., Mann, F. C., McLoughlin, Q., and Warwick, D. P. (1965). *Shift Work.* Ann Arbor, University of Michigan Press.

Nicholson, A. N. (1970). Sleep patterns of an airline pilot operating world-wide East-West routes. *Aerospace Medicine* 41, 626–632.

Nicholson, A. N. (1972). Duty hours and sleep patterns in aircrew operating world-wide routes. *Aerospace Medicine* **43**, 138–141.

Nicholson, A. N. and Stone, B. N. (1981). Hypnotics and shiftwork. In: *The Twenty-Four Hour Workday: Proceedings of a Symposium on Variations in Work-Sleep Schedules*. L. C. Johnson, D. I. Tepas, W. P. Colquhoun, and M. J. Colligan (Eds.). Cincinnati, DHHS (NIOSH) 467–492.

Ostberg, O. (1973). Interindividual differences in circadian fatigue patterns of shift workers. *British Journal of Industrial Medicine* **30**, 341–351.

Patkai, P., Akerstedt, T., and Pettersson, K. (1977). Field studies of shiftwork: I. Temporal patterns in psychophysiological activation in permanent night workers. *Ergonomics* **20**, 611–619.

Preston, F. S. (1974). Physiological problems in air cabin crew. *Proceedings of the Royal Society of Medicine* **67**, 23–27.

Preston, F. S. (1978). Temporal discord. *Journal of Psychosomatic Research* **22**, 377–383.

Preston, F. S. and Bateman, S. C. (1970). Effect of time zone changes on the sleep patterns of BOAC B. 707 crews on world-wide schedules. *Aerospace Medicine* **41**, 1409–1415.

Preston, F. S., Bateman, S. C., Short, R. V., and Wilkinson, R. T. (1973). Effects of flying and of time changes on menstrual cycle length and on performance in airline stewardesses. *Aerospace Medicine* **44**, 438–443.

Ray, J. T., Martin, O. E. Jr., and Alluisi, E. A. (1961). *Human performance as a function of the work-rest cycle*. Washington, National Academy of Sciences—National Research Council Publication No. 882.

Reinberg, A. (1970). Evaluation of circadian dyschronism during transmeridian flights. *Life Sciences and Space Research* **8**, 172–174.

Reinberg, A., Vieux, N., Ghata, J., Chaumont, A., and Laporte, A. (1978). Is the rhythm amplitude related to the ability to phase-shift circadian rhythms of shift-workers? *Journal of Physiology (Paris)* **74**, 405–409.

Rutenfranz, J. and Colquhoun, W. P. (1979). Circadian rhythms in human performance. *Scandinavian Journal of Work Environment and Health* **5**, 167–177.

Rutenfranz, J., Colquhoun, W. P., Knauth, P., and Ghata, J. N. (1977). Biomedical and psychosocial aspects of shift work. *Scandinavian Journal of Work Environment and Health* **3**, 165–182.

Rutenfranz, J., Knauth, P., and Angersbach, D. (1981). Shift work research issues. In: *The Twenty-Four Hour Workday: Proceedings of a Symposium on Variations in Work-Sleep Schedules*. L. C. Johnson, D. I. Tepas, W. P. Colquhoun, and M. J. Colligan (Eds.). Cincinnati, DHHS (NIOSH) 221–260.

Strughold, H. (1952). Physiological day–night cycle in global flights. *Aviation Medicine* **23**, 464–473.

Tasto, D. L. and Colligan, M. J. (1977). *Shift Work Practices in the United States*. Washington, HEW (NIOSH) No. 77-148.

Tasto, D. L., Colligan, M. J., Skjei, E. W., and Polly, S. J. (1978). *Health Consequences of Shift Work*. Washington, HEW (NIOSH) 78-154.

Taub, J. M. and Berger, R. J. (1973a). Performance and mood following variations in the length and timing of sleep. *Psychophysiology* **10**, 559–570.

Haub, J. M. and Berger, R. J. (1973b). Sleep stage patterns associated with acute shifts in the sleep–wakefulness cycle. *Electroencephalography and Clinical Neurophysiology* **35**, 613–619.

Taub, J. M. and Berger, R. J. (1974a). Acute shifts in sleep–wakefulness cycle: Effects on performance and mood. *Psychosomatic Medicine* **36**, 164–173.

Taub, J. M. and Berger, R. J. (1974b). Effects of acute shifts in circadian rhythms of sleep and wakefulness on performance and mood. In: *Chronobiology*. L. E. Scheving, F. Halberg, and J. E. Pauly (Eds.). Tokyo, Igaku Shoin.

Taub, J. M. and Berger, R. J. (1976a). The effects of changing the phase and duration of sleep. *Journal of Experimental Psychology: Human Perception and Performance* 2, 30–41.

Taub, J. M. and Berger, R. J. (1976b). Effects of acute sleep pattern alternation depend upon sleep duration. *Physiological Psychology* 4, 412–420.

Taub, J. M. and Berger, R. J. (1976c). Altered sleep duration and sleep period time displacement: Effects on performance in habitual long sleepers. *Physiology and Behavior* 16, 177–184.

Tepas, D. I. (1969). Are stages of sleep really necessary? *Activas Nervosa Superior (Prague)* 11, 82–89.

Tepas, D. I. (1976). Methodological pitfalls of shift work research. In: *Shift Work and Health*. P. G. Rentos and R. D. Shepard (Eds.). Washington, HEW (NIOSH) No. 76-203.

Tepas, D. I. (1979). Methodological approaches to the study of shiftwork: Introduction. *Behavior Research Methods and Instrumentation* 11, 3–4.

Tepas, D. I., Walsh, J. K., and Armstrong, D. (1981). Comprehensive study of the sleep of shift workers. In: *The Twenty-Four Hour Workday: Proceedings of a Symposium on Variations in Work–Sleep Schedules*. L. C. Johnson, D. I. Tepas, W. P. Colquhoun, and M. J. Colligan (Eds.). Cincinnati, DHHS (NIOSH) 419–434.

Tepas, D. I., Walsh, J. K., Moss, P. D., and Armstrong, D. (1981). Polysomnographic correlates of shift worker performance in the laboratory. In: *Night and Shift Work: Biological and Social Aspects*. A. Reinberg, N. Vieux, and P. Andlauer (Eds.). Oxford, Pergamon.

Van Loon, J. H. (1963). Diurnal body temperature curves in shift workers. *Ergonomics* 6, 267–273.

Walsh, J. K., Tepas, D. I., and Moss, P. D. (1981). The EEG sleep of night and rotating shift workers. In: *The Twenty-Four Hour Workday: Proceedings of a Symposium on Variations in Work–Sleep Schedules*. L. C. Johnson, D. I. Tepas, W. P. Colquhoun, and M. J. Colligan (Eds.). Cincinnati, DHHS (NIOSH) 451–466.

Webb, W. B. (1977). Schedules of work and sleep. In: *Sleep 1976*. W. D. Koella and P. Levin (Eds.). Basel/New York, S. Karger.

Webb, W. B. (1978). The forty-eight hour day. *Sleep* 1, 191–197.

Webb, W. B. and Agnew, H. W. Jr. (1975). Are we chronically sleep deprived? *Bulletin of the Psychonomic Society* 6, 47–48.

Webb, W. B. and Agnew, H. W. Jr. (1978). Effects of rapidly rotating shifts on sleep patterns and sleep structures. *Aviation, Space, and Environmental Medicine* 49, 384–389.

Webb, W. B., Agnew, H. W. Jr., and Williams, R. L. (1971). Effect on sleep of a sleep period time displacement. *Aerospace Medicine* 42, 152–155.

Wedderburn, A. A. I. (1975). EEG and self-recorded sleep of two shiftworkers over four weeks of real and synthetic work. In: *Experimental Studies of Shiftwork*. W. P. Colquhoun, S. Folkard, P. Knauth, and J. Rutenfranz (Eds.). Opladen, Westdeutscher Verlag.

Weitzman, E. D., Kripke, D. F., Goldmacher, D., McGregor, P., and Nogeire, C. (1970). Acute reversal of the sleep-waking cycle in man: Effect on sleep stage patterns. *Archives of Neurology* 22, 438–489.

Wilkinson, R. T. (1968). Sleep deprivation: Performance tests for partial and selective sleep deprivation. *Progress in Clinical Psychology* 8, 28–43.

Williams, H. L., Lubin, A., and Goodnow, J. J. (1959). Impaired performance with acute sleep loss. *Psychological Monographs* 73, No. 14.

Chapter 8

Performance during Sleep

Michael Bonnet

The eye—it cannot choose but see;
We cannot bid the ear be still;
Our bodies feel, where'er they be
Against or with our will.

William Wordsworth

INTRODUCTION

This chapter is concerned with the capacity of humans to perform during sleep. It will present data indicating that persons are differentially sensitive to stimulation and that their thresholds are modified by the characteristics of the stimulus and a wide range of variables such as the sensory modality and sleep level, age, and individual differences. This constitutes the first half of the chapter. The second half treats the differentiation and modifiability of responding while asleep and considers the topics of discrimination, generalization, habituation, and extinction, as well as such higher order variables as stimulus meaningfulness, learning, and memory.

Finally, in light of the findings on perception and learning, speculation on the reasons for performance change and the range of possible performances during sleep will be made.

REACTION TO STIMULI

The experimental study of sleep can be dated to 1862 when Kohlschutter, a student of Fechner, questioned his master concerning his statement that it was not possible to measure the depth of sleep (Wohlisch, 1957). Kohlschutter (1862), using a sound pendulum, determined auditory thresholds during sleep on a single subject. This curve, based on 74 arousals over eight experimental nights, was a very good approximation of the prior description of the trend of 'general unconsciousness' given by Fechner. Selected data points (Swan, 1929) showed an early maximum threshold followed by a logarithmic curve of threshold decay.

In the next 40 years, four threshold studies were reported. The studies included replication of the auditory threshold results (Moenninghoff and Piesbergen, 1883; Michelson, 1897), threshold to electric shock in children (Czerny, 1896), and an elegant study of pressure thresholds (DeSanctis and Neyroz, 1902) in which there was a clear 90–120 minute rhythmicity.

Kleitman and his students in the 1930s studied the relationships between time asleep, motility, and auditory thresholds (Mullin, Kleitman, and Cooperman, 1933, 1937; Mullin, 1937; Mullin and Kleitman, 1938). Movement time per hour showed an increase across the night which inversely paralleled Kohlschutter's degree of sleep curve. There was an initial rise of threshold for the first 25 minutes after sleep onset which was maintained for some 25 minutes followed by a rapid decrease. Thresholds were found related to body movements, increasing as a function of elapsed time after a body movement.

During the 1930s the electroencephalogram was first used as a measure of sleep behaviour by Blake and Gerard (1937). They published the initial paper relating EEG 'stages' to thresholds. They presented a constant intensity, 1000 Hz tone for one minute during episodes of different brain rhythms, verbally asked subjects if they were awake and measured response times. Their conclusions set the standards which were to hold for more than 20 years. At a relatively high level of excitation (awake, resting) thresholds were low, and relatively fast frequency alpha was seen. The relationship of delta activity (slow wave activity) to sleep depth was quite striking. A curve of data averaged from five subjects across ten nights showed an almost perfect correspondence between the predominance of delta in each hour and the response rate to a tone presented at various times across the night. Both curves corresponded well with Kohlschutter's hypothesized curve of the depth of sleep. There was a smooth decline and no secondary peak. Blake and Gerard did not convincingly deal with the low voltage sleep EEG (presently associated with both stage 1 light sleep and REM sleep) but stated that it was to be considered a transition between the alpha and delta states and, therefore, that the awakening thresholds also fell in the middle ranges between waking and deep sleep.

The ensuing years have resulted in intensive and extensive experimentation on threshold values during sleep in terms of stimulus parameters, response dimensions, and such within subject variables as sleep stage, drugs, prior wakefulness, time of night, circadian effects and individual differences. These will be examined in turn.

Audition. The great majority of sleep threshold studies have used auditory stimuli, and there are representative studies in each of the classes listed above. Several studies have used an ascending method of limits (Rechtschaffen and

Lentzner, 1960; Shapiro, Goodenough, and Gryler, 1963; Goodenough *et al.*, 1965; Watson and Rechtschaffen 1969; Zimmerman, 1970; Keefe, Johnson, and Hunter, 1971; Bonnet, Johnson, and Webb, 1978). As a representative example, Rechtschaffen and Lentzner (1960) presented a 500 Hz tone for 5 seconds at assumed waking threshold. If the subject did not respond, the tone was repeated at an intensity 5 dB greater after a pause of 10 seconds. Intensity was increased until the subject responded. The results indicated that sleep stages are monotonically related to sleep depth in terms of intensity (stage 4 deepest; stage 1 lightest). Unfortunately, perhaps because background noise differs among sleep labs, reported threshold values differ greatly from lab to lab (from 36 dB to 91 dB in stage 4, for example). However, as an indication of the typical magnitude of threshold values, the average values in one study using an ascending series of 1000 Hz tones (30 seconds apart) were: stage 2, 70 dB; stage 4, 92 dB; REM 83 dB (Bonnet, Johnson, and Webb, 1978).

Some studies have employed the method of constant stimuli (Williams *et al.*, 1964; Rechtschaffen, Hauri, and Zeitlin, 1966). The results with this method of stimulus presentation agreed well with the studies using the method of limits. The overall response threshold was 65 dB. Fewest responses at a specific intensity were seen in stages 3 and 4, and more were seen in REM and stage 2, which did not differ.

Another primary aspect of an auditory signal is its frequency. Ashton (1971) examined infants' responsivity (several different body movements) to an 85 dB tone at the frequencies of 75, 95, 115, and 135 Hz. There were no obvious differences due to frequency. Weir (1976) examined responsiveness to 75 dB tones over six frequencies ranging from 70 to 2000 Hz, and found increased responsiveness at 120 and 250 Hz irrespective of sleep state. The author speculated that such special sensitivity might occur because infant and adult speech sound load primarily within the range of these two frequencies. A pair of studies on adults by Levere *et al.* (1973, 1974) also found greater responsiveness to lower frequencies, but only in slow wave sleep.

The few studies of the effects of stimulus rise time have given contradicting results. Oswald, Taylor, and Treisman (1960) found slow rise times more effective in producing responses while Rechtschaffen, Hauri, and Zeitlin (1966) found high thresholds with slowly increasing stimuli due to dream incorporation. Levere *et al.* (1976) found fast rise time stimuli more effective in producing increased cortical desynchronization than slow rise stimuli, but only in slow wave sleep.

A final stimulus parameter area is complexity, which refers to other than pure tone stimuli. It is possible to mathematically equate sounds that vary along several dimensions. For example, intensity (dB) may be weighted for the approximate sensitivity of the human ear to to different frequencies (dBA), for the frequency band (weighted) intensity or noiseness (PNdB), for the duration of the stimulus (E), or for the impulse characteristics (ic) of a sound among other things (Kryter, 1970). Using these various definitions of sound intensity, Lukas (1973) constructed several correlation matrices from his own and other data to try to find which particular measures related most highly to various forms of sleep disruption. In his initial results, it was concluded that the measures of maximum dBA, and PNdB, and the measures with impulse correction added were the best predictors, but those results were based on only six subjects and did not agree completely with the results of other studies from which Lukas had been able to extract appropriate data. In a 1975 paper (Lukas, Peeler, and Davis, 1975), in which there were twelve subjects, the highest correlations were again seen with maximum dBA and PNdB. The response measure which was correlated most highly with the stimulus parameters in both studies was the percentage of responses which involved less than a sleep stage shift, and the corresponding correlations were greater than 0.9 in all cases.

In a recent review of the effects of noise on sleep, Lukas (1975) has collected data from several investigators and plotted dBA and PNdB level against percentage of subjects awakened or aroused and also against the probability of no sleep disruption. Perhaps, the most impressive finding by Lukas is the relation between sound level in EPNdB and probability of no sleep disruption. Data from seven separate studies were plotted, showing an obviously linear relationship (the correlation was −0.77). No sleep disruption was seen below 70 EPNdB and 50% disruption was seen around 93 EPNdB.

Studies using words or speech sound combinations will be reviewed under the topic of discrimination.

Tactile. In the tactile sense, three types of threshold—pain, pressure, and temperature—have been measured. Pisano *et al.* (1966) studied responsiveness to a shock on the arm. Both long duration pulses (7–10 seconds) and one second trains of brief pulses were used, but no differential results as a function of stimulus duration were reported. Threshold in stage 1 was significantly lower than threshold in stages 2, 3–4, or REM. Wolff (1967) measured infant responsivity to pain (tickling), touch, and sound stimuli. The tickling that Wolff classified as 'pain' was induced by 'stroking a cotton wisp three times across the nasolabial fold'; touch by moving the finger three times across the umbilicus; and sound by ringing a bell three times. Infants were more responsive (in terms of mobility change) to the pain than to the touch, and more sensitive to the touch than to the sound in both 'quiet' and 'active' (REM) sleep (Chapter III). Since differences in the response to the different stimuli were almost non-existent during waking, the implication is that the infant, at least, is predisposed to respond to the tickling pain differentially over sound and touch during sleep as compared to waking.

Temperature. The single study involving temperature as a stimulus was reported by Schmidt and Birns (1971) and involved the applications of a chilled coin to the abdomen of a sleeping infant. No differences were found between 'quiet' and 'active' sleep, although a general trend of less responsiveness during quiet sleep is seen in the data.

Visual. Four studies have examined the effect of visual stimuli on threshold during sleep. Unfortunately, across study comparisons are impossible because only one study (Johnson and Lockwood, 1972) reports anything corresponding to an intensity or duration of the visual stimulus (a 15 watt light bulb was used). Fischgold and Schwartz (1960) employed a single flash from a stroboscope, while Okuma *et al.* (1966) presented 3–6 flashes from a stroboscopic bulb at a rate of one per second. Nakamura, Iwahara, and Fulisawa (1966) presented 5–10 flashes per trial but no further details were specified. The studies are in agreement, however, that responsiveness to constant level stimuli generally diminishes from wake to stage 4. Responsiveness was as great or greater in REM than in stage 2 in the three studies testing REM sleep thresholds.

Olfaction. Murray and Campbell (1970) have reported olfactory thresholds during sleep in infants. Amyl acetate was used in a geometric progression of concentrations ranging from 1.56% to 100% in an ascending series with a 60 second interstimulus interval. The distribution of responses was quite amazing. In 'active' sleep, the peak response was to the lowest concentration, while during 'quiet' sleep it was to the highest. There was no overlap in distribution.

Vestibular. Reding and Fernandez (1968) reported the single study of vestibular stimulation during sleep. Children sleeping in a chair were rotated one complete revolution every ten minutes throughout the night. The normal waking response to this stimulus is nystagmus. The results showed nystagmus (as measured by EOG) to be greatly suppressed in all stages of NREM sleep (less than 1% of the trials), but present in about 50% of REM trials.

While our knowledge of the effects of various auditory stimulus parameters upon arousal threshold is fairly extensive, very little is known concerning other sensory modalities. No one has seriously attempted to collect multi-modality threshold data in waking and sleeping subjects to test for differential threshold shifts as a function of state.

Response Variables

Perception and performance are virtually always defined in terms of production of appropriate responses. Many different types of response have been recorded from sleeping subjects. Their major categories are the cortical responses, averaged and ongoing EEG changes, and behavioural responses such as button pushes.

Evoked potentials. The early work of Davis *et al.* (1939) showed the possibility of obtaining discrete cortical response during sleep to an auditory stimulus. The development of computer summating techniques has permitted detailed analysis of this evoked brain activity to stimuli. Components of auditory evoked potentials are generally defined in terms of their latency. The components of the first 50 milliseconds after the stimulus are the brief latency components and those of more than 50 milliseconds the middle and long latency components.

The short latency components trace the path of the signal from the ear to the brain. Studies by Amadeo and Shagass (1973), Mendel (1974), and Kupperman and Mendal (1974) have consistently concluded that sleep does not affect the latency or the amplitude of the early components of the averaged auditory evoked potential.

The middle and long latency components are thought to reflect central processing factors. The initial reports on these components were made by Williams, Tepas, and Morlock (1962) and Weitzman and Kremen (1965) and showed that sleep did indeed alter the configuration of these components in systematic ways. Several studies of auditory thresholds have focused on the longer latency potentials. The studies can be summarized in two points:

(1) There is no general threshold elevation for the appearance of the longer latency potentials during sleep (Price and Goldstein, 1966; Davis *et al.*, 1967; Hrbek, Hrbkova, and Lenard, 1969; Mendel *et al.*, 1975); but
(2) the form and latency of the potentials do change during sleep.

EEG changes. A number of studies have used as criteria one or several gross changes in ongoing EEG. These responses, of course, are evoked but are visible without averaging.

The early study of Davis *et al.* (1939), reported that K-complexes (Chapter III) could be evoked by several types of stimuli during sleep. Two studies have used K-complex production as a criterion for discrimination of stimuli. Oswald, Taylor, and Treisman (1960) and Frazier, McDonald, and Edwards (1968) found that K-complexes were elicited significantly more often to one's own name than to other control names or to a designated different 'important' name or to 500 Hz tones.

Several studies have used a 'change' in ongoing EEG as a criterion for response. Levere *et al.* (1973, 1974) have used 'overall cortical desynchronization' (a measure based on the most common EEG frequencies in different sleep stages) and found that presentation of stimuli resulted in greater shifts in synchrony during slow wave sleep than during REM sleep—possibly because overall synchrony is greater during slow wave sleep. Williams *et al.* (1964), basing their procedure on a system pioneered by Derbyshire and Farley (1959), used six specific EEG changes to derive a score of responsiveness. Stimuli were presented in the various stages of sleep and the number of responses totalled within states. The number of EEG events were found to be greater in stages 2 and 3 than in stage 4 and REM.

However, several major problems arise as a result of scoring variations in voltage and frequency from different stages of sleep. For example, a frequency increase has a different probability of occurrence in REM than in stage 4. Also, because the stimuli used in these studies often did not result in awakening and were not remembered by subjects, the significance of EEG shifts is not apparent, even if such shifts can be reliably produced.

Keefe, Johnson, and Hunter (1971) examined a range of physiological response measures in addition to EEG shifts. During sleep, significant EEG responses to tones were first seen at a level 25–30 dB below arousal threshold (assessed by a button push response or by the occurrence of waking EEG). Significant finger pulse volume changes were seen 15–20 dB and heart rate acceleration at 5–20 dB below arousal threshold, but skin potential change, skin resistance change, and respiration decreases were found at arousal threshold (during normal waking, all of these responses tend to occur simultaneously).

Behavioural responses. Several types of different behavioural responses have been examined including reflexes, muscle movements, button pushes, and verbal responses.

Kleitman (1929, 1963) has reviewed the course of reflex responsivity during sleep. Reflexes such as tendon reflexes (Miller, 1926; Bass, 1931) and cutaneous reflexes (Kleitman, 1963) generally have been shown to weaken and become longer in latency during sleep in a fashion which may be correlated to depth of sleep (Kleitman, 1963).

Two studies (Ferrari and Messina, 1972; Kimura and Harada, 1972) have examined reflex activity in humans in conjunction with the recording of EEG activity. In both studies, the threshold of the electromyographic response of the mimetic muscles, which control the blink reflex, was assessed under varying shock intensities to the fifth cranial nerve. In the Ferrari and Messina (1972) study, the muscle response showed a definite increase in threshold from waking to slow wave sleep, and, although data were not presented, was said to increase from stage 1 to stage 4. Thresholds during REM, however, did not differ from waking thresholds obtained before and after sleep. The Kimura and Harada (1972) study is basically a replication of Ferrari and Messina. Though data were not given for waking responses, the response was present as often in stage 1 as it was in REM. Response probability decreased through stages 1, REM, 2, 3, and 4, but responsiveness differed significantly only between stages 1 and REM and the other sleep stages. However, Ferrari and Messina (1972) also presented evidence that, during waking, increases in vigilance level increased the response. Such varying reflex responsiveness as a result of degree of muscular relaxation even while awake is supported by Miller (1926), and casts some doubts on the validity of attempts to measure sleep depth by any sort of muscular response. Further, the fairly selective muscle atonia associated with REM sleep might raise response levels in some but not all muscle groups regardless of sleep depth.

The most common types of muscular response measures used are voluntary. Studies of several types of such responses have been made. The simplest and most common response has been a previously agreed signal by the subject that he is aware of the stimulus. For example, Oswald, Taylor, and Treisman (1960) had subjects clench their fist in response to a stimulus, while Williams *et al.* (Williams *et al.*, 1964; Williams, Morlock, and Morlock, 1966), Keefe, Johnson, and Hunter (1971), and Johnson and Lockwood (1972) had subjects push a button. Such methodology seems straightforward, but these responses can be made accidentally, and also by subjects who remain in what is electro-encephalographically stage 2 sleep so that it may be difficult to use such a response to define 'wakefulness'. The latter problem is a continuing one in this research, but the former was overcome by simply having the subject push the button two or three times (Fishchgold and Schwartz, 1960; Rechtschaffen and Lentzner, 1960). Two studies (Nakamura, Iwahara, and Fulisawa, 1966; Okuma *et al.*, 1966) examined such responsiveness even more closely by awakening subjects either when they did not respond following a stimulus or when they responded incorrectly by pushing the button too few times. The studies found that if subjects were awakened and asked the number of stimuli after an incorrect non-zero motor response, they made the correct verbal response about 27% of the time. After no motor response, subjects reported the correct number of stimuli only 12% of the time and this is what would be expected by chance. However, when the individual stage data was examined, about half of the correct verbal responses, whether the motor response was not attempted or was incorrect, were seen in REM. This is considerably more than chance, and presents evidence for the possibility that discrimination takes place during REM but that the actual motor response is difficult. Subjective reports indicated that dream incorporation may account for the finding.

Another way of using the button push response is to measure its latency. Generally a rather loud tone is presented and continues until turned off by the button push. Okuma *et al.* (1966) presented 90 dB, 800 Hz tones and found latencies increased from about 0.35 seconds in restful waking to about 1.2 seconds in stage 2 to about 2.5 seconds in stage 4. The latency was about 1.5 seconds in REM. Goodenough *et al.* (1965) used an 80 dB bell as a stimulus. The latency in stage 3 and 4 was about 27 seconds and in REM varied between

4 and 10 seconds depending on the length of the REM period at the time of stimulation. These are about 10 times as long as the Japanese results, in part because the required response was picking up a telephone receiver (which included finding it in the dark). However, it is possible that there is a non-linear relation between latency and tone intensity and that there is an asymptote between 80 and 90 dB. Also, many cultural and motivational variables may have differed in the experiments. In a study using the subject's name played forward or backward at a level of about 50 dB, Langford, Meddis, and Pearson (1974) found a striking latency difference. When the name was played backward, the mean response latency in REM was 50 seconds and in stage 2 was 76 seconds. When the names were played forward, the reaction times were 11 and 28 seconds respectively. Disregarding the many other variables involved, data for the four studies described above are plotted in Figure 1.

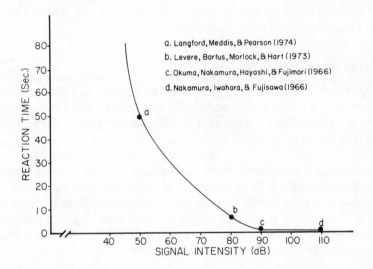

Figure 1   Reaction time as a function of stimulus tone intensity during sleep

Another popular response is a verbal one; i.e. when the subject says, 'I am awake'. Pilot work in our laboratory has tended to show that verbal responses are not as easy to elicit as a simple button push and tend to be better remembered by the subject. Several investigators have used this response (Shapiro, Goodenough, and Gryler, 1963; Goodenough *et al.*, 1965; Pisano *et al.*, 1966; Zimmerman, 1970). The findings are in general agreement with responsiveness being least in stages 3 and 4 and most in stage 1.

In this forest of possible responses, a few generalizations are possible. In terms of sensitivity to external stimuli, a rough rank ordering of responses would be evoked potentials, transient EEG events such as K-complexes, major EEG events such as stage changes or jumps, body movements, various cardio-vascular and electrodermal responses, simple muscular or behavioural response, vocalization, EEG defined awakening and complex response. This hierarchy appears clearly adaptive. Basic information processing continues at near waking threshold level. This implies that cortical control at some level might serve to drive responsiveness in the other systems. The first non-cortical system driven, according to Keefe, Johnson, and Hunter (1971), is the cardio-vascular system, a logical choice in the beginning of bodily activation. At arousal intensities, all systems, of necessity, must respond in preparation for action.

Regardless of the response hierarchy, a response must be chosen within the light of the purpose of the study at hand. If one is interested in a consciously remembered awakening, a complex motor response or verbal response may be necessary. Some measure of sleep disruption may be defined by a stage change. Assessment of simple information input or simple discrimination might require only evoked potential responses.

Variables Which Modify Thresholds

A majority of threshold studies have considered threshold values as a function of other than the stimulus or modality. These have included sleep stage, age, drugs, prior wakefulness, time of night (placement during sleep), circadian phase position, and individual differences.

Sleep stage. As noted above many studies have focused on sleep stages as a threshold determinant. Table 1 depicts the rough percentage of studies which found increasing thresholds as sleep stages progressed from stage 1 through stage 4. Data from 16 studies have been summarized and the differences indicated were not always statistically significant. The thresholds in REM sleep were approximately equal to those in stage 2 sleep.

Age. A few studies have examined responsiveness across age groups. All have been concerned with the effects of aircraft noise and sonic booms. Remarkably, only one of these studies reported any sort of threshold data within sleep stage for the various age groups studied. Lukas and Kryter (1970) studied subjects at about 8, 45, and 70 years of age. Approximate awakening percentages for sonic boom and aircraft noise are summarized in Table 2. As can be seen from the table, the 45 year old and 8 year old subjects awoke to booms only about 2% of the time, whereas the 70 year olds awoke 70% of the time, despite the fact that the latter subjects had some hearing loss and were not even exposed to the most intense boom and flyover sound level. These results, unfortunately, were based on only two subjects in each group and,

Table 1   Percentage of between study agreement of sleep stage and sleep depth in studies of human sleep

	Stage 2	Stage 3	Stage 4	REM
Stage 1	92	100	100	88
Stage 2		87	83	33
				42*
				25
Stage 3			86	27
Stage 4				20

Note: With the starred exception, the table is read 'stage listed at top of table was found to be deeper than stage in left vertical column of table in 00% of studies'. For example, stage 2 was found deeper than stage 1 in 92% of studies.
*REM was found deeper than stage 2 in 33% of the studies, as deep as stage 2 in 42% and lighter than stage 2 in 25%.

therefore should be replicated. Kramer *et al.* (1971), Roth, Kramer, and Trinder (1972) and Collins and Iampietro (1972) each studied the effects of noise on the sleep of subjects in each of three age groups: 25, 50, and 75 years of age. General findings indicated that noises sufficient to cause only a stage change in younger subjects were sufficient to cause awakenings in the older subjects. The older subjects either had a different sleep stage distribution, had lower thresholds within stages, or had had a shift in characteristic response pattern to noise ('fragile' sleep).

Drugs. Five studies have examined the effect of drugs on arousal threshold during or at the conclusion of sleep. Johnson *et al.* (1979) measured auditory arousal thresholds in various sleep stages after 30 mg of flurazepam and found an increase in stage 4 thresholds in their drug subjects as compared to placebo subjects. Bonnet, Webb, and Barnard (1979) studied multiple arousals in stage 2 sleep and sketched a drug time course effect. They found highest thresholds during the second hour of sleep at the same time Johnson *et al.* (1979) found maximum effects. Bonnet, Webb, and Barnard (1979) also studied pento-

Table 2   Sleep stage threshold (percentage awakening response) as a function of age and stimulus

Age (years)	Sonic boom			Flyover noise		
	REM	Stage 2	Delta	REM	Stage 2	Delta
70	93	70	48	36	29	18
45	4	3	2	11	9	3
8	3	0	0	7	1	3

barbital, a depressant, and caffeine, a stimulant. The time course for these drugs and placebo, as measured by auditory arousal threshold referenced to prior evening threshold when awake, can be seen in Figure 2. Itil (1976) reported a series of three studies in which subjects were awakened in the morning with a threshold procedure after taking one of five different drugs. Significant auditory threshold elevation (as compared to placebo) was found after 2 mg of triazolam and 30 mg of flurazepam in one of two studies.

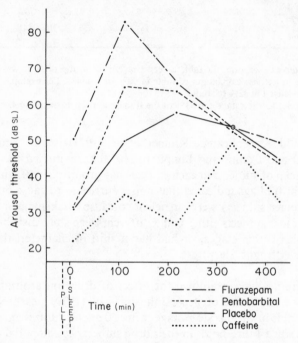

Figure 2   Auditory arousal threshold from stage 2 sleep across the sleep period after administration of flurazepam, pentobarbital, caffeine, or placebo. (From Bonnet, Webb, and Barnard, 1979)

Prior wakefulness. Three human studies have considered the effects of prior wakefulness on responsiveness during sleep. Williams *et al.* (1964) measured responsiveness (button press to one of several tone intensities) on two baseline nights and then again on two recovery nights after 64 hours of sleep deprivation. Percent of correct button push responses to a 35 dB above background noise burst ranged from about 24% in stage 2 to about 10% in stage 4 on the control nights. After 64 hours of deprivation, the percentage of correct responses ranged from 4% in stage 2 to 1% in stage 4.

Similarly, Snyder and Scott (1972) found a significant increase in reaction time to a stimulus in all stages of sleep during a night which followed a preceding night of only 4 hours of sleep. Lindsley (1957) employed a constantly increasing tone which could be decreased in intensity by a button push response. The subjects averaged about 1500 responses on control nights but only produced about 600 after 38 hours of sleep deprivation.

Time of night. Either time of night or prior sleep has also appeared to affect thresholds within sleep stage. Shapiro, Goodenough, and Gryler (1963) found that the first REM period had higher thresholds than later REM periods and the effect was later replicated (Goodenough *et al.*, 1965). Rechtschaffen's group reported similar threshold shifts occurred across the night in REM and in stage 2 (Rechtschaffen, Hauri, and Zeitlin, 1966). These results have been replicated by Watson and Rechtschaffen (1969), Zimmerman (1970), and Keefe, Johnson, and Hunter (1971).

Three studies did not support these results. Williams *et al.* (1964) traced thresholds in stage 2 across the night and found a response decrement in their button push response. However, because a very large number of stimuli were presented (100+ per night), response decrement might have come from habituation to the experimental situation. More recently, Bonnet, Johnson, and Webb (1978) hypothesized that time of night effects might be a dual function of the facts that spontaneous body movements increase in frequency across the night (page 206 above) (Mullin, Kleitman, and Cooperman, 1933) and that thresholds are lower in temporal proximity to body movements (Kleitman, Cooperman, and Mullin, 1936; Mullin, Kleitman, and Cooperman, 1937). They analysed their data two ways—including all arousals as they occurred in proximity to body movements, and excluding an awakening which occurred less than 10 minutes after a body movement. A significant time of night effect was found when all threshold observations were included, but the effect disappeared when threshold determinations within ten minutes after a body movement were eliminated. Wills and Trinder (1978) also found no significant time of night effect.

Circadian effects. All of the studies cited in the preceding section reported data collected from sleep periods occurring from about 11 PM to 7 AM. For this reason, it cannot be concluded whether the effects reported were due to the prior amount of sleep or to diurnal rhythms. Corvalan and Hayden (unpublished abstract) determined awakening thresholds for subjects in sleep periods beginning at 10 PM, 8:15 AM, 9:15 AM, 10:15 AM, and noon. The threshold values from REM and stage 4 showed a circadian effect with the highest values at 10 PM and 8 AM. Corvalan (1969) reported reaction time to a constant level stimulus during sleep across day and night. Reaction time during REM appeared to show a circadian effect decreasing with absolute time across the 24 hours. From the brief information reported, there appear to be many problems with these experiments, and further carefully controlled studies in this area are needed. Keefe, Johnson, and Hunter (1971) gave threshold data involving subjects sleeping at a non-normal time, but these were collected at least seven days after a rhythm shift. They found, paradoxically, thresholds in stage 2 were higher in their adjusted day sleepers than in another group of normal night sleepers. It should be noted that threshold data were collected on the first night in the laboratory and may demonstrate a first night effect of lowered within stage thresholds.

Individual differences. Thresholds during sleep display large individual differences in responsiveness. Several investigators have mentioned this, e.g., Corvalan and Hayden (unpublished) and Schmidt and Birns (1971). However, wide individual threshold differences are also seen in waking subjects (Stone, Pryor, and Colwell, 1967). Schmidt and Birns (1971), who worked with babies, speculated on a possible relation of threshold to personality. Zimmerman (1968, 1970) made awakening threshold his major independent variable. Groups of 'light' sleepers and 'deep' sleepers were chosen on the basis of normal thresholds above or below an average awakening value of 65 dB (groups corresponded approximately to upper and lower thirds of all subjects tested). The light sleepers had more stage 1, awakenings, and body movements than the deep sleepers and tended to be generally more 'aroused' than the deep sleepers. The deep sleepers gave more reports of dreams during NREM sleep and fewer reports of thinking than the light sleep group.

Bonnet, Johnson, and Webb (1978) examined the reliability of auditory threshold measurements taken during sleep and found:

(1) significant reliability from night to night and within night;
(2) people who had high thresholds in stage 4 also tended to have high thresholds in stage 2 and REM;
(3) threshold when awake was not significantly correlated with threshold when asleep.

Six studies have hypothesized differences in sleep depth for different types of people. Boyd (1960) tested the hypothesis that enuretic children were deeper sleepers than normal children. More than 100 enuretics were tested during sleep for responsiveness to their name followed by gentle shaking. Sleep EEG was not recorded, and no difference was seen in threshold between the enuretics and the controls. Zung, Wilson, and Dodson (1964) found that clinically depressed patients had lower thresholds in all stages of sleep (REM was not scored) than control subjects. As the patients improved clinically, their awakening thresholds increased so that they no longer differed significantly from the controls.

Cobb *et al.* (1965) tested responsiveness during sleep as a function of hypnotic susceptability. Subjects were given a post-hypnotic suggestion to move their pillow when the word 'pillow' was heard. When the suggestion was given during REM, the hypnotizable subjects responded to the suggestion during that and succeeding REM periods. The low hypnotizable subjects did not respond to the suggestion in any stage of sleep. A later study (Perry *et al.*, 1978) concluded that the difference was probably one of rapport because 'interested' subjects who could not be hypnotized could produce the same responses.

Nan'no *et al.* (1970) studied REM thresholds in narcoleptics and controls. Both EEG response and a button push response were studied in the narcoleptics' onset REM period and in the first normally placed nocturnal REM period in both groups. The sleep onset REM period was characterized by elevation in both types of response threshold above the thresholds of the first REM period for the control group, and the second REM period for the narcoleptics which did not differ from the control. The narcoleptics maintained that they perceived the stimuli during the onset REM period but had been incapable of responding.

In brief summary, the data reviewed reveal that sensory signal reception during sleep is complex and by no means fully explored. This is not surprising when considering the complexity of waking sensations and thresholds. Not unexpectedly, variations in the stimulus dimension and the modality of reception have been found to be significant as well as the substantial presence of individual differences, age, and drug effects. The studies have used a wide variety of response criteria that have ranged from evoked potentials to verbal affirmations of wakefulness. This makes cross-comparisons of conditions difficult but often explicates and specifies a relationship under study. The presence of sleep itself is clearly a significant factor. While the length of sleep, *per se* is questionable as a variable, the specific sleep stage certainly affects threshold levels. While depth of sleep measured by thresholds shows some evidence of a curvilinear relationship e.g. Johnson and Lockwood, 1972 the untangling of a circadian *vs* 'sleep' influence has barely begun.

All in all, the filling in of the complex matrix of variables and their interactions which will be necessary to speak definitively of sensory reception of signals while asleep has barely begun.

LEARNING DURING SLEEP

The production of the correct response in a given situation based on past experiences is defined as a learned response. Using such a definition, learned responses during sleep to relevant signals, or the habituation of responses to signals, are obviously common occurrences. Learning within the period of sleep will be examined in three sections—the basic capabilities of discrimination or habituation, short term memory, and long term memory.

Discrimination

The early studies of discrimination during sleep were animal studies involving classical tone/shock conditioning learned while the animal was awake and tested when it was asleep. Rowland (1957) presented a 10 second tone followed by a shock to awake cats for about 50 trials. All the cats were then tested during sleep under extinction. Both neutral and test tones initially produced cortical desynchronization, but while the response to the neutral tone lessened and disappeared in about four trials, the latency and the length of desynchronization to the conditioned stimulus increased over the first few trials and did not extinguish completely for 30–50 trials.

Later studies with rats (Cornwell, 1967) and humans (Buendia *et al.*, 1963; Beh and Barratt, 1965; McDonald *et al.*, 1975) extended and replicated the findings of Rowland. Cornwell (1967) allowed 10 seconds between the end of the CS (a tone) and the beginning of the UCS (a shock). Arousal did not occur to the presentation of the CS, but tended to follow after about ten seconds during extinction trials in sleep. Beh and Barratt (1965) demonstrated that the classical conditioning could itself take place while the animal was asleep.

Williams, Morlock, and Morlock (1966) used a simpler learning design. They told their human subjects that either an 800 or 1200 Hz tone was a 'critical' tone and the other was not. Under one condition, non-response to the critical tone was punished by a fire alarm, flashing light, and threat of shock. Subjects displayed an ability to push a microswitch proportionally better to the critical tone than to the neutral tone in stages 1, 2, and REM, with the best discrimination seen in stage 1. Response to the neutral tone was uniformly low (under 20%) in all stages under all conditions, while responses to the critical tone averaged abou 70% across all conditions in stage 1, 30% in stage 2, and 35% in REM. Response rate in stages 3 and 4 was very low in all conditions.

Several studies have used meaningful sounds and have asked subjects to differentiate among them. Zung and Wilson (1961) presented sounds from several sources (including cars, doors, chimes, trains, bagpipes, and monkey howls) to sleeping subjects. While no attempt was made to examine the effect of individual stimuli, familiarity on the whole had no effect. Some of the subjects were paid according to their ability to awaken to specific sounds (a telephone and a bagpipe). The subjects motivated to make a discrimination responded almost perfectly to the designated sounds in all stages of sleep (REM was not scored in this study), and the increase in response rate was significant in all stages except stage 4. Zung and Wilson also found that the motivated subjects responded more often to the signal stimuli than did the control subjects in all stages of sleep, except in stage 1, in which both groups had a high response rate. The motivated subjects responded less often to non-signal stimuli than did the control group, except in stage 4. Wilson and Zung (1966) used the same methodology in a study designed to test for sex differences in response probability during sleep. Again in this study, the response rate to signal stimuli was close to perfect for all stages. Both sexes responded more to signal than to non-signal stimuli in all stages of sleep, including REM. The largest increase in response rate due to motivaton occurred in stage 4, in which males jumped from 14% to 92% correct. All of the other increases were bounded by perfect response on one side and a response rate to non-signal stimuli larger than that for stage 4 on the other. Also, the females responded significantly more than the males to neutral stimuli in all stages of sleep except REM. These two studies supply impelling evidence that simple experimental instructions could greatly influence responsiveness during sleep and that subjects were capable of making rather large modification of their responsiveness during sleep. Further, the responses were clearly signal specific, except perhaps in stage 4. The data give indications that higher cortical control can override reticular deactivation.

Two studies have examined the ability of mothers to discriminate differentially the cries of infants. Poitras *et al.* (1973) studied auditory arousal thresholds to infant cries in pregnant females before and after delivery and found thresholds significantly lower about 34 days after giving birth. While the authors concluded that physiological changes based on delivery were responsible, there was no control for possible learning effects, and such learning effects from night to night may be significant by themselves (Watson and Rechtschaffen, 1969). Formby (1967) examined the ability of new mothers at a hospital to discriminate their own baby's cry from the cries of other babies over the first four postnatal nights. For the first three nights, about 58% of the mothers' awakenings were to their own children's cries; this rose to 96% on the fourth night. This study apparently tracks the development of a subtle, relevant discrimination, which is learned in both sleep and waking and expressed during sleep.

Several studies have used known words or names as the basis for discrimination during sleep. Some words (a subject's name, for example) hold more relevance for the subject than others and, thus, could be termed signal stimuli. Oswald, Taylor, and Treisman (1960) found that subjects responded more often (hand clasp response) to their own name than to other names. The production of a K-complex response to the names was also scored. A K-complex was significantly more likely to follow the presentation of the subject's name than other names. A study by Howarth and Ellis (1961) employed a methodology similar with *awake* subjects. Percentages of correct response for each study are presented in Table 3. While absolute percentage correct depends on overall intensity levels, the difference between 'own' and 'other' does not.

Minard *et al.* (1968) presented evidence for increased differential responsiveness to signal versus non-signal stimuli during sleep. They found that individually selected, personally significant words such as 'dumb' or 'sin'

Table 3   Responsiveness to name in a waking study and a sleep study

	Waking	Sleep	
	Howarth and Ellis (1961) % correct	Oswald, Taylor, and Treisman (1960) Hand clasp response %	K-complex response %
Own name	77	25	66
Other name	51	12	35
Difference	26	13	31

elicited EOG changes and heart rate accelerations during sleep, as compared to control stimuli such as 'drum' or 'sit'. Differential responsiveness to the two sets of stimuli was not seen when the subjects were awake.

Habituation

An experiment by Sommer-Smith *et al.* (1962) demonstrated the effects of signal relevance and habituation. Sleeping cats were shocked shortly after the termination of a long, habituated conditioned stimulus tone. Initial response was greater at tone onset than offset, but the response to the tone offset increased while the response to tone onset habituated over trials. Arousal became a function of tone offset in expectancy of shock. Weinberger and Lindsley (1964) produced either a 3 second burst of noise or noise which otherwise was constant. A similar cortical synchrony was found in both conditions. An expectancy/habituation framework can explain such results.

The germinal habituation study was that of Sharpless and Jasper (1956). Sleeping cats were presented with a tone loud enough to cause arousal. The length of the cortical desynchrony was recorded and the animal was allowed to sleep again. The procedure was repeated until the tone failed to cause any loss of cortical synchrony; this occurred after about 30 presentations within about a 2 hour period. A change in frequency, intensity, or duration of the tone resulted in a return of the arousal response. Some generalization and spontaneous recovery after an hour (also see Glickman and Feldman, 1961) was noted. Leaton and Buck (1971) found much more rapid habituation (2 or 4 trials) than was found earlier studies and no spontaneous recovery for at least 30 days; Leaton and Jordan (1978) replicated the 1971 study and added that habituation even appeared with a 24 hour interstimulus interval between test stimuli. They also found that habituation during waking (in terms of EEG arousal response) continued to be effective during sleep.

In human subjects, virtually all sleep researchers allow for the phenomenon of habituation during sleep by discarding data from a subject's first night in the laboratory recording. A noticeable modification of sleep patterns is seen between the first night of recording and subsequent or 'habituated' nights

(Agnew, Webb, and Williams, 1966). Several manipulations can extend or reinstate (dishabituation) such a first night effect by creating novel environments (Scott, 1972; Bonnet and Webb, 1976). However, where detailed habituation studies using human subjects have been done, they have produced results neither as simple nor as straightforward as those reported by Sharpless and Jaspter with cats. Johnson and Lubin (1967) briefly reviewed disparate findings from several studies investigating varied responses and themselves attempted to examine several types of response to a 3 second tone 30–35 dB above threshold, presented every 30–45 seconds throughout a night beginning at bedtime. EEG, EOG, skin potential, skin resistance, heart rate, respiration rate, and finger vasoconstriction were recorded. During a day control, the stimulus elicited an orienting response which habituated with repetition for all variables. However, no evidence for habituation of any variable was seen during sleep in this study. Disagreement has been the rule in this area. Roth, Shaw, and Green (1956) reported no habituation of the K-complex to stimuli presented during sleep. Oswald, Taylor, and Treisman (1960) reported habituation of the K-complex. While Johnson and Lubin (1967) and Townsend, Johnson, and Muzet (1973) reported no habituation, Ackner and Pampiglione (1957) did. In response to the many disagreements, Johnson, Townsend, and Wilson (1975) examined the topic once again. Specifically, sets of 20 tones were presented at 75 dB in stage 2 or in REM, measures being recorded as in the 1967 Johnson and Lubin study. In the new study habituation was found for finger vasoconstriction and heart rate response during stage 2 but not during REM. These results, of course, did not agree with the earlier ones. In the face of many different experimental findings Johnson, Townsend, and Wilson (1975) concluded that wide within and between subject differences exist during sleep and that such individual variance could greatly affect outcomes in studies with a small number of subjects.

There have been three other recent studies of habituation during sleep. McDonald and Carpenter (1975) studied 46 subjects. Their study differed from that of Johnson, Townsend, and Wilson (1975) in that they used less intense stimuli at a shorter interstimulus interval. They found habituation of the finger vasoconstriction and heart rate response in REM sleep while Johnson, Townsend, and Wilson did not. Another very similar study was done by Firth (1973) on three subjects; he found habitation of the skin potential response in all stages of sleep. These data do not agree with any other report and might be a consequence of large individual differences and a very small *N*. The third study (Berg, Jackson, and Graham, 1975) noted that the heart rate acceleration is characteristic of a defensive response (not the orienting response the other studies have claimed to examine) and defensive responses habituate very slowly.

In short, attempts to measure habituation autonomically during sleep have been disappointing. The lack of habituation in all variables may be a function of the disassociation of autonomic events during sleep. From the most recent data, it looks as if the lack of agreement in results has come mainly from insensitive procedures and the probability that habituation during sleep is not as strong as during waking. The use of more meaningful stimuli or different measures of habituation (say an EEG response such as alpha production) might be more rewarding.

The lack of evidence for habituation in autonomic systems is unsettling if it is accepted (as it appears generally to be) that habituation does take place. However, evidence for this broad generality is harder to find than might be supposed. Miller (1971) remarked on the relative lack of consistency of reports of lessening responsivity even when the response was behavioural awakening. Thiessen (1970) found no statistically significant adaption to truck noises over 12 nights, and Collins and Iampietro (1972) found no adaptation to sonic booms over the same period. Lukas, Peeler, and Davis (1975), however, have found some evidence for adaptation in their experiments. Lukas (1972) found that in response to flyover noise, there was a significant reduction in awake response (a drop from 59% to 18%) from the first two nights to the fifth and sixth. Adaptation to sonic booms was less, possibly because only 22% of the booms resulted in awakening initially. Lukas (1972) found non-significant trends for adaptation to pink noise and treated (filtered) jet noise but not to untreated jet noise over nine nights. Lukas, Peeler, and Davis (1975) again found only trends for adaptation, and these trends appeared primarily for softer stimuli of all sorts and pink noise (over nine nights). These data together implied that minimal adaptation did take place but that it was less likely (at least in terms of response/non-response) to intense stimuli and unlikely at all if experimental manipulations initially caused only minor disruption of the sleep process or there were only a few trials. These latter criticisms apply to virtually all of the noise and boom studies. Miller (1971) suggested that the adaptation which is commonly thought to take place to common non-signal stimuli might be due more to habituation in memory (increased amnesia for awakenings) rather than in actual responsiveness.

Short Term Memory

The discrimination of a single baby's cry or one's own name during sleep implies transfer of discrimination training from wakefulness to sleep. Further studies have placed both the conditioning for the discrimination and tests for discrimination during sleep. Both conditioning and discrimination appear to function over a long period during sleep once such abilities have been established.

The third possible area of inquiry is the study of transfer of acquisition during sleep to wakefulness and studies have examined both short term and long term waking memory for events occurring during sleep.

Four studies have examined short term recall for material presented during sleep and tested for after an arousal which followed the stimulus from a few seconds to 30 minutes. Okuma *et al.* (1966) instructed subjects to press a button for each of a varying number of stroboscopic flashes. They were then awakened. If subjects had pressed the button the correct number of times, they could always report that same correct number to the experimenter. However, on some occasions during REM, subjects made no response, but, when awakened, could report the correct number of flashes (which usually had been incorporated into a dream). In NREM sleep, when subjects pushed the button an incorrect number of times, it was always less than the actual number of flashes and they tended to report as many flashes as pushes. The implication was that either attention or a lightening of sleep was necessary for the complete number of flashes to register and be remembered shortly thereafter in NREM but that dreams might serve to hold information in REM.

Lasaga and Lasaga (1973) presented numbers during various stages of sleep and aroused subjects 15 seconds later to test for recall. Several of the stimulus numbers themselves caused an arousal or sleep stage shift, which increased the probability of recall. Even when stimuli were presented in stage 3–4 sleep (with only 3 of 22 trials resuling in stage shifts to stage 1), all eight subjects showed better than chance probability of recognizing the correct stimulus. As might be predicted from threshold data, the probability of a correct response decreased in the usual order: stage 1, REM, stage 2, stage 3, and stage 4.

Oltman *et al.* (1977) habituated their subjects to numbers repeated every 30 seconds all night so that no EEG changes occurred in response to them. They then awakened the subjects from stage 2 sleep, 1–10 seconds after the presentation of a number and tested for recall. Although they did not get a drop in recall as the interval increased from 1 to 10 seconds (as could be expected on the basis of waking short term memory work for unattended recall by Glucksberg and Cowen, 1970 and Eriksen and Johnson, 1964), they did find significantly better recall than could be expected by chance. It is possible that a recall curve was not found because the average response time for the shortest arousal was 1 second to beginning of awakenig plus 9.7 seconds for the subject to pick up a phone and report the number. This recall period of 10.7 seconds is longer than 10 seconds by itself, by which time the effect may have disappeared.

Shimizu *et al.* (1977) presented either tape recorded names (50–60 dB) or 1–10 stroboscopic flashes during stage 2 or REM and woke subjects up 5 seconds to 30 minutes after the stimulations to test recall. The authors stated that when stimuli elicited less than 5 seconds of alpha there was 'usually' no recall even after an immediate arousal. When evoked alpha was 5–20 seconds in duration, correct recall for names was 100% in REM for 2 minutes after stimulation and fell to 50% in about 11 minutes. In stage 2, 100% correct recall lasted less than a minute after stimulation and fell below 50% within 2 minutes. Similar results were found with photic stimulation.

By testing at very short intervals and with a non-auditory (non-interfering) arousal, Oltman *et al.* (1977) and Lasaga and Lasaga (1973) may have been tapping a different type of memory store than Shimizu *et al.* (1977). Of more importance, both results imply that a short term memory function for external stimuli during sleep does exist for at least 10 seconds and perhaps as long as 2 minutes.

Long Term Memory

It appears that the idea of learning complex material during sleep for later use during the day had its roots in the science fiction of the early 1900s (first Hugo Gernsback in 1911 and later Huxley in *Brave New World*), a literature which has been cited by Russian investigators as the first studies (Kulikov, 1968). Actual experiments began as early as 1916, when Thurstone supplemented the training of Navy men by presenting Morse code during their sleep. Between 1916 and the early 1950s, about 10 studies of sleep learning (hypnopaedia) were done (reviewed by Simon and Emmons, 1955). Seven concluded that some learning had occurred during sleep. However, in the three studies in which the subjects' sleep was carefully monitored to prevent learning during transient arousals, no sleep learning was reported.

The Russian hypnopaedia literature is quite extensive. Several Russian papers were translated and published in books by Rubin (1968, 1971) and reviewed by Aarons (1976); in general, results were quite favourable. In a typical Russian experiment (Zukhar *et al.*, 1968), a large number of subjects were exposed to tape recorded Russian–English or Russian–Latin word pairs during the time period 23 00 to 0 30 and 6 00 to 6 30 over a loudspeaker system. Although EEG was not recorded, the number of words remembered after the sleep learning procedure was two or three times as many as the number remembered from a control list given for one trial in the morning. The times of presentation, clearly, were chosen to maximize periods of wakefulness and light sleep, when the probability of learning might be greatest.

Besides time of night differences between the Russian studies and American studies, learning set, suggestibility of subjects, and extent of both pretraining and within sleep training were variables also maximized in Soviet experiments. A study by Hoskovec and Coper (1967) is illustrative of a western attempt to duplicate Russian findings. In it, eleven highly hypnotically susceptible subjects were told to remember the Russian–English pairs they heard during the night. In the waking (control) condition, subjects remembered about 90% of the material but remembered only 30% when tested immediately after presentation of the words during sleep. Parenthetically, the authors report studying three pilot subjects. Two subjects remembered none of the words and the third subject, who later reported having awakened during the presentations, remembered 90% of the words. Average recall for these three subjects, then, was also 30%.

The major pitfall of the Russian work is that no EEG recordings were done and it is impossible to tell how much learning occurred when subjects were awake. One eastern European study which did record ongoing EEG (Hradecky *et al.*, 1968) found no instance in 990 trials of learning of an unknown word during EEG defined sleep.

The western EEG literature on hypnopaedia has been almost as discouraging as the Hradecky *et al.* (1968) study. While learning has been reported in all of the eleven studies that have been done, that learning was virtually always traced back to alpha production after presentation. The landmark work was that of Simon and Emmons (1956) and Emmons and Simon (1956). The first paper found learning decreased as drowsiness increased up to the point of what is presently defined as stage 2 sleep; at this point, probability of recall fell to chance control levels. The second paper showed that the lack of learning during normally defined sleep was not a function of stimulus repetition. The papers together were so convincing that hypnopaedia was not studied by similar procedures in the United States for 12 years.

Several learning experiments were done in the late 1960s and early 1970s. Of them, many reported, with increasing conviction, that the probability of recall was enhanced by longer periods of alpha, and that if periods of alpha of 5–10 seconds did not appear there would be no above chance recall (Pieper and Kugler, 1966; Koukkou and Lehmann, 1968; Tani and Yoshii, 1970; Jus and Jus, 1972; Lehmann and Koukkou, 1973). In addition, other findings from Simon and Emmons were replicated. In two studies (Hoskovec and Cooper, 1967; Levy, Coolidge, and Staab, 1972) better than chance learning during EEG defined sleep were reported. The actual number of alpha trials and the chance response rate is difficult to calculate in both studies, so that an actual claim for learning during non-alpha sleep is still very difficult to sustain.

The failure to find convincing evidence for long term memory of complex material presented during sleep when tested in wakefulness may be of importance for understanding sleep as a state as well as for understanding performance properties. It is possible that the failure of recall is a state dependent effect. But, if this were the case, discrimination of signal stimuli (i.e. names) learned in wakefulness should not be expected during sleep. Alternatively, the failure could be a function of attention during sleep—that is, material cannot be focused and rehearsed a sufficient number of times to move it from short to long term memory. This argument is weakened though, because discrimination/habituation has been reported even in rats during sleep. However, the animal data must be qualified because it is not completely certain that the learning did not take place during transient arousals after stimulus presentation. Unfortunately, tests of these possible explanations have not been made.

MAGNITUDE OF PERFORMANCE DECREMENT DURING SLEEP

We have seen that performance during sleep is poorer than waking performance on a large number of tasks, ranging from sensory–motor response to list learning. While it would be simple to conclude that those differences were the state specific differences assumed to accompany sleep, at least three other variables—fatigue, circadian tendencies, and relaxation—must be considered as contributing to performance loss during sleep.

Fatigue

A primary cause of fatigue at bed time is sleep deprivation. A large number of studies have examined threshold or performance under this condition. Williams, Lubin, and Goodnow (1959) used a reaction time paradigm in which a subject pressed a response key when one of two lights lit. With sleep loss and accompanying fatigue, mean reaction time slowly increased so that after 78 hours of deprivation, reaction times were twice the base line values. Only a small increase in reaction time was seen in subjects' best trials, but a large increase was seen in the worst trials. Okuma *et al.* (1966) and Nakamura, Iwahara, and Fulisawa (1966) report reaction times in sleeping and waking subjects. Their waking values agree well with Williams and his colleagues and are about 0.35 seconds. After 78 hours of sleep deprivation, the Williams subjects (awake) had a reaction time of about 0.90 seconds. In normal stage 2 sleep, the Nakamura subjects responded in 0.82 seconds and the Okuma *et al.* subjects in 1.2 seconds. Variability measures are not available, stimulus characteristics differed, and the motivational surround probably was not the same in the studies; but with these notable objections in mind, reaction time lengths appear similar in stage 2 sleep and after 78 hours of sleep deprivation.

Two other studies allow comparison between waking and sleeping responsiveness. Wilkinson, Morlock, and Williams (1966) reported changes in components of evoked potentials over the course of a 2 hour vigilance task. Williams, Tepas, and Morlock (1962) reported evoked potential changes during sleep. Three evoked components are reported in both sets of data. If the waking evoked potential amplitudes of the Williams *et al.* (1962) study are set equal to the amplitude of the evoked potentials seen in the first half hour of the Wilkinson *et al.* (1966) study, the following comparisons can be made. The amplitude of P2 falls as the vigilance task lengthens and as the subject falls asleep and moves toward stage 4. With the waking P2s equated at 6.9 microvolts (μV), the fall of P2 during the vigilance task is only to 5.3μv, a level slightly greater than seen in stage 1 (non-Rem) sleep (4.8μV). N2 also decreased across both studies. In the equated figures, it fell in the vigilance task from -3.7 to -6.6 μV, a level indicative of stage 4 sleep in the sleep study. The N1 response shifted in the vigilance task from about -4.0 μV to about

–3.3 μV, a level closest to that seen in stage 1 sleep in the sleep study. In short, although an assumption of adjusted means was necessary to arrive at the figures quoted, even the process of extended vigilance performance resulted in a corical responsiveness shift (gross EEG changes were not reported) similar to that seen in sleep.

The general conclusion is that sleep deprivation or 'fatigue' can be related to the response decrements noted in some measures which are equivalent to decrements seen in stage 1 or stage 2 sleep. Obviously, the factors involved in such experiments are complex and may differ from those seen during sleep. Also, the possibility of subjects actually falling asleep for a few seconds during the experiments cannot be discounted. This would imply occasional very long response times as encountered by Williams, Lubin, and Goodnow (1959).

Circadian Effects

A second factor possibly accounting for response decrements during sleep may be circadian determined impairments. As noted in Chapters III and VII performance during the usually scheduled sleep period, e.g. during shift work periods, is typically depressed on a wide range of tasks. While many of these findings are compounded by sleep loss (see Bonnet and Webb, 1978) or by disturbed prior sleep, as in shift word designs, an increasing body of evidence demonstrates a decrement in performance during the original sleep period, when the amounts of prior wakefulness are controlled. From this one may infer an inherent circadian peak and trough influencing performance which is itself associated with but independent of the sleep processes.

Relaxation

The third variable associated with sleep which in itself could modify responsiveness is muscular relaxation. Kleitman (1929, 1963) briefly reviewed results of the early relaxation studies. Miller (1926) found that in subjects taught to relax (awake) there was decreased flexion, increased reaction time, and a diminished subjective intensity of a finger shock which normally resulted in flexion of the arm at the elbow. In some subjects, the response disappeared completely. This last finding was replicated by Jacobson and Carlson (in Kleitman, 1929). Since relaxation is a fundamental characteristic of sleep (Kleitman, 1963, Chapter 2) at least some aspects of performance decrements may be attributable to relaxation rather than sleep. A few recent studies report the effects of relaxation on several responses. For example, Wilkinson (1961) recorded muscle tension in subjects before and during a vigilance test after a night of sleep deprivation. Although a statistical treatment was not given, those subjects whose muscle tension increased the most during the task performed best on it. Ham and Edmonston (1971) compared the effects of of relaxation, hypnotic relaxation, and hypnotic alertness on a reaction time measure. The relaxed group was told that they would not be hypnotized but did hear a 13 minute tape recorded trance induction. Simple reaction time to an auditory signal was recorded. The reaction time in the alert induction group was about 0.36 seconds, which is equivalent to general waking reaction time. Both relaxation groups had significantly longer reaction time (both about 0.63 seconds) than the alert group. These values are still less than those found in stage 2 sleep or 78 hours of sleep deprivation (about 0.9 seconds).

Ferrari and Messina (1972) examined habituation of the blink reflex during relaxed waking. They found that the response dishabituated if a light or a sound occurred or was expected by the subject. They interpreted the return of the response to an increase in vigilance. This data fits well with much provided by Sokolov (1963). It is conceivable that relaxation interacts with habituation. But it is also possible that habituation is state dependent and these experiments alter state.

Envoi

It is clear that the presence of sleep raises a screen between our ordinary and waking ways of sensing and responding to the world around us. But it is equally clear that this is not a solid impenetrable barrier erected between the individual world of waking and the world of sleep. Sleep does not bring a 'little death' or a state of unconsciousness. The screen is penetrable and the systematic elements of that process have begun to emerge relative to signal properties, modalities, and state variables such as individual differences, sleep stages, drugs, age, and time asleep. Response dimensions are apparent — from cortical 'acknowledgements' to full arousal. Processing is present — descrimination and short term memory are certain and habituation and more complex processing are topics of relevance.

Indeed this understanding of the capacity for performance by the ostensibly 'absent' sleeper will provide us with some of the most intriguing and functional knowledge about sleep and a better comprehension of the 'whole' person in a 24 hour world.

SUMMARY

This chapter has reviewed the responsivity of subjects while asleep.

First, the sensitivity of subjects to stimulation is examined relative to sensory modalities, response measures used and modifier variables such as sleep stage, age, drugs, time of night and individual differences. The modifiability of responding during sleep is considered under the topics of discrimination and habituation and higher order variables such as learning and memory. The reduced response levels associated with sleep are discussed in terms of the concepts of fatigue, circadian effects and relaxation.

REFERENCES

Aarons, L. (1976). Sleep assisted instruction. *Psychological Bulletin* 83, 1–40.

Ackner, B. and Pampiglione, G. (1957). Some relationships between peripheral vasomotor and electroencephalographic changes. *Journal of Neurology, Neurosurgery, and Psychiatry* 20, 58–64.

Agnew, H., Webb, W., and Williams, R. (1966). The first night effect: an EEG study of sleep. *Psychophysiology* 2, 263–266.

Amadeo, M. and Shagass, C. (1973). Brief latency click-evoked potentials during waking and sleep in man. *Psychophysiology* 10, 244–250.

Ashton, R. (1971). State and the auditory reactivity of the human neonate. *Journal of Experimental Child Psychology* 12, 339–346.

Bass, M. J. (1931). Differentiation of the hypnotic trance from normal sleep. *Journal of Experimental Psychology* 14, 382–399.

Beh, J. C. and Barratt, P. (1965). Discrimination and conditioning during sleep as indicated by electroencephalogram. *Science* 147, 1470–1471.

Berg, W. K., Jackson, L. C., and Graham, F. K. (1975). Tone intensity and rise-decay time effects on cardiac responses during sleep. *Psychophysiology* 12, 254–261.

Blake, H. and Gerard, R. (1937). Brain potentials during sleep. *American Journal of Physiology* 119, 692–703.

Bonnet, M. H., Johnson, L. C., and Webb, W. B. (1978). The reliability of arousal threshold during sleep. *Psychophysiology* 14, 412–416.

Bonnet, M. H. and Webb, W. B. (1976). Effect of two experimental sets on sleep structure. *Perceptual and Motor Skills* 42, 343–350.

Bonnet, M. H. and Webb, W. B. (1978). The effect of repetition of relevant and irrelevant tasks over day and night work periods. *Ergonomics* 21, 999–1005.

Bonnet, M. H., Webb, W. B., and Barnard, G. (1979). The effect of flurazepam, pentobarbital, and caffeine on arousal threshold. *Sleep* 1, 271–280.

Boyd, M. M. M. (1960). The depth of sleep in enuretic school-children and in non-enuretic controls. *Journal of Psychosomatic Research* 4, 274–281.

Buendia, N., Sierra, G., Goode, M., and Segundo, J. P. (1963). Conditioned and discriminatory responses in wakeful and in sleeping cats. *Electroencephalography and Clinical Neurophysiology* Supplement 24, 199–218.

Cobb, J. C., Evans, F. J., Gustafson, L. A., O'Connel, O. N., Orne, M. T., and Shor, R. E. (1965). Specific motor responses during sleep to sleep-administered meaningful suggestion: an exploratory investigation. *Perceptual and Motor Skills* 20, 629–635.

Collins, W. E. and Iampietro, P. F. (1972). *Simulated Sonic Booms and Sleep Effects of Repeated Booms of 1.0 PSf (FAA-AM-72-35)*. Washington D.C., Department of Transportation.

Cornwell, A. C. (1967). Temporal conditioning of the arousal response. *Physiology and Behavior* 2, 65–71.

Corvalan, J. C. (1969). Correlation of electroencephalographic, reaction time, and auditory thresholds on 24 hour recordings. *Electroencephalography and Clinical Neurophysiology* 27, 696.

Corvalan, J. C. and Hayden, M. P. Depth of sleep and auditory thresholds during 24-hour recording. Unpublished abstract.

Czerny, A. (1896). Zurkenntnis des physiologischen Schlafes. *Jahrb. Kinderheilk.* **41**, 331–342.

Davis, H., Davis, P. A., Loomis, A. C., Harvey, E. N., and Hobart, G. (1939). Electrical reactions of the human brain to auditory stimulation during sleep. *Journal of Neurophysiology* **2**, 500–514.

Davis, H., Hirsch, S. K., Shelnutt, J., and Bowers, C. (1967). Further validation of evoked response audiometry (ERA). *Journal of Speech and Hearing Research* **10**, 717–727.

Derbyshire, A. J. and Farley, J. C. (1959). Sampling auditory responses at the cortical level. *Annals of Otology* **68**, 675–697.

De Sanctis, S. and Neyroz, U. (1902). Experimental investigations concerning the depth of sleep. *Physiological Review* **9**, 254–282.

Emmons, W. and Simon, W. (1956). The non-recall of material presented during sleep. *American Journal of Psychology* **69**, 76–81.

Eriksen, C. W. and Johnson, H. J. (1964). Storage and decay characteristics of nonattended auditory stimuli. *Journal of Experimental Psychology* **68**, 28–36.

Ferrari, E. and Messina, C. (1972). Blink reflexes during sleep and wakefulness in man. *Electroencephalography and Clinical Neurophysiology* **32**, 55–62.

Firth, H. (1973). Habituation during sleep. *Psychophysiology* **10**, 43–51.

Fischgold, H. and Schwartz, B. A. (1960). A clinical, electroencephalographic, and polygraphic study of sleep in the human adult. In *Ciba Foundation Symposium on the Nature of Sleep*. G. E. W. Wolstenholme and M. O'Connor (Eds.). Boston, Little, Brown.

Formby, D. (1967). Maternal recognition of infant's cry. *Developmental Medicine and Child Neurology* **9**, 293–298.

Frazier, R., McDonald, D. G., and Edwards, D. (1968). Discrimination between signal and non-signal stimuli during sleep. *Psychophysiology* **4**, 369 (abstract).

Glickman, S. E. and Feldman, S. M. (1961). Habituation of the arousal response to direct stimulation of the brainstem. *Electroencephalography and Clinical Neurophysiology* **13**, 703–709.

Glucksberg, S. and Cowen, G. (1970). Memory for nonattended auditory material. *Cognitive Psychology* **1**, 149–156.

Goodenough, D. R., Lewis, H. B., Shapiro, A., and Sieser, I. (1965). Some correlates of dream reporting following laboratory awakenings. *Journal of Nervous and Mental Disease* **140**, 365–373.

Ham, M. W. and Edmonston, W. E., Jr. (1971). Hypnosis, relaxation and motor retardation. *Journal of Abnormal Psychology* **77**, 329–331.

Hoskovec, J. and Cooper, L. (1967). Comparison of recent experimental trends concerning sleep learning in the U.S.A. and the Soviet Union. *Activitas Nervosa Superior* **9**, 93–98.

Howarth, C. I. and Ellis, K. (1961). The relative intelligibility threshold for one's own name compared with other names. *Quarterly Journal of Experimental Psychology* **13**, 236–239.

Hradecky, M., Barton, V., Brezinova, V., Burian, M., Stepanek, S., and Mikuleckz, M. (1968). Report on the problem of absorbing ideas during sleep. In: *Current Research in Hypnopaedia*. F. Rubin (Ed.). New York, American Elsevier.

Hrbek, A., Hrbkova, M., and Lenard, H. (1969). Somato-sensory, auditory and visual evoked responses in newborn infants during sleep and wakefulness. *Electroencephalography and Clinical Neurophysiology* **26**, 597–603.

Itil, T. M. (1976). Discrimination between some hypnotic and anxiolytic drugs by computerized analyzed sleep. In: *Pharmacology of Sleep*, R. L. Williams and I. Karacan (Eds.). pp.225–238. New York, John Wiley and Sons.

Johnson, J. and Lockwood, P. (1972). *Reactivity to Intermittent Light Stimulus during Sleep.* Paper presented at the meeting of the Electrophysiological Technologists Association, Manchester.

Johnson, L. C. and Lubin, A. (1967). The orienting reflex during waking and sleeping. *Electroencephalography and Clinical Neurophysiology* 22, 11–21.

Johnson, L. C., Church, M. W., Seales, D. M., and Rossiter, V. S. (1979). Auditory arousal thresholds of good sleepers and poor sleepers with and without flurazepam. *Sleep* 1, 259–270.

Johnson, L. C., Townsend, R. E., and Wilson, M. R. (1975). Habituation during sleeping and waking. *Psychophysiology* 12, 574–584.

Jus, A. and Jus, A. (1972). Experimental studies in memory distsurbances in humans in pathological and physiological conditions. *International Journal of Psychobiology* 2, 205–218.

Keefe, F. B., Johnson, L. C., and Hunter, E. J. (1971). Electroencephalographic and autonomic response patterns during waking and sleep stages. *Psychophysiology* 8, 198–212.

Kimura, J. and Harada, O. (1972). Excitability of the orbicularis oculi reflex in all night sleep: its suppression in non-rapid eye movement and recovery in rapid eye movement sleep. *Electroencephalography and Clinical Neurophysiology* 33, 369–377.

Kleitman, N. (1929). Sleep. *Physiological Reviews* 9, 624–665.

Kleitman, N. (1963). *Sleep and Wakefulness.* Chicago, University of Chicago Press.

Kleitman, N., Cooperman, N. R., and Mullin, F. J. (1936). Is there a continuous curve of the depth of sleep? *American Journal of Physiology* 116, 92–93.

Kohlschutter, E. (1862). Messungen der Festigheit des Schalfes. *Zeitschriftfur Rechtsmedezin* 17, 209–253.

Koukkou, M. and Lehmann, D. (1968). EEG and memory storage in sleep experiments with humans. *Electroencephalography and Clinical Neurophysiology* 25, 455–462.

Kramer, M., Roth, T., Trinder, J., and Cohen, A. (1971). *Noise Disturbance and Sleep.* (FAA-NO-70-16). Washington D.C., Department of Transportation.

Kryter, E. D. (1970). *The Effects of Noise on Man.* New York, Academic Press.

Kulikov, V. N. (1968). The question of hypnopaedia. In: *Current Research in Hypnopaedia.* F. Rubin (Ed.). New York, American Elsevier.

Kupperman, G. L. and Mendel, M. I. (1974). Threshold of the early components of the averaged electroencephalic response determined with tone pips and clicks during drug-induced sleep. *Audiology* 13, 379–390.

Langford, G. W., Meddis, R., and Pearson, A. J. D. (1974). Awakening latency from sleep for meaningful and nonmeaningful stimuli. *Psychophysiology* 11, 1–5.

Lasaga, J. and Lasaga, A. (1973). Sleep learning and progressive blurring of perception during sleep. *Perceptual and Motor Skills* 37, 51–62.

Leaton, R. N. and Buck, R. L. (1971). Habituation of the arousal response in rats. *Journal of Comparative and Physiological Psychology* 75, 430–434.

Leaton, R. and Jordan, W. (1978). Habituation of the EEG arousal response in rats: short- and long-term effects, frequency specificity, and wake–sleep transfer. *Journal of Comparative and Physiological Psychology* 2, 803–814.

Lehman, D. and Koukkou, M. (1973). Learning and EEG during sleep in humans: *Sleep: Physiology, Biochemistry, Psychology, Pharmacology, Clinical Implications.* 1st European Congress on Sleep Research, Basel 1972, 43–47. Basel, Karger.

Levere, T. E., Bartus, R. T., Morlock, G. W., and Hart, F. D. (1973). Arousal from sleep: responsiveness to different auditory frequencies equated for loudness. *Physiology and Behavior* 10, 53–57.

Levere, T., Davis, N., Mills, J., Berger, E., and Reiter, W. (1976). Arousal from sleep: the effects at the rise time of auditory stimuli, *Physiological Psychology* 4, 213–218.

Levere, T. E., Morlock, G. W., Thomas, L. P., and Hart, F. D. (1974). Arousal from sleep: the differential effect of frequencies equated for loudness. *Physiology and Behavior* 12, 573–582.

Levy, C., Coolidge, F., and Staab, L. (1972). Paired associate learning during EEG-defined sleep: a preliminary study. *Australian Journal of Psychology* 24, 219–225.

Lindsley, O. R. (1957). Operant behavior during sleep: a measure of depth of sleep. *Science* 126, 1290–1291.

Lukas, J. S. (1972). *Effects of Aircraft Noises on the Sleep of Women.* (NASA Report Number CR-2041). Menlo Park, California, Stanford Research Institute.

Lukas, J. S. (1973). Predicting the response to noise during sleep. In: *Proceedings of the International Congress on Noise as a Public Health Problem.* W. D. Ward (Ed.). Washington D.C., US Environmental Protection Agency.

Lukas, J. S. (1975). *Assessment of Noise Effects on Human Sleep.* Paper presented at American Psychological Association, Chicago, August, 1975.

Lukas, J. S. and Kryter, K. D. (1970). Awakening effects of simulated sonic booms and subsonic aircraft noise. In: *Psychological Effects of Noise.* B. L. Welch and A. S. Welch (Eds.). New York, Plenum Press.

Lukas, J. S., Peeler, D. J., and Davis, J. E. (1975). *Effects on Sleep of Noise from Two Proposed STOL Aircraft.* (NASA Report Number CR-132564). Menlo Park, California, Stanford Research Institute.

McDonald, D. G. and Carpenter, F. A. (1975). Habituation of the orienting response in sleep. *Psychophysiology* 12, 618–623.

McDonald, D., Schicht, W., Frazier, R., Shallenberger, H., and Edwards, D. (1975). Studies of information processing in sleep. *Psychophysiology* 12, 624–629.

Mendel, M. I. (1974). Influence of stimulus level and sleep stage on the early components of the averaged electroencephalic response to clicks during all-night sleep. *Journal of Speech and Hearing Research* 17, 5–17.

Mendel, M. I., Hosick, E. C., Windman, T. R., Davis, H., Hirsch, S. K., and Dinges, D. F. (1975). Audiometric comparison of the middle and late components of the adult auditory evoked potentials awake and asleep. *Electroencephalography and Clinical Neurophysiology* 38, 27–33.

Michelson, E. (1897). Intersuchungen ueber die Tiefe des Schlafes. *Psychologic Arbeiten* 2, 84–117.

Miller, J. D. (1971). *Effects of Noise on People* (NTID 300.7). Washington D.C., US Government Printing Office.

Miller, M. (1926). Changes in the response to electric shock produced by varying muscular conditions. *Journal of Experimental Psychology* 9, 26–44.

Minard, J., Loiselle, R., Ingledue, E., and Dautlich, C. (1968). Discriminative electro-culogram deflections (EOGDs) and heart-rate pauses elicited during maintained sleep by stimulus significance. *Psychophysiology* 5, 232 (abstract).

Moenninghoff, O. and Piesbergen, F. (1883). Meisungen ueber die Tiefe des Schlafes. *Zeitschrift fur Biologie* 19, 114–128.

Mullin, F. J. (1937). Changes in irritability to auditory stimuli on falling asleep. *American Journal of Physiology* 119, 377–378.

Mullin, F. J. and Kleitman, N. (1938). Variation in threshold of auditory stimuli necessary to awaken the sleeper. *American Journal of Physiology* 123, 477–481.

Mullin, F. J., Kleitman, K., and Cooperman, N. R. (1933). The effect of alcohol and caffeine on motility and body temperature during sleep. *American Journal of Physiology* 106, 478–487.

Mullin, F. J., Kleitman, N., and Cooperman, N. R. (1937). Studies on the physiology of sleep changes in irritability to auditory stimuli during sleep. *Journal of Experimental Psychology* **21**, 88–96.

Murray, B. and Campbell, D. (1970). Difference between olfactory thresholds in two sleep states in the newborn infant. *Psychonomic Science* **18**, 313–314.

Nakamura K., Iwahara, S., and Fulisawa, K. (1966). A psychophysiological study of the depth of sleep. *Japanese Psychological Research* **8**, 179–191.

Nan'no, H., Hishikawa, Y., Koida, H., Takashashi, H., and Kaneko, Z. (1970). A neurophysiological stsudy of sleep paralysis in narcoleptic patients. *Electroencephalography and Clinical Neurophysiology* **28**, 382–390.

Okuma, T., Nakamura, K., Hayashi, A., and Fujimori, M. (1966). Psychophysiological study on the depth of sleep in normal human subjects. *Electroencephalography and Clinical Neurophysiology* **21**, 140–147.

Oltman, P., Goodenough, D., Koulack, D., Maclin, E., Schroeder, R., and Flannigan, M. (1977). Short term memory during stage 2 sleep. *Psychophysiology* **14**, 439–444.

Oswald, I., Taylor, A. M., and Treisman, M. (1960). Discriminative responses to stimulation during human sleep. *Brain* **83**, 440–453.

Perry, C. W., Evans, F. J., O'Connell, D. N., Orne, E. C., and Orne, M. T. (1978). Behavioral response to verbal stimuli administered and tested during REM sleep: a further investigation. *Waking and Sleeping* **2**, 35–42.

Pieper, E. and Kugler, J. (1966). Learning during sleep. *Electroencephalography and Clinical Neurophysiology* **21**, 204–206.

Pisano, M., Rosadini, G., Rossi, G. F., and Zattoni, J. (1966). Relations between threshold of arousal and electroencephalographic patterns during sleep in man. *Physiology and Behavior* **1**, 55–58.

Poitras, A., Thorkildsen, A., Gagnon, M., and Naiman, J. (1973). Auditory discrimination during REM and non-REM sleep in women before and after delivery. *Canadian Psychiatric Association Journal* **8**, 519–526.

Price, L. L. and Goldstein, R. (1966). Averaged evoked reponses for measuring auditory sensitivity in children. *Journal of Speech and Hearing Disorders* **31**, 248–255.

Rechtschaffen, A., Hauri, P., and Zeitlin, M. (1966). Auditory awakening thresholds in REM and NREM sleep stages. *Perceptual and Motor Skills* **22**, 927–942.

Rechtschaffen, A. and Lentzner, R. (1960). *A Comparison of Auditory Thresholds during Dreaming and Non-dreaming Sleep.* Paper presented at the meeting of the Illinois Psychological Association, Chicago, October, 1960.

Reding, G. R. and Fernandez, C. (1968). Effects of vestibular stimulation during sleep. *Electroencephalography and Clinical Neurophysiology* **24**, 75–79.

Roth, M., Shaw, J., and Green, J. (1956). The form, voltage distribution and physiological significance of the K-complex. *Electroencephalography and Clinical Neurophysiology* **8**, 385–399.

Roth, T., Kramer, M., and Trinder, J. (1972). The effect of noise during sleep on the sleep patterns of different age groups. *Canadian Psychiatric Association Journal* **17**, 197–201.

Rowland, V. (1957). Differential electroencephalographic response to conditioned auditory stimuli in arousal from sleep. *Electroencephalography and Clinical Neurophysiology* **9**, 585–594.

Rubin, F. (Ed.) (1968). *Current Research in Hypnopaedia.* New York, American Elsevier.

Rubin, F. (1971). *Learning and Sleep: the Theory and Practice of Hypnopaedia.* Bristol, England, John Wright.

Schmidt, K. and Birns, B. (1971). The behavioral arousal threshold in infant sleep as a function of time and sleep state. *Child Development* 269-277.

Scott, T. D. (1972). The effects of continuous, high intensity, white noise on the human sleep cycle. *Psychophysiology* 9, 227-232.

Shapiro, A., Goodenough, D. R., and Gryler, R. B. (1963). Dream recall as a function of method of awakening. *Psychosomatic Medicine* 25, 174-180.

Sharpless, S. and Jasper, H. (1956). Habituation of the arousal reaction. *Brain* 79, 655-680.

Shimizu, A., Takahashi, H., Sumitsuji, N., Tanaka, M., Yoshida, I., and Kaneko, Z. (1977). Memory retention of stimulations during REM and NREM stages of sleep. *Electroencephalography and Clinical Neurophysiology* 43, 658-665.

Simon, C. and Emmons, W. (1955). Learning during sleep? *Psychological Bulletin* 52, 328-343.

Simon, C. and Emmons, W. (1956). Responses to material presented during various levels of sleep. *Journal of Experimental Psychology* 51, 81-97.

Snyder, F. and Scott, J. (1972). The psychophysiology of sleep. In: *Handbook of Psychophysiology*. N. S. Greenfield and R. A. Sternback (Eds.). New York, Holt, Rinehard and Winston.

Sokolov, E. N. (1963). *Perception and the Conditioned Reflex*. New York, Macmillan.

Sommer-Smith, J. A., Galeano, C., Pineyrua, M., Roig, J. A., and Segundo, J. P. (1962). Tone cessation as a conditioned signal. *Electroencephalography and Clinical Neurophysiology* 14, 869-877.

Stone, H., Pryor, G., and Colwell, J. (1967). Olfactory detection thresholds in man under conditions of rest and exercise. *Perception and Psychophysics* 2, 167-170.

Swan, T. H. (1929). A note on Kohlschutter's curve of the 'depth of sleep'. *Psychological Bulletin* 26, 607-610.

Tani, K. and Yoshii, N. (1970). Efficiency of verbal Learning during sleep as related to the EEG pattern. *Brain Research* 17, 277-285.

Thiessen, G. J. (1970). Effects of noise during sleep. In: *Physiological effects of noise*. B. L. Welch and A. S. Welch (Eds.). New York, Plenum Press.

Townsend, R. E., Johnson, L. C., and Muzet, A. (1973). Effects of long term exposure to tone pulse noise on human sleep. *Psychophysiology* 10, 369-375.

Watson, R. and Rechtschaffen, A. (1969). Auditory awakening thresholds and dream recall in NREM sleep. *Perceptual and Motor Skills* 29, 635-644.

Weinberger, N. M. and Lindsley, D. B. (1964). Behavioral and electroencephalographic arousal to contrasting novel stimulation. *Science* 144, 1357-1359.

Weir, C. (1976). Auditory frequency sensitivity in the neonate: a signal detection analysis. *Journal of Experimental Child Psychology* 21, 219-225.

Weitzman, E. D. and Kremen, H. (1965). Auditory evoked responses during different stages of sleep in man. *Electroencephalography and Clinical Neurophysiology* 18, 65-70.

Wilkinson, R. T. (1961). Interaction of lack of sleep with knowledge of results, repeated testing, and individual differences. *Journal of Experimental Psychology* 62, 263-271.

Wilkinson, R. T., Morlock, H. C., and Williams, H. L. (1966). Evoked cortical response during vigilance. *Psychonomic Science* 4, 221-222.

Williams, H. L., Hammack, J. T., Daly, R. L., Dement, W. C., and Lubin, A. L. (1964). Responses to auditory stimulation, sleep loss, and the EEG stages of sleep. *Electroencephalography and Clinical Neurophysiology* 16, 269-279.

Williams, H. L., Lubin, A., and Goodnow, J. J. (1959). Impaired performance with acute sleep loss. *Psychological Monographs*, 73, No. 14 (Whole No. 484), p.26.

Williams, H. L., Morlock, H. C., and Morlock, J. V. (1966). Instrumental behavior during sleep. *Psychophysiology* 2, 208-216.

Williams, H. L., Tepas, D. I., and Morlock, H. C. (1962). Evoked responses to clicks and electroencaphalographic stages of sleep in man. *Science* **138**, 685-686.

Wills, N. and Trinder, J. (1978). Influence of response criterion on the awakening thresholds of sleep stage. *Waking and Sleeping* **2**, 57-62.

Wilson, W. P. and Zung, W. K. (1966). Attention, discrimination, and arousal during sleep. *Archives of General Psychiatry* **15**, 523-528.

Wohlisch, E. (1957). The course of the depth of sleep and its recovery equivalent. *Klinische Wochenschrift* **35**, 705-714.

Wolff, P. H. (1967). The sleep of infants. *Psychological Issues* **5**, 1-105.

Zimmerman, W. B. (1968). Psychological and physiological differences between 'light' and 'deep' sleepers. *Psychophysiology* **4**, 387 (abstract).

Zimmerman, W. B. (1970). Sleep mentation and auditory awakening thresholds. *Psychophysiology* **6**, 540-549.

Zukhar, V. T., Kaplan, Y. Y., Maksimov, Y. A., and Pushkina, I. P. (1968). A collective experiment on hypnopaedia. In: *Current Research in Hypnopaeia*. F. Rubin (Ed.). New York, American Elsevier.

Zung, W. K. and Wilson, W. P. (1961). Response to auditory stimulation during sleep. *Archives of General Psychiatry* **4**, 548-552.

Zung, W. K., Wilson, W. P., and Dodson, W. E. (1964). Effect of depressive disorders on sleep electroencephalographic responses. *Archives of General Psychiatry* **10**, 439-445.

Biological Rhythms, Sleep, and Performance
Edited by Wilse B. Webb
©1982 John Wiley & Sons Ltd.

Chapter 9

Ultradian Rhythms in Human Sleep and Wakefulness

Peretz Lavie

BACKGROUND

Common sense would predict that over long periods performance of well practised tasks should decline monotonically as a function of 'fatigue'. However, recent research indicates that the quality of the performance of some tasks varies in cycles whose period is approximately 90 minutes, remarkably like the period of the REM–NONREM sleep cycle described in Chapter II. Such cycles have been called ultradian rhythms by Halberg (1967). Any cycle whose period is shorter than half a day is an ultradian cycle.

This chapter reviews the data on the appearance of 90 min ultradian rhythms in the waking human. Some of the rhythms have been observed in physiological functions, others in measures of performance. The possible relationship of these rhythms to the cyclic appearance of REM periods in sleep and theoretical and practical implications for human performance will be discussed.

Rhythms in Human Performance

Thorndike (1900), Kraepelin (1893), and others investigated the daily course of 'mental fatigue'. They concluded that there may be natural rhythms in performance, independent of the amount of work done (for a recent review see Lavie, 1980).

Subsequently, interest in cyclic variations in performance waned. The revival of interest in this problem, that was accelerated in recent years, may be attributed to the accumulation of evidence about the rhythmicity of many biological phenomena.

Interest in the psychophysiology and mechanisms of sleep, triggered by the

239

discovery of rapid eye movement (REM) sleep by Aserinsky and Kleitman (1953) also encouraged research into performance rhythms, particularly those related to the sleep–wake cycle. Ultimately, as will be described shortly, speculations about the sleep cycles led to the study of ultradian fluctuations, which are the subject of the present chapter.

Until recently, however, most if not all experimental interest in behavioural cyclicity in humans focused on circadian variations. The voluminous data on endogenous circadian rhythms in biological processes implied the possible existence of comparable rhythms in behaviour. Thus, for example, Kleitman (1963) studied the relation between diurnal changes in body temperature and mental function. In addition to the endogenous circadian pacemakers, environmental stimuli provide numerous exogenous circadian *Zeitgebers* ('time givers') which may influence behaviour. In contrast, we know of no such *Zeitgebers* with 'natural' periodicities within the ultradian range of 70–140 min. Some of the interest in circadian rhythms arose within the context of attempts to solve human engineering problems presented by the growth of air travel and by the increasing awareness of the psychobiological and medical aspects of shift work.

Interest in circadian variations, and short term changes in vigilance performance led to experimental designs which obscured ultradian variability. Studies of circadian fluctuations generally sample behaviour less than once per hour. These sampling rates are obviously too slow to detect the ultradian variations. Studies of vigilance do employ sampling rates which are sufficiently fast to enable registration of ultradian rhythms. Yet these experiments generally last for, at most, a 1–2 hour period, too short, of course, for detection of 90 min ultradian cycles. Furthermore, it has been assumed that 'the most characteristic feature of long term performance on monotonous perceptual tasks is that it deteriorates with the passage of time' (Jerison, 1967); consequently, in studies of vigilance, data are averaged across subjects, a design which would hide any time related variability in the data. Thus, the theoretical interest in changes unrelated to ultradian rhythms led to assumptions in experimental design and inference which tended to mask the latter phenomena.

Early Evidence of Ultradian Rhythms in Human Behaviour

Nevertheless, there is abundant evidence that the direction of change in human performance and perception over extended periods is not uniform; such phenomena can represent regular ultradian rhythmicity in behaviour, though none of the theoretical interpretations previously offered for these data have considered this possibility. Thus, Murrell (1967) tested subjects for 3.5 hours on a task simulating the checking of electrical components. He observed that 'after work had continued for a period of time, there was a phase of irregularity in the performance, this was followed by an improvement in regularity and a second deterioration' (Murrell, 1967, p.428). Though Murrell did not specify the time course of these changes, if we assume that the variations in performance reflected a fragment of an ongoing rhythm, we can estimate that the period of this rhythm was within the ultradian range.

Murrell was unable to attribute his findings to any experimental variable. In support of his data, he presented additional examples of such changes from the data of Dordeno (1959) and Ross *et al.* (1959) (quoted by Murrell, 1967). His analysis indicated that grouped data usually presented in vigilance studies may mask little noticed, but striking, differences in variations in performance of individuals over time. Murrell attributed these differences to fluctuations in arousal, which are partly under the subject's control.

Studies of perception of apparent motion using the spiral after-effect and phi phenomenon present further evidence of possible ultradian changes. As early as 1894, Hoppe reported that the magnitude of the 'spiral after-effect', an apparent motion experienced following the fixation of a rotating spiral, tends to wax and wane without apparent reason. According to Gilbert (1939), Wertheimer, who conducted extensive investigations of this problem, argued that changes in the magnitude of the apparent motion resulted from fluctuations in attention and motivation. Gilbert himself observed 'violent fluctuations' in the perception of the phi phenomenon, an apparent motion illusion in which a spot of light is flashed successively at two different points, but is perceived as a continuous stimulus moving across the field. Gilbert believed that these variations were too large to be attributable to motivational or attentional fluctuations, as Wertheimer has argued, and proposed instead that they might be due to unknown metabolic changes at the level of the receptors. Spectral analysis of data retrieved from the figures presented by Gilbert, revealed a 95 min periodicity in the results of one of two subjects who had been tested continuously for 4 hours (Lavie and Sutter, 1975).

Rapoport (1963) and Andersson (1969) studied changes in perception of the spiral after-effect in tests administered on two different days. In each study, it was found that during the first test there were progressive increases in the duration of the illusion for some subjects, whereas others showed a constant duration of the illusion. A third group showed a decrease. On the second test, some subjects displayed the pattern as they had shown initially, while in other subjects the illusion decreased over the second test series while it had increased over the first series and vice versa. Both investigators attributed these changes to personality differences. However, although it well may be that variations in illusionary perceptual process are related to personality, the subsequent demonstration (Lavie, Lord, and Frank, 1974) of 90 min ultradian rhythms in perception of this apparent motion can also account for these observations.

The Basic Rest-Activity Cycle (BRAC) Hypothesis

Interest in ultradian rhythms in human physiology and performance was reawakened with the discovery that the appearance of paradoxical sleep or rapid eye movement (REM) sleep alternates cyclically with NONREM sleep (Aserinsky and Kleitman, 1953), each mode being characterized by a distinct set of psychophysiological correlates (see Chapter II of the present volume).

Kleitman, who with Aserinsky first described the REM state, postulated that the rhythmic occurrence of REM in sleep is only a fragment of a broader biological alertness rhythm which operates continuously in both sleep and wakefulness, and which he termed the basic rest-activity cycle (BRAC) (Kleitman, 1963).

Kleitman maintained that the adult diurnal sleep–wakefulness cycle is an advanced complex state which develops from briefer sleep–wakefulness cycles evident in infants. According to Kleitman, these more primitive rhythms, with a periodicity of 2–4 hours, represent a coalescence of shorter 50–60 minute rest–activity cycles, which is also the dominant periodicity of the infant REM cycles, and can be detected in fetal motility cycles as well (Sterman, 1972; Granat *et al.*, 1979). As the adult diurnal sleep cycle develops, the basic period is lengthened from 50–60 minutes to 80–100 minutes. Kleitman predicted that this basic cycle which appears in sleep as the REM and NONREM cycles would be manifested during the waking hours in periodic fluctuations in alertness.

ULTRADIAN CYCLES DURING WAKEFULNESS

Kleitman (1963) believed that the BRAC developed from a more primitive rhythm in digestive function, which was adjusted to the organism's nutritional needs. Accordingly, one would expect to find ultradian rhythms in ingestive, digestive, and excretory functions of humans, as well as rhythms in waking performance and psychophysiological measures attributable to fluctuations in alertness. However, before turning to the experimental evidence, some methodological comments are in order.

Research and statistical methodology of biological rhythms research has been discussed in detail in the first chapter of this volume, so they need not be described here. However, the types of data collected in ultradian rhythm experiments do not easily lend themselves to statistical analysis, because of short experimental sessions. Hence, various techniques have been used, from 'Eyeballing' peaks and troughs in the data to the sophisticated complex demodulation technique (see Chapter 2). In many studies the statistical significance of the observed rhythmicity was not indicated, nor was the relative contribution of the rhythm to the total variance in the data. In such cases, it is difficult to assess the importance of the observed rhythmicity, since even through consistent rhythmicity may exist in specific behaviours or physiological processes, its contribution to the total variability may be so small that its influence on ongoing behaviour can be ignored. Thus, the following review will emphasize reports in which the magnitude and significance of the ultradian rhythmicity were indicated.

Digestion, Ingestion, and Excretion

Friedman and Fisher (1967) reported that humans allowed free access to food will display an 80–100 minute ultradian cycle in their eating behaviour. These findings were confirmed by Oswald, Merrington, and Lewis (1970) and by Kripke (1972).

In cats, Sterman, Lucas, and Macdonald (1972) found ultradian eating rhythms with periods of approximately 20 minutes, corresponding to the length of the REM cycle in that species. Significant ultradian fluctuations in hand–mouth behaviour of rhesus monkeys have also been observed (Lewis, Kripke, and Bowden, 1977). Later, Bowden, Kripke and Wyborney (1978) reported that in the same species, locomotion, exploration, ingestion, and resting all varied in an ultradian manner; resting was inversely related to the other behaviours. The ultradian rhythmicities accounted for approximately 10–15% of the total variance.

Mandell *et al.* (1966) suggested the existence of ultradian rhythms in urine flow in catheterized sleeping patients which were correlated with the REM–NONREM cycles, but did not present statistical analyses. Subsequently, Lavie and Kripke (1977) demonstrated significant 90 minute cyclicity in urine flow of waking subjects, and found that concentrations of Na^+ and K^+ ions fluctuated in a similar rhythm, 180° out of phase with changes in volume. The rhythms in volume and solute excretion were of large amplitudes and accounted for approximately 20% of the total variance. In recumbent, catheterized subjects Luboshitzky *et al.* (1978) found significant ultradian rhythms in urinary osmolality and cation concentrations of waking subjects, which accounted for a similar portion of the total variance, but did not observe cyclic variation in volume of urine flow as had Lavie and Kripke (1977). Recent results from our laboratory demonstrated rhythms of similar periodicity and magnitude in urine flow and osmolality of sleeping and waking catheterized dogs (Gordon and Lavie, in press).

Also in accordance with Kleitman's hypothesis, both waking fasting humans (Hiatt and Kripke, 1975) and sleeping subjects (Tassinari *et al.*, 1973; Lavie *et al.*, 1978) apparently display rhythms in gastric contraction activity with a period of approximately 100 minutes. It is interesting to note that the 1.5 hour rhythmicity in gastric activity was first described in 1922 by Wada, long before the recognition of the REM–NONREM cycles.

Psychophysiological Measures

A number of recent studies have reported ultradian changes in psychological measures of alertness and in psychophysiological indices which are thought to be related to alertness, lending direct support to the BRAC hypothesis (Kleitman, 1963).

In isolated subjects under partial sensory deprivation, Kripke (1972) reported significant ultradian rhythms in eating, and rhythms in electro-encephalographic activity at various frequencies that were most prominent in the delta frequency band (0.5–3 cps).

Othmer, Heyden, and Segelbaum (1969) reported cyclic changes in rapid eye movement activity in waking subjects, which resembled REM cycles in sleep. No statistical analysis accompanied their conclusion, however. Horne and Whitehead (1976) reported on approximately 90 min rhythms in respiratory rate of isolated subjects. Earlier, West *et al.* (1962) were impressed that subjects undergoing prolonged sleep deprivation showed periodic episodes of 'psychotic-like' hallucinatory behaviour with a frequency similar to that of the sleep REM cycle, but they did not statistically analyse this behaviour. Kripke and Sonnenschein (1978) studied the relation between waking rapid eye movements, electroencephalographic activity and episodes of daydreaming in isolated subjects or in subjects in their natural social environment. Daydreaming, characterized by vivid sensory imagery and bizarre symbolic or autistic content, resembling the hypnagogic hallucinations of sleep onset, occurred at 90 minute intervals, and were correlated with continuous alpha EEG activity and diminution of rapid eye movements. These effects were most pronounced in the isolated condition.

Pupillary diameter, stability, and reactivity to light are well established indices of sleepiness and fatigue (Lowenstein, Feinberg, and Lowenfeld, 1963; Yoss, Mayer, and Hollenhorst, 1969). Recently, Lavie (1979) demonstrated ultradian rhythms in pupillary size and in an index of pupillary stability under constant illumination conditions. In this study, pupillary measures were sampled every 15 minutes for 10 hours, and significant 70–90 minute rhythms in the two pupillary indices were evident, which accounted for 17–20% of the total variance. Figure 1 illustrates ultradian rhythms in pupillary diameter and in the index of pupillary stability, which were clearly out of phase with each other. That is, pupillary dilation was associated with increased stability of pupillary diameter. As is evident from Figure 1 the ultradian rhythms in pupillary diameter are superimposed on a linear trend, which probably reflects circadian changes (Doring and Schaefers, 1950).

Lavie and Scherson (1981) postulated that ultradian rhythms in alertness, if present, should be reflected in subjects' ability to fall asleep at different times in the day. Nine subjects were instructed to close their eyes and to fall asleep during 5 minute periods of darkness at 15 minute intervals for 12 hours.

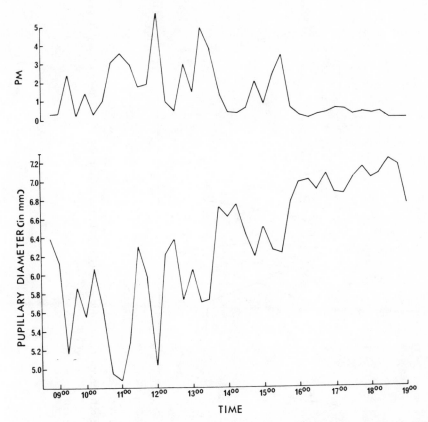

Figure 1   Ultradian rhythms in pupillary diameter (in mm) and inverse ultradian
rhythms in pupillary stability (in units of pupillary motility, PM)

Sleep and wakefulness were defined electroencephalographically. Significant
ultradian 90 minute periodic fluctuations in stage 1 sleep measured in this way
were evident. Figure 2 gives the percentages of theta and alpha activity in each
5 minute dark period in one subject; the reciprocal ultradian fluctuations in
these variables are clearly evident. As one might expect, ability to fall asleep
was also modulated by circadian rhythmicity with increased awake time
toward afternoon and early evening hours, and increased sleep stage 2 around
midday. Interestingly enough, in the second part of the study, when subjects
were sleep deprived, the ultradian rhythmicity disappeared.

The results of studies using human subjects have been confirmed by animal
experimentation. Kripke *et al.* (1976) made continuous 24 h electrophysiological
recordings in rhesus monkeys maintained on 12 h light 12 h dark cycles, and
observed ultradian rhythms in several electroencephalographic frequency

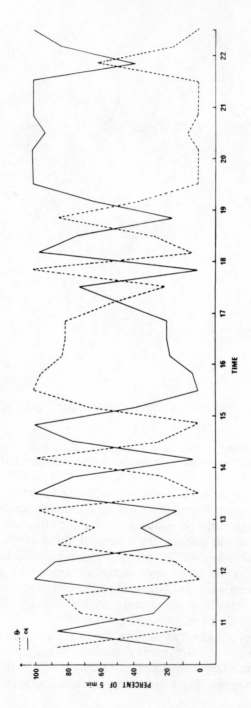

Figure 2   Ultradian rhythms in alpha and theta electroencephalographic activity in subjects attempting to fall asleep every 20 min for 5 min

bands during both periods. During the light-on period, however, the rhythms were considerably slower, 120 min/cycle *vs* 60 min/cycle during lights-off period, suggesting a circadian modulation of the ultradian frequency. Since the phase relationships among the variables were preserved from lights-on to lights-off, Kripke *et al.* suggested a joint mechanism for the sleep and wakefulness rhythms. In cats that were sleep deprived by brain stem electrical stimulation, Lucas and Harper (1976) reported 24 h, 3 h, and 20 min periods in the rate of brain stimulation required to maintain arousal. The latter period of 20 min is identical to that of cat REM–NONREM cycle.

Perceptual Phenomena

As previously noted, variations in perception of apparent motion had been attributed to personality differences (Rapoport, 1963; Andersson, 1969) or to variations in subject's motivation or receptor sensitivity (Gilbert, 1939). Lavie, Levy, and Coolidge (1975) tested perception of the spiral after-effect at 5 minute intervals in 8 hour day and 8 hour night periods. They found that fluctuations in the duration of the illusion describe a clear 90 minute rhythm, an effect which was independent of individual differences in the duration of the illusion. These findings are shown in Figure 3 which also gives the autocorrelation function calculated up to 40 lags (200 minutes). These results were confirmed by Lavie, Lord, and Frank (1974) in subjects tested on two consecutive evenings from 1600 to 2400 hours. Similar rhythms have been found in the phi phenomenon, and these were synchronized with those observed for the spiral after-effect illusion (Lavie, 1976). In all these studies the rhythms were of remarkably large amplitude. More recently, Klein and Armitage (1979) tested Broughton's (1975) suggestion that the BRAC involves an alternation in the relative efficiency of the two cerebral hemispheres, and reported 180° out of phase 90 min oscillations in verbal and spatial matching tasks, supporting Broughton's hypothesis.

Vigilance and Perceptual–motor Performance

Though it would be logical to look for rhythms in vigilance in the light of the BRAC hypothesis, there has been suprisingly little work in this direction. Globus *et al.* (1971) reported equivocal 100 minute cycles in performance of a 6 hour continuous vigilance task. However, these rhythms were rather weak and accounted for a negligible portion of the total variability. Evidence of fluctuations at other frequencies was apparent in the data as well. Orr, Hoffman, and Hegge (1974) studied prolonged complex vigilance and concomitantly monitored heart rate. Complex demodulation revealed a 90 minute periodicity in performance, which was weakly and inconsistently related to changes in heart rate. The statistical technique, however, did

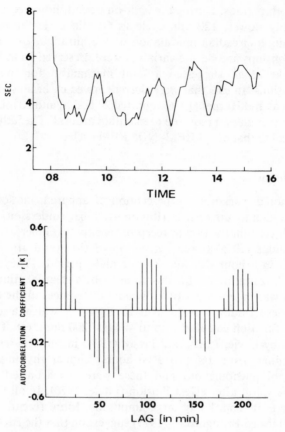

Figure 3   Ultradian rhythms in the duration of the spiral after-effect (upper panel) and corresponding autocorrelation function (lower panel)

not permit evaluation of the statistical significance of the performance rhythms.

In our laboratory we have employed perceptual–motor rather than vigilance tasks because the former are more easily controlled and can be administered for breif periods spread out over many hours, preventing the confounding of possible ultradian rhythms with fatigue effects which occur in continuous vigilance tasks.

We first investigated the linear positioning task (Gopher and Lavie, 1980), in which subjects were required to move a lever to a distance of 20 cm along a metal rod, relying only on auditory and proprioceptive stimuli. These were provided by an audio signal whose frequency varied with the displacement of the rod, and by a weight attached to the spring of the lever. The task is illustrated in Figure 4.

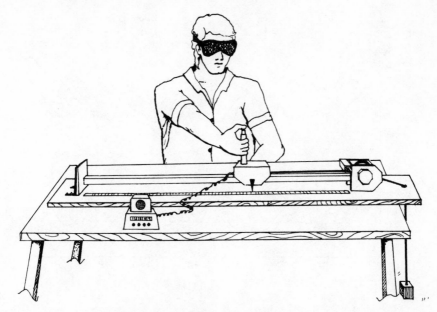

Figure 4   The linear positioning task (see explanation in the text)

Eight subjects were tested at 20 minute intervals, and 8 others at 10 minute intervals. Testing continued from 8 AM to 6 PM. Each test consisted of 5 trials with knowledge of results (KR) and 5 without (NKR). For both groups, positioning errors in the NKR condition varied in a 100 minute ultradian rhythm. The rhythms were of large amplitude and accounted for approximately 20% of the variance, but in some subjects as much as 30% of the total variability was accounted for by ultradian rhythmicity. No significant periodicity was found in speed of performance in either condition, and no rhythms in accuracy were found in the KR 'feedback' condition. Spectral analysis revealed rapid 20–40 minute fluctuations in accuracy in the KR conditions, as opposed to the significant 100 minute periodicity evident in the NKR condition. Records of one subject shown in Figure 5 illustrate these findings. Between trials urine volume was also sampled. This varied in an ultradian rhythm, but these cycles were not consistently related to performance rhythms.

Though the positioning task did not reveal cyclic changes in movement time, we hoped that such rhythms in reaction time might be evident in another type of task. In that study (Lavie *et al.*, in press), an adaptive serial reaction time test, subjects responded to random numbers appearing on a CRT by pressing the appropriate button before display termination; failures to respond before termination of the display and incorrect responses were scored as errors. A correct response on a given trial shortened display time by 20 msec on the

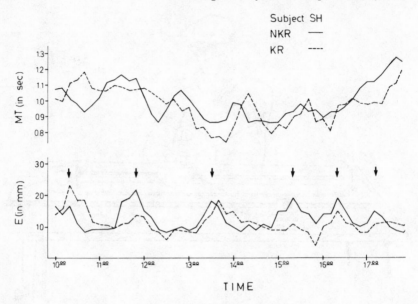

Figure 5   Ultradian rhythms in the error (E) of the positioning task, arrows indicate peaks in errors. Note that there are small variations in movement time (MT) superimposed on slow trend that probably reflect circadian trend

following trial. Conversely, an error lengthened display time on the next trial by 20 msec.

Eight subjects were tested initially from 0800 to 2000 hours, and retested from 2000 to 0800 hours in a separate session. Tests lasting 1.0 to 1.5 minutes and consisting of 40 trials were given at 15 minute intervals. Initial trials of each test began with a display duration which was the modal duration of the previous session. Spectral analyses of mean and modal display times in each session revealed no ultradian performance rhythms in either day or night sessions. Most spectral variance was in the low frequency range, suggesting possible circadian fluctuations. This effect was particularly evident in the night time series.

The results of the linear positioning and adaptive serial reaction time tasks are summarized in Figure 6 which displays the curves for each dependent variable in each task. The curves were peak synchronized, a procedure intended to enhance major trends; this would tend to emphasize any rhythmicity common to all subjects, and cancel out random fluctuations. It is evident from the figure that while accuracy of performance did display ultradian rhythmicity, no such effect was evident in reaction time scores in either study. Perhaps reaction time tasks are too simple or insensitive to

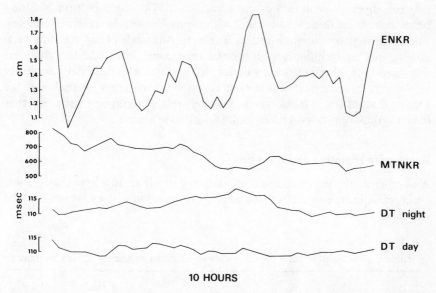

Figure 6 Peak synchronized curves for error (ENKR) and movement time (MTNKR) in positioning task, and display time of the adaptive serial reaction time task (DT), during day and night periods

reflect ultradian rhythmicity. Hiatt, Kripke, and Lavie (1975) also failed to find ultradian rhythmicity in reaction time tasks.

RELATIONS BETWEEN WAKING CYCLICITIES

The findings presented in the previous section indicate that, as proposed by Kleitman (1963) ultradian rhythms are evident in various aspects of digestive activity and in measures related to variations in arousal. It is perhaps logical to ask at this point whether, as would appear to follow from Kleitman's hypothesis, these various rhythms are related to each other. The strongest evidence in favour of this hypothesis would be the demonstration of a common neural or metabolic mechanism underlying these rhythms, but given the present state of knowledge, such data are not forthcoming. In the absence of such information, we must base our evaluation of the relationship between these rhythmic phenomena, upon correlations between them and similarity of periods, an approach whose obvious weaknesses will be discussed after reviewing the evidence.

Rhythms in 'Arousal'

As previously noted (page 244), a number of studies have found correlations between rhythmicity in two or more variables. With the exception of eating behaviour, all of these studies dealt with arousal or arousal related variables. These findings are summarized in Table 1. Although eating has not been investigated concomitantly with arousal related measures, the fact that cats displayed both 20 minute eating cycles and rhythms with a similar periodicity in the rate of electrical stimulation required to maintain arousal and the finding that resting in monkeys was inversely related to ingestion suggests that these rhythms may be correlated with variations in arousal.

Rhythms in Digestion and Excretion

A number of findings indicate that, contrary to Kleitman's hypothesis, some cyclic variations, especially those related to digestion and excretion, may be unrelated to arousal.

Table 1   Indices of arousal shown to vary in ultradian manner in waking humans

Measure	Investigator	High arousal	Low arousal
Delta EEG activity	Kripke (1972)	↓	↑
Theta EEG activity	Lavie and Scherson (1981)	↓	↑
Fantasies and daydreaming	Kripke and Sonnenschein (1978)	↓	↑
Ocular activity	Othmer, Hayden, and Segelbaum (1969)	↑	↓
Pupillary diameter	Lavie (1979)	↑	↓
Pupillary motility	Lavie (1979)	↓	↑
Vigilance performance	Orr, Hoffman, and Hegge (1976)	↑	↓
Perceptual–motor performance	Gopher and Lavie (1980)	↑	↓
Heart rate	Orr, Hoffman, and Hegge (1976)	↑	↓
Eating related behaviour	Friedman and Fisher (1967) Oswald, Merrington, and Lewis (1970) Kripke (1972) Sterman, Lucas, and Macdonald (1972)	↑	↓
Respiratory rate	Horne and Whitehead (1976)	↑	↓

Though occurrence of daydreaming has been shown to be related to electro-encephalographic and eye movement activity in waking subjects, Hiatt, Kripke, and Lavie (1975) did not find a correlation between rhythms in gastric contractions and those observed in daydreaming. Gopher and Lavie (1980) did not find a correlation between rhythms in performance of a linear positioning task and cycles of similar periodicity in volume of urine excretion.

Problems in Inference

Obviously, similar periodicity in various rhythms, or even correlations between them, do not prove that they are under the control of a single mechanism. Correlation can be due to synchronization by some external entrainment mechanism. This is illustrated by findings of research into circadian rhythms. Circadian rhythms in performance, subjective arousal, and physiological measures such as body temperature, which are normally in close synchrony (Colquhoun, 1971) are apparently not causally related (Moses *et al.*, 1978). Circadian rhythms in sleep and body temperature, which normally share the same periodicity and are closely correlated, show different periodicities when all external time cues are eliminated (Aschoff, Genecke, and Wever, 1967). Evidence based upon similar periodicity in ultradian rhythms is even weaker than such evidence in circadian rhythms, since the signal to noise ratio appears lower in ultradian rhythms than in circadian rhythms.

On the other hand, rhythmicity may be modulated by various factors, and such modulation may obscure the correlation between rhythms by selectively altering the phase of one of them, or even eliminate cyclic changes entirely. Thus for example, in the study of Lavie and Scherson (1981), ability to fall asleep was dependent upon both circadian and ultradian rhythms. Similarly, ultradian rhythms in pupillary diameter were modulated by circadian rhythms, while stability measures were less affected (Lavie, 1979). Lavie (1977) concluded that the period of ultradian fluctuations in perception of the spiral after-effect was modulated by circadian rhythms and was shorter in the morning and noontime than in the afternoon and evening hours. Kripke *et al.* (1976) reported on lengthening of the ultradian rhythmicity in monkeys during light on period. Such non-stationarity would tend to obscure the phase relationships of these rhythms with fluctuations whose period is not affected by circadian variation.

Other studies (Gopher and Lavie, 1980) indicate that the appearance of ultradian cyclicity may depend on task parameters and details of experimental design. The dependence of the ultradian phenomena on variations in experimental procedure is not restricted to psychological variables. As noted above, ultradian rhythms in urine flow were evident in subjects allowed to stand or sit (Lavie and Kripke, 1977) but not in waking recumbent subjects (Luboshitzky *et al.*, 1978). However, ultradian cyclicity in osmolality and cation concentrations were evident in both cases.

One Waking Rhythm or Many?

The hypothesis of a basic rest-activity cycle (Kleitman, 1963) would predict that all the daytime ultradian rhythms should be correlated with each other. Despite similar periodicity, it appears that rhythms in gastric contractions and urinary flow are not correlated with rhythms in performance, indices of arousal, and eating.

In inferring the relationship between these variables from correlations, we must be aware of a number of reservations. Lack of correlation could be due to use of a poor measure, with little variability, as appears to be the case for adaptive reaction time; it could be due to selective modulation of the period of one of the rhythms by circadian variation, or to difficulties in selecting appropriate tasks and experimental designs. Thus, for example, ultradian variation in performance may be eliminated or modified by knowledge of results. Conversely, studies which have shown correlation between arousal related indices have never examined more than three or four variables at a time, and were usually restricted to two. Of course, if A correlates with B and B correlates with C, one cannot necessarily infer that A correlates with C.

None the less, I would like, tentatively, to offer the hypothesis that all the arousal related indices reflect the activity of a common mechanism, or mechanisms; despite their similar periodicities, rhythms in renal and gastric function are under different controls. Traditionally, arousal has been seen in psychological literature as a measure of how wide awake the organism is, or of its response readiness (Duffy, 1957). Arousal has been viewed as a continuum ranging from sleep, or coma, at one pole, to excited behaviour at the other pole. Others suggested the existence of a dual arousal system, regulating tonic and phasic arousal (Ruttenberg, 1968). Control of cortical arousal is done by the brain stem ascending reticular activating system (ARAS), which receives simultaneously stimulation from all sensory pathways. ARAS stimulation produces cortical desynchronization and vegetative changes indicative of sympathetic activation.

An ultradian rhythm in arousal may reflect at least one of the following

(1) periodic, endogenously produced ARAS activation,
   superimposed on a tonic state of moderate arousal level;
(2) periodic, endogenously produced ARAS inactivation, superimposed on similarly tonic state of moderate arousal level; and
(3) the mutual coexistence of endogenously produced ARAS activation and inactivation.

It is not necessary to assume that the neuroanatomical clock, or clocks, resides in the ARAS, it may be located elsewhere and the ARAS participates as a servo mechanism.

Experimental evidence clearly supports possibility (2), the existence of periodic, endogenously produced ARAS inactivation, or in other words, the existence of daytime ultradian 'sleepiness' cycles. When provided conditions for sleep, humans show ultradian rhythms in the appearance of sleep stage 1 (Lavie and Scherson, 1981). Similar rhythms were shown in the appearance of electroencephalographic delta activity (Kripke, 1972), and in pupillary diameter and stability (Lavie, 1979). Hence, throughout the waking day there are multiple 'gates' of increased physiological readiness for sleep. During these 'gates' modifications of cognitive as well as perceptual processes can be expected.

Though limited, experimental evidence may suggest that rhythms in ARAS inactivation, indeed alternate with periodic ARAS activation rather than with a moderate state of tonic arousal, as stated above in (3). Bowden, Kripke, and Wyborney (1978) reported that in rhesus monkeys ultradian rhythms in resting were inversely related to rhythms of similar periodicity in locomotion, exploration, and ingestion. If these non-human behaviours are comparable to the human rhythms in eating (Friedman and Fisher, 1967; Oswald, Merrington, and Lewis, 1970; Kripke, 1972) a dual rhythmic system can be envisioned, with states of increased sleepiness alternating with states of increased arousal, the latter accompanied by eating behaviour probably mediated by activation of limbic structures. Although it is most logical to assume reciprocal relationships between the 'sleepiness' and 'activation' phases of the ultradian rhythm, I would like to hypothesize that these relationships are not obligatory and desynchronization may occur, which may have physiological and behavioural implications.

Further experimentation is needed to determine how the rhythms in alternating arousal states are related to the rhythms in perception and lateralization. Do periodic lengthenings of visual illusions indicate increased cortical arousal, or perhaps perceptual modifications are not associated with the 'ups' and 'downs' in arousal, but with the shifts in arousal from one state to the other. It well may be that shifts in arousal states are associated with changes in relative cerebral dominance. No doubt simultaneous investigations of several variables are required to resolve these questions.

After discussing the data on the relationships among the waking rhythms, it would be worthwhile to review the data relating REM cycles to waking rhythms; as shall become apparent, these data seem to indicate that the REM cycle actually may be composed of several different rhythms which are synchronized with each other, and may be related to similarly synchronized rhythms in CNS activity, but not to gastric or renal rhythms.

RELATION BETWEEN SLEEP AND WAKING RHYTHMS

As we have seen, research has borne out Kleitman's prediction of daytime cyclicity similar to that observed in REM–NONREM fluctuations in sleep, and, apparently, at least some of these daytime rhythms are related to each other. Presently, we shall examine the possible relationship between rhythmicity observed in sleep and wakefulness. As is the case with waking rhythms, there are several possible approaches to the experimental study of relations between REM rhythms in sleep and daytime fluctuations in performance and physiological functions. Demonstration of similar periodicity does not, of course, constitute evidence for relationship between the phenomena, but demonstration of widely different periodicities might constitute a valid argument against the hypothesis that two types of variations are related. Correlational studies are possible only between sleep states and ongoing physiological functions such as gastric or renal activity. In studying the relation between REM sleep cycles and behavioural fluctuations, two kinds of evidence may be substituted for correlational influence. One may examine the functional similarity between the two phenomena by showing, for example, that behavioural variation similar to that shown during the day is evident in subjects wakened from REM or NONREM sleep respectively; such evidence is complemented by attempts to show phase continuity between REM–NONREM cycles in sleep and those evident in waking behaviour.

Correlational Evidence; Gastrointestinal, Renal Cycles, and REM

We have already noted that neither gastric motility nor urine flow cycles appear to be related to waking performance rhythms (Hiatt, Kripke, and Lavie, 1975; Gopher and Lavie, 1980). In sleeping subjects, gastric cycles were found with a periodicity similar to that observed during waking, but these were not correlated with rhythms in REM–NONREM sleep (Lavie *et al.*, 1978; Tassinari *et al.*, 1973). Moreover, unlike eating, species whose REM cycles are much shorter than 90 minutes, such as rabbits, sheep, and dogs, none the less display gastric motility rhythms with periods approximating 90 minutes (Grivel and Ruckebusch, 1972).

We recently repeated the study of Mandell *et al.* (1966) on urinary flow in sleeping subjects (Lavie *et al.*, 1979). In agreement with the Mandell *et al.* findings, we observed that REM periods were associated with a biphasic variation in urine flow; however overall fluctuations in urine volume of most subjects were arrhythmic and episodic, and were not related to the periodicity in sleep stages. The biphasic variation in urine flow during REM may be due to flow inhibition by sympathetic activation during initiation of REM. Furthermore, in recent results from our laboratory (Gopher and Lavie, in press), we demonstrated significant ultradian rhythms in urine flow, osmolality, and cation concentrations in dogs unrelated to the dogs' REM–NONREM cycles. Urine sampling in dogs whose sleep was monitored electrophysiologically revealed no phase relationship between the rhythms in renal excretion and the REM–NONREM cycles.

The data accumulated to date suggest that both renal and gastric rhythms are independent of cyclity in REM sleep, just as they are apparently unrelated to waking rhythms in performance and daydreaming.

Functional Similarity of REM and Waking Rhythms

Waking rhythms in arousal and eating and the sleep REM–NONREM cycles all have periods of about 90 minutes, a similarity which is both suggestive and misleading. Gastric and renal variations also show 90 minute periodicity, but are apparently unrelated to either REM or arousal variations.

Resemblance in functional states may be more convincing evidence for the relationship between REM and arousal cyclicity. Both rhythms are composed of periodic increases in instinctive behaviour. The synchronized cyclicity of eating and oral behaviour and of arousal in the waking state has been discussed earlier in this chapter. REM sleep is accompanied by intense neuronal firing rates in occipital and other cortical areas and in the brain stem (e.g. Evarts, 1962; Huttenlocher, 1961). Certain brain stem neurons exhibit a distinct discharge pattern during waking motor behaviour, and a similar pattern during REM sleep, indicating, perhaps, the covert expression of waking movement patterns in REM (McGinty and Siegel, 1977). In cats suffering restricted dorsolateral pontine lesions the muscular flaccidity normally characteristic of REM sleep is absent; the REM sleep of such animals is marked by episodes of motor activity suggesting aggression and flight (Jouvet, 1962). These findings seem to indicate the covert activation of instinct related neural circuitry during REM sleep, a surmise which is also supported by the finding that in men such sleep is accompanied by penile erection (Karacan *et al.*, 1966).

Periodic instinctual activation in sleep may be advantageous to animals whose sleep must be interrupted frequently to allow feeding, as implied by Kleitman (1963). Conceivably, tonic muscular inhibition during REM evolved to prevent the overt appearance of instinctual motor patterns during uninterrupted sleep where such behaviour would be maladaptive.

If REM and NONREM sleep represent different levels of activation analogous to those observed in waking alertness, then perhaps subjects awakened from either REM or NONREM sleep should show performance differences analogous to those seen in different phases of the daytime waking arousal cycle. This prediction is borne out by a number of findings. Subjects awakened from REM sleep showed longer duration of apparent motion illusions than did those aroused during NONREM sleep (Lavie and Giora, 1973; Lavie, 1974a; Lavie and Sutter, 1975). As will be demonstrated shortly, these differences persisted for extended periods following the awakening, precluding the possibility that they reflect differences in the awakening process from the two types of sleep. Fiss, Klein, and Bokert (1966) reported that subjects awakened from REM sleep responded to the Thematic Apperception Test more vividly and loquaciously than when arising from NONREM sleep. Feltin and Broughton (1968) reported that choice reaction times were faster after REM than after NONREM sleep; this may indicate greater arousal in former state, though it should be noted that no ultradian rhythms in reaction time have been found in waking subjects tested during the day. Broughton (1968) reported that visual evoked potentials recorded prior to sleep or following REM sleep were similar, while those recorded following NONREM sleep incorporated the frequency characteristics of the EEG of the preceding sleep state. Meier-Ewert and Broughton (1967) reported that in photosensitive epileptic patients sudden arousal from NONREM sleep initiates myoclonic episodes, which may last up to 40 minutes following the awakening. Arousal from REM sleep, however, never provoked such episodes. Taken together, these findings imply that REM–NONREM cycles may be linked to functional variations similar to those observed in waking arousal rhythms.

Continuity Between Sleep and Waking Rhythms

Perhaps the most convincing evidence that REM sleep and some of the waking rhythms in waking subjects may be controlled by the same mechanism is that of phase continuity, which is at least a necessary condition for the assumption that they are generated by a single mechanism. Such continuity does not necessarily require strict time locking. Subjects awakened from REM sleep may not show rhythms 180° out of phase with those of subjects awakened from NONREM sleep throughout the day, since time locking may be obscured by alteration of the phase of the continuous rhythms through environmental and circadian influences.

Lavie and Giora (1973), Lavie (1974a), and Lavie and Sutter (1975) reported consistent phase differences in perception of apparent motions in subjects awakened from REM or NONREM sleep. These findings are illustrated in Figure 7, which shows the average duration of the spiral after-effect sampled at 5 minute intervals for 3 hours in 4 subjects awakened from REM and NONREM sleep on separate nights. While variations in post-awakening perception in both cases are rhythmic, subjects awakened from REM sleep showed the longest duration of illusions 40–50 minutes later than when arising from NONREM, suggesting that subjects were in opposite phases of a single rhythm. The initial decrease in the duration of the after-effect in both conditions may have been a learning effect, since tests were conducted on different nights spaced approximately one week apart (Lavie, 1974b).

One study has produced evidence for continuity of sleep cycles with waking behaviour in non-humans. Sterman, Lucas, and Macdonald (1972) reported that rhythms in food rewarded operant behaviour in cats were continuous with REM cyclicity.

Continuity and REM Sleep Latency

If REM sleep cycles are continuous with waking ultradian rhythms, one would expect that the latency of initial REM period onset would be determined by the phase of the ultradian rhythms at which subjects retire; this latency should vary from zero to at most 90 minutes. However, in normal humans going to sleep at habitual sleep time, latency of REM sleep onset is seldom less than 60 minutes and may be as long as 120 minutes. Furthermore REM occurring close to sleep onset is a pathological sign indicative of narcolepsy (Dement, Rechtschffen, and Gulevich, 1966). Arguments based on such considerations were presented by Moses *et al.* (1977) to contradict the 24 hour BRAC notion. They argued that the REM–NONREM cycle is sleep dependent, and that the clock regulating those cycles run only during sleep. Lavie and Scherson (1981), however, demonstrated that REM sleep can occur in short naps spaced 2-3 hours apart, with minimal amounts of intervening NONREM sleep.

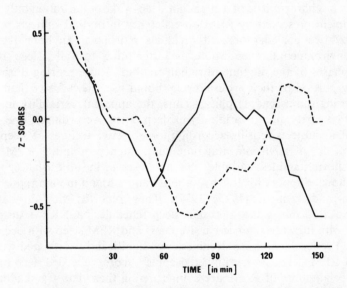

Figure 7 Continuation of the spiral after-effect rhythms with the REM–NONREM cycle. Time indicates time from the awakening. Broken line: REM awakening, continuous line: NONREM awakening

Several researchers have addressed themselves to the question regarding the phasing of the REM–NONREM cycles. Globus (1966) investigated the time of the first REM sleep as a function of the onset of daytime nap sleep, and concluded that the occurrence of REM sleep is dependent, at least in part, on clock time. Schulz, Dirlich, and Zulley (1975) reported that in the same subject the phasing of the REM–NONREM cycle systematically varies from night to night, suggesting perhaps that the diurnal and nocturnal fragments of the BRAC are not an integral subharmonic of 24 h. These findings were not replicated, however, by Mealey and Carman (1978) and by McPortland and

Kupfer (1978) in depressive patients. These latter investigators reported that the phase of the REM sleep rhythm in nocturnal recordings was dependent on both clock time and on the time of sleep onset. They further concluded that the similarity of REM times across subjects suggests environmental synchronization of the REM–NONREM cycle.

Other investigators studying altered sleep–wake schedules reported changes in first REM latency when sleep occurred at times other than habitual sleep time (Webb, Agnew, and Sternthal, 1966; Weitzman *et al.*, 1974; Webb and Agnew, 1977). REM sleep occurs earlier when sleep takes place at early morning hours than when sleep occurs at early evening hours. Furthermore, in ultradian sleep–wake schedules, such as 30 min sleep–60 min wake and in infants sleep, REM periods may be observed immediately after falling asleep (Carskadon and Dement, 1977). Thus it may be that the initial NONREM period may be characteristic of a circadian sleep–wake organization only.

The problem presented by REM onset latency in normal subjects may be resolved by two considerations. Individuals retiring at an hour fixed by external environmental cues would be attempting to fall asleep during different phases of the daytime ultradian rhythm. Those retiring during the descending portion of their arousal cycle should fall asleep faster than those retiring during the ascending phase. Thus, the apparent variability in REM onset may be partly due to variability in sleep onset. Accordingly, one might expect that in subjects retiring according to subjective feelings of sleepiness, without the use of environmental time cues, latency of initial REM onset should be shorter, and less variable than that observed in subjects going to bed at a fixed hour. Support for this hypothesis can be found in data reported by Carskadon and Dement (1975, 1977). They reported that in subjects maintaining a 30 min wake – 60 min sleep schedule, NONREM sleep was associated with increased subjective sleepiness and REM sleep with decreased sleepiness. Presleep subjective sleepiness was significantly correlated with the amount of REM sleep, so that higher sleepiness scores preceded sleep periods with greater amounts of REM sleep. Interpreting their data Carskadon and Dement concluded that: 'It is difficult to rule out the possibility of an underlying ultradian rhythm in sleepiness that independently affects the appearance of the two states of sleep and favors slow wave sleep or NONREM sleep on the upswing of the cycle and REM sleep on the downswing' (p.131). However, this explanation does not account for the minimum initial lag of 60 minutes normally observed in REM sleep onset. Broughton (1975) has suggested that deep NONREM sleep which precedes the initial REM period may be a major factor in the entrainment of the endogenous circadian rhythm, which has a period longer than 24 hours, to 24 hour geophysical cyclicity. This initial NONREM phase at sleep onset may also operate as a phase resetting mechanism for the various ultradian rhythms associated with the REM–NONREM cycle itself. The suggestion that the first NONREM may have a special role in sleep organization is further supported by the finding that REM can be triggered in humans shortly after sleep onset by physiotygmine infusion (Sitaram *et al.*, 1976) without interfering with the periodicity of the subsequent REM cycles. This suggests that a specific neurochemical mechanism may influence the initial onset of REM; but once initiated, appearance of REM may be controlled by an independent oscillatory mechanism which would produce continuity with the arousal cycles of the following day. Schulz, Dirlich, and Zulley (1975) also concluded that the first REM period is tied to sleep onset and is not drifting in time like subsequent REM periods.

However, the orderly alternation of REM and NONREM periods normally observed during sleep may be composed of rhythmic fluctuations in several different, potentially independent mechanisms which are synchronized by the phase resetting mechanism. Criteria for scoring REM depend upon three indices: EEG, EOG, and EMG (Rechtschaffen and Kales, 1968). In addition several other physiological measures such as penile erection (Karacan *et al.*, 1966), blood pressure (Coccagna *et al.*, 1971), metabolic rate (Brebbia and Altshuler, 1968) and brain temperature (Kawamura, Whitmoyer, and Sawyer, 1966) are normally synchronized with the REM cycles, at least some of these normally synchronized rhythms may be dissociable. Dement and Kleitman (1957) observed that subjects sometimes displayed low voltage fast EEG activity at the appropriate time of REM sleep, in the absence of rapid eye movements and EMG suppression; such 'missed' REM periods were accompanied by penile erections, even in subjects deprived of REM sleep (Karacan *et al.*, 1966; 1972). In a developmental study, Karacan *et al.* (1976) found different ontogenetic trends in the total duration of REM sleep and total duration of penile tumescence, and in latency of initial REM and tumescence periods. Taken together, these findings suggest that the various indices of REM sleep, which are normally synchronized, may be controlled by different, potentially independent regulatory mechanisms.

The importance of the proposed synchronization function of the initial NONREM period may be indicated by findings regarding narcoleptic patients who are subject to sudden sleep attacks during the waking hours. These patients display REM immediately after falling asleep at night, and subsequent occurrence of REM sleep is episodic and irregular, lacking the orderly cyclicity characteristic of normal subjects (Hishikawa *et al.*, 1976).

REM Rebound Phenomenon

Subjects deprived of REM sleep show shorter latency of REM onset and longer duration of REM episodes on subsequent nights (Dement, 1960). Such compensation or rebound phenomena should not occur if appearance of REM sleep is locked into an ultradian rhythm which is continuous with daytime arousal rhythms. However, it has been pointed out (Kripke, 1974) that such compensation may be limited to only some components of the REM state, which may be only tangentially related to the 24 hour BRAC. In humans, Cartwright, Monroe, and Palmer (1967) reported that subjects having a greater number of daydream experiences during waking show less compensation following REM deprivation. Actively ill schizophrenics, who hallucinate during daytime hours also show less REM rebound (Zarcone *et al.*, 1968). These findings suggest that compensation phenomena may be related to the hallucinatory component of REM only. However, the relationship between daydreams which occur during the low phases of the daytime arousal cycle, and REM dreaming, which occurs during the high phase of the nocturnal arousal cycle is not completely understood.

In animals, a characteristic component of REM is the occurrence of EEG spike activity along the visual pathways in the pons, geniculate nucleus, and occipital cortex (PGO spikes) which may be related to dream hallucinations. Dement *et al.* (1969) compared the effect of suppression of PGO spike activity on spike activity rebound to suppression of REM sleep in general upon REM compensation, and found the former effect to be greater. These findings may support the proposition that various components of REM are potentially independent, and that compensation phenomena may be limited to only some of them.

The survey presented in this section indicates that REM cyclicity, like waking arousal rhythms, are apparently unrelated to cycles of similar periodicity in gastric and renal function. There are several similarities, however, between functioning in different phases of the waking arousal cycle a and variations in functional state of the organism in REM and NONREM phases of sleep, as evident both from animal experiments and behaviour of humans awakened from different sleep phases. There also appears to be continuity between sleep and waking in rhythms appearing in perception of apparent movement and other phenomena. However, continuity between waking and sleep cycles is apparently interrupted by a delay in the appearance of the initial REM period. This may be due to the operation of a phase reset or entraining mechanism. In the absence of this delay, as in narcolepsy, both ultradian rhythms and circadian sleep–wake behaviour lacks cyclicity and is chaotic and maladaptive (Hishikawa *et al.*, 1976). One function of this reset mechanism may be to synchronize different aspects of the REM cycle, which, rather than being due to oscillation of a single functional state or clock, may be composed of several potentially independent components. It will be recalled that various aspects of circadian rhythmicity are dissociable even though they are usually synchronized, and that a similar hypothesis was offered in the previous section with regard to relations between various components of the arousal rhythm. The next section will discuss possible mechanisms and features of ultradian variation and synchrony in ultradian cycles, and consider the practical implications of the phenomena.

A MULTIOSCILLATORY CONCEPT

The present analysis suggests that the sructure and organization of ultradian rhythms in physiological functions and behavioural performance are considerably more complex than one might have predicted from Kleitman's BRAC model. In addition to arousal cycles, there are at least two independent rhythms in renal excretion and gastric motility. While NON–NONREM cyclicity may be continuous with cyclic variations in perception of apparent motions on the following day, the daytime portion of the hypothetical BRAC is apparently not continuous with REM cycles of the following night. Both day and night rhythms may be influenced by circadian variation and by environmental factors of various kinds, which may alter their periods or attenuate their amplitude.

It also appears that the arousal and REM–NONREM cycles are themselves composed of fluctuations in several different variables, which are potentially independent. If all the variations represented in the activity of a single rhythm, or the hands of a single clock, one would expect consistent and rigid phase relations between the various components, which should be evident both in sleep and waking. However, the different components of the REM–NONREM cycle are apparently dissociable, and there is no evidence that the daytime cycle components which may be normally synchronized are not dissociable under various conditions. It is clearly obvious that while some measures, such as perception of after-effect illusions may be continuous with the night phase of the BRAC on the following day, other measures having a different significance when measured in sleeping and in waking subjects are not. During sleep, REM periods, which are supposed to be indicative of relatively high arousal, are accompanied by dreaming and electroencephalographic theta activity. In waking subjects, daydreaming and EEG theta are characteristic of low arousal. Thus we would expect at least some measures to show phase reversal in the transition from night time to daytime BRAC.

These considerations indicate that both sleep and waking ultradian rhythms in arousal may best be viewed as the end-products of a synchronized multioscillatory system. Each of the several rhythms may be due to the operation of separate oscillators; this allows for the possibility that sleep rhythms incorporate different components, in different combinations, from those which make up the daytime arousal cycle.

The 90 Minute Enigma

I have already noted that gastric activity and renal function rhythms are apparently unrelated to the 24 hour BRAC. If so, one may be tempted to ask why all these rhythms share a common periodicity of 90 minutes. Furthermore, the 24 hours BRAC itself may be a multioscillatory system composed of several independent clocks having 90 minute periods.

It has also been mentioned that a similar dissociation has been found in research into circadian rhythms; that is, several rhythms having in normal conditions periods of about 24 hours which are normally synchronized have been shown to be unrelated. However, while the synchronized circadian periodicity normally observed in various measures may be attributed to the existence of prominent 24 hour geophysical *Zeitgebers*, there is as yet no explanation for the 90 minute periodicity. The fact that it appears in so many biological and behavioural functions may imply that it is due to time parameters a rather general and basic intracellular process, such as rate of protein synthesis, or time constants related to such synthesis, or the time required to transport a particular protein from the ribosomes of one cell to specific targets in other cells or organs.

The 90 minute period may be due to the activity of specific pacemaker cells or ganglia at various sites. Oscillations with a period of about 2–3 hours in the response thresholds of single units in the brain stem to sensory stimuli have been shown by Scheibel and Scheibel (1965) and 24 hour periodicity in pacemaker cells has been found in the primitive nervous system of the *Aplysia* (Strumwasser, 1965).

A third possibility which cannot be excluded is that the various rhythms may be under hormonal control. Though research on periodicity in endocrine functions has focused primarily on circadian rhythms, recent studies have shown 80–100 minute ultradian rhythms in nocturnal and diurnal secretion of parathyroid hormone (Kripke *et al.*, 1978) antidiuretic hormone (Lavie *et al.*, 1980) and luteinizing hormone (Yen *et al.*, 1974). These rhythms might be due to various factors. For example they could reflect fluctuations in the neuronal and neurosecretory functions of the hypothalamus, which partially controls secretion of these hormones, or they might reflect the time constant or lag in the homoeostatic mechanism responsible for maintaining more or less fixed levels of these substances during a given period in the life of the organism. One may speculate that the independent 90 minute rhythms evident in various behavioural measures may each reflect the influence of rhythms in different endocrine systems.

Certainly, the '90 minute enigma' is a formidable research problem; given the complex nature of the oscillatory system or systems, the enigma will probably yield only to a multidisciplinary effort.

Possible Adaptive Value of Ultradian Variation

At present, suggestions as to the mechanisms which may be responsible for the periodicity and synchronization of ultradian variation must remain speculative. The adaptive value, if any, of ultradian fluctuations is another problem whose conclusive solution requires further research.

The proposal that ultradian rhythmicity may have some adaptive significance is supported by clinical findings. As noted in the previous section narcoleptic patients show neither the initial synchronizing NONREM sleep stage, nor orderly cyclicity alternation of nocturnal sleep phases. It is conceivable that this disorganization of ultradian variation is in some way partly responsible for the involuntary daytime sleep attacks suffered by these patients. Depressive patients fail to show the normal synchrony between sleep REM–NONREM cycles and body motility rhythms (Foster and Kupfer, 1975).

The obvious variability in the thresholds for production of instinct related behaviours has led several authors to propose that the BRAC may be related to satisfaction of appetitive drives (Kleitman, 1963; Morruzi, 1969; Kripke, 1974). However, the lack of synchrony between arousal rhythms and gastric and renal activity cycles indicates that the BRAC did not develop from a digestive cycle in the manner first proposed by Kleitman. Jouvet (1962) has suggested that REM sleep may program neural circuits related to instinctual behaviours.

Ethologists have proposed that spontaneous fluctuations in thresholds of instinctual responses to environmental releasing stimuli may be due to the influence of internal releasing mechanisms (Lorenz, 1937). These internal releasing mechanisms might be activated periodically by the sleep and waking ultradian rhythms.

The synchronous activation of drive related mechanisms may allow superior performance of complex behaviours such as hunting and foraging for food for short periods, followed by a recuperation interval. Such an arrangement may have proven more adaptive than a 'steady state' mechanism, which would have provided for unchanging rates of anabolism and catabolism throughout the day, allowing only average performance at all times.

Implications for Research

The proposal that ultradian variations may be controlled by a multioscillatory system suggests the need for research along several lines. Attempts should be made to measure as many arousal indicators as is possible simultaneously, to determine which variables normally display synchronized rhythmicity. Other studies are needed to determine which measures are dissociable under certain conditions, and which rhythms are non-dissociable and might therefore, be causally related. More information is also required on the problem of continuity between various ultradian phenomena during waking and sleep, and the mechanism of entrainment and synchronization. The possible functions of ultradian variation and synchronization of rhythmic variations may be further elucidated by assessing the effects of experimental disruption of ultradian rhythms in normal subjects. Studies of alterations in ultradian variation in various pathological states may be of both theoretical and clinical interest.

Ultradian variation may be an important factor to consider in designing studies in other fields of experimental psychology as well. Such phenomena might account for the often puzzling results of vigilance studies noted by Loeb and Alluisi (1977) and by others, especially since not all measures of arousal may display synchronized rhythmicity under all conditions. Ultradian variation may also explain perceptual differences perviously attributed to personality variables, as discussed on page 241. An intriguing possibility is that inidividual differences in the period, synchrony orderliness, or amplitude of arousal rhythms may be related to personality differences.

Practical Implications

In addition to their possible clinical importance, ultradian variation may be a factor to be considered in human engineering applications. For example, it has been suggested that in tasks requiring high alertness for long periods, arousal could be maintained by giving the operator feedback from psycho-physiological indices such as EEG, galvanic skin response, or characteristics of the evoked potential (Donchin, 1978). However, since various measures of alertness may not be causally related to each other or to capacities required for performing the task, maintenance of a steady state in a given psychophysical measure by use of biofeedback may have no affect whatever on performance abilities. Even if such feedback is effective for short periods, it might produce a disruption of normal rhythms which could prove debilitating in the long run. It is possible, however, that continuous recording of physiological measures that are synchronized with ultradian variation in performance can provide information on the phase of the rhythm and hence anticipate decrease in performance and alert the operator.

It is well known that assembly line tasks are associated with boredom, high employee turnover, and poor morale. In some cases, self-paced work, allowing for ultradian variations in performance levels, may be more efficient than constant assembly line pacing. Some people may be more suited to assembly line or machine-paced work than others, due to individual differences in the magnitude of ultradian fluctuations. Thus, some problems in the design of man–machine systems might be solved by selection of appropriate personnel, others may be solved by changing the pace of the machine to fit the varying arousal levels of the operator, while in other applications it may be necessary to maintain performance artificially by knowledge of results or biofeedback.

SUMMARY

This chapter has reviewed the evidence for ultradian rhythms. These include rhythms of ingestion, digestion, excretion, psychophysiological, perceptual and vigilance, and perceptual–motor performance. These, in turn, are considered in relationship to the ultradian of REM or activated sleep rhythm. A multioscillatory concept for these rhythms is proposed and the research and practical implications are noted.

ACKNOWLEDGMENTS

The support of the Israeli Center for Psychobiology and the USA Army Grant No. DA-ERO-77-G-057 are gratefully acknowledged. Drs. A. Isseroff and E. Donchin made helpful comments on the manuscript.

REFERENCES

Andersson, A. L. (1969). Adaptive regulation of visual aftereffect duration and social-emotional adjustment. *Acta Psychologia* 29, 1–34.

Aschoff, J., Genecke, V., and Wever, R. (1967). Desynchronization of human circadian rhythms. *Japanese Journal of Physiology* 17, 450–457.

Aserinsky, E. an Kleitman, N. (1953). Regularly occurring periods of eye motility and concomitant phenomena during sleep. *Science* 118, 273–274.

Bowden, D. M., Kripke, D. F., and Wyborney, V. G. (1978). Ultradian rhythms in waking behavior of rhesus monkeys. *Physiology and Behavior* 21, 929–933.

Brebbia, D. R. and Altshuler, K. Z. (1968). Stage related patterns and nightly trends of energy exchange during sleep. In *Computers and Electronic Devices in Psychiatry* pp.319–355. N. Kline and E. Laska, (Eds.). New York, Grune and Stratton.

Broughton, R. J. (1968). Sleep disorders: Disorders of arousal. *Science* 159, 1070–1098.

Broughton, R. J. (1975). Biorhythmic variations in consciousness and psychological functions. *Canadian Psychological Review* 16, 217–239.

Carskadon, M. A. and Dement, W. C. (1975). Sleep studies on a 90 minute day. *Electroencephalography and Clinical Neurophysiology* 39, 145–155.

Carskadon, M. A. and Dement, W. C. (1977). Sleepiness and sleep state on a 90-min schedule. *Psychophysiology* 14, 127–133.

Cartwright, R. D., Monroe, L. J., and Palmer, C. (1967). Individual differences in response to REM deprivation. *Archives of General Psychiatry* 16, 297–303.

Coccagna, G., Mantovani, M., Brignani, F. *et al.* (1971). Arterial pressure changes during spontaneous sleep in man. *Electroencephalography and Clinical Neurophysiology* 31, 277–281.

Colquhoun, W. F. (1971). Circadian variations in mental efficiency. In: *Biological Rhythms and Human Performance*. W. P. Colquhoun (Ed.). London, Academic Press.

Dement, W. (1960). The effect of dream deprivation. *Science* 131, 1705–1707.

Dement, W., Cohen, H., Ferguson, H., and Zarcone, V. (1969). A sleep researcher's odyssey: The function and clinical significance of REM sleep. In: *The Psychodynamic Implications of the Physiological Studies on Dreams*, pp.47–71. L. Madow and L. H. Snow (Eds.). Springfield, Ill., Charles C. Thomas.

Dement, W. and Kleitman, N. (1957). Cyclic variations in EEG during sleep and their relation to eye movements, body motility and dreaming. *Electroencephalography and Clinical Neurophysiology* 9, 673–690.

Dement, W., Rechtschaffen, A., and Gulevich, G. (1966). The nature of the narcoleptic sleep attack. *Neurology* 16, 18–33.

Donchin, E. (1978). Brain electrical activity as an index of mental work load in man-machine systems *Proceedings of the Symposium on Man-System Interface: Advances in Work Load Study*. Washington, Airline Pilot Association.

Doring, G. K. and Schaefers, E. (1950). Uber die Tagesrhythmik der Pupillen weite Bein Menschen. *Pfluegers Archiv: European Journal of Physiology* **252**, 537–541.

Duffy, E. (1957). The psychological significance of the concept of 'arousal' or 'activation'. *Psychological Review* **64**, 265–275.

Evarts, E. V. (1962). Activity of neurons in visual cortex of the cat during sleep with low voltage fast EEG activity. *Journal of Neurophysiology* **25**, 812–816.

Feltin, M. and Broughton, R. (1968). Differential effects of arousal from slow wave sleep versus REM sleep. *Psychophysiology* **5**, 231 (Abst).

Fiss, H., Klein, G. S., and Bokert, E. (1966). Waking fantasies following interruptions of two types of sleep. *Archives of General Psychiatry* **19**, 543–551.

Foster, G. F. and Kupfer, D. J. (1975). Psychomotor activity as a correlate of depression and sleep in acutely disturbed psychiatric in-patients. *American Journal of Psychiatry* **132**, 928–931.

Friedman, S. and Fisher, C. (1967). On the presence of a rhythmic, diurnal, oral instinctive drive cycle in man. *Journal of the American Psychoanalysis Association* **15**, 317–343.

Gilbert, G. M. (1939). Dynamic psychophysics and the phi phenomenon. *Archives of Psychology* No. 237.

Globus, G. G. (1966). Rapid eye movement cycles in real time. *Archives of General Psychiatry* **15**, 654–659.

Globus, G. G., Drury, R. L., Phoebus, E. C., and Boyd, R. (1971). Ultradian rhythms in human performance. *Perceptual and Motor Skills* **33**, 1171–1174.

Gopher, D. and Lavie, P. (1980). Short term rhythms in the performance of a simple motor task. *Journal of Motor Behavior* **12**, 207–219.

Gordon, C. R. and Lavie, P. (1982). Ultradian rhythms in urine excretion in dogs. Role of sympathetic innervation. *Sleep Research*, in press.

Granat, M., Lavie, P., Adar, D., and Sharf, M. (1979). Short term cycles in human fetal activity. I. Normal pregnancies. *American Journal of Obstetrics and Gynecology* **134**, 696–701.

Grivel, M. L. and Ruckebusch, Y. (1972). The propagation of segmental contractions along the small intestines. *Journal of Physiology* **227**, 611–625.

Halberg, F. (1967). Physiologic consideration underlying rhythmometry, with special reference to emotional illness. In: *Cycles Biologiques et Psychiatrie*, pp.73–126. J. Ajuriaguerra (Ed.). Geneve, Symposium Bel-Air II.

Hiatt, J. F. and Kripke, D. F. (1975). Ultradian rhythms in waking gastric activity. *Psychosomatic Medicine* **37**, 320–325.

Hiatt, J. F., Kripke, D. F., and Lavie, P. (1975). Relationships among psychophysiologic ultradian rhythms. *Chronobiologia* Supp. 1, 43.

Hishikawa, Y., Wakamatsu, H., Furuya, E., Sugits, Y., Masaoka, S., Kaneda, H., Sato, M., Nan'no, H., and Kaneko, Z. (1976). Sleep satiation in narcoleptic patients. *Electroencephalography and Clinical Neurophysiology* **41**, 1–18.

Hoddes, E., Zarcone, V., Smythes, H., Phillips, R., and Dement, W. C. (1973). Quantification of sleepiness: A new approach. *Psychophysiology* **10**, 431–436.

Hoppe, J. J. (1894). Studien zur Erklärung Gewisser Scheinbewegungen. *Z. Psychol. Physiol. Sinnesorg* **7**, 29–37.

Horne, J. and Whitehead, M. (1976). Ultradian and other rhythms in human respiration rate. *Experimentia* **32**, 1165–1167.

Huttenlocher, P. R. (1961). Evoked and spontaneous activity in single units of medial brain stem during natural sleep and waking. *Journal of Neurophysiology* **29**, 451–468.

Jerison, H. J. (1967). Activation and long term performance. In: *Attention and Performance. I. Proceedings of a Symposium on Attention and Performance*, pp.373–388. A. F. Sanders (Ed.). Amsterdam, North Holland Pub. Comp.

Jouvet, M. (1962). Recherches sur les structures nerveuses et les mechanismes responsables des différentes phases du sommeil physiologique. *Archives Italiennes de Biologie* **100**, 125–206.

Karacan, I., Goodenough, D. R., Shapiro, A., and Starker, S. (1966). Erection cycle during sleep in relation to dream anxiety. *Archives of General Psychiatry* **15**, 183–189.

Karacan, I., Hursch, C. J., Williams, R. L., and Thornby, J. I. (1972). Some characteristics of nocturnal penile tumescence in young adults. *Archives of General Psychiatry* **26**, 351–356.

Karacan, I., Salis, P. F., Thornby, J. E., and Williams, R. L. (1976). The ontogeny of nocturnal penile tumescence. *Waking and Sleeping* **1**, 27–44.

Kawamura, H., Whitmoyer, D. I., and Sawyer, C. H. (1966). Temperature changes in the rabbit brain during paradoxical sleep. *Electroencephalography and Clinical Neurophysiology* **21**, 469–477.

Klein, R. and Armitage, R. (1979). Rhythms in human performance: 1–1½ hour oscillations in cognitive style. *Science* **204**, 1326–1328.

Kleitman, N. (1963). *Sleep and Wakefulness* (2nd Edn). Chicago, University of Chicago Press.

Kraepelin, E. (1893). Ueber psychische disposition. *Arch. J. Psychiat.* **25**, 593–594.

Kripke, D. F. (1972). An ultradian biological rhythm associated with perceptual deprivation and REM sleep. *Psychosomatic Medicine* **3**, 221–234.

Kripke, D. F. (1974). Ultradian rhythms in sleep and wakefulness. In: *Advances in Sleep Research*, Vol. I, pp.305–325. E. D. Weitzman (Ed.). New York, Spectrum Pub.

Kripke, D. F., Halberg, F., Crowley, T. J., and Pegram, V. (1976). Ultradian spectra in monkeys. *International Journal of Chronobiology* **3**, 193–204.

Kripke, D. F., Lavie, P., Parker, P., Huey, L., and Deftos, L. J. (1978). Plasma parathyroid hormones and calcium are related to sleep stage cycles. *Journal of Clinical Endocrinology and Metabolism* **47**, 1021–1027.

Kripke, D. F. and Sonnenschein, D. (1978). A biologic rhythm in waking fantasy. In: *The Stream of Consciousness*, pp.321–32. D. Pope and J. L. Singer (Eds.). New York, Plenum Pub.

Lavie, P. (1974a). Differential effects of REM and NONREM awakenings on the spiral aftereffect. *Physiological Psychology* **2**, 107–108.

Lavie, P. (1974b). *Aspects of Ultradian Rhythms in Man*. Unpublished Doctoral Dissertation.

Lavie, P. (1976). Ultradian rhythms in the perception of two apparent motions. *Chronobiologia* **3**, 214–218.

Lavie, P. (1977). Nonstationarity in human perceptual ultradian rhythms. *Chronobiologia* **4**, 38–48.

Lavie, P. (1979). Ultradian rhythms in alertness—a pupillographic study. *Biological Psychology* **9**, 49–62.

Lavie, P. (1980). The search for cycles in mental performance—From Lombard to Kleitman. *Chronobiologia* **7**, 247–256.

Lavie, P. and Giora, Z. (1973). Spiral aftereffect durations following awakening from REM sleep and NONREM sleep. *Perception and Psychophysics* **1**, 19–20.

Lavie, P., Gopher, D., Fogel, R., and Zomer, J. (1981). Ultradian rhythms in perceptual motor tasks. In: The twenty-four hour workday: *Proceedings of the Symposium on Variations in Work-Sleep Schedules*. Johnson, L. C., Tepas, D. I., Colquhoun, W. P. (Eds.), 1979, Cincinnati: HHS (NIDSH), p.181–196.

Lavie, P. and Kripke, D. F. (1977). Ultradian rhythms in urine flow in waking humans. *Nature* **269**, 142–144.

Lavie, P., Kripke, D. F., Hiatt, J. F., and Morrison, J. (1978). Gastric rhythms during sleep. *Behavioral Biology* **23**, 526–530.

Lavie, P., Levy, C. M., and Coolidge, F. L. (1975). Ultradian rhythms in the perception of the spiral aftereffect. *Physiological Psychology* **3**, 144–146.

Lavie, P., Lord, J. W., and Frank, A. R. (1974). Basic rest-activity cycle in the perception of the spiral aftereffect: A sensitive detector of a basic biological rhythm. *Behavioral Biology* **11**, 373–379.

Lavie, P., Luboshitzky, R., Kleinhaus, N., Shen-Orr, Z., Barzilai, D., Glick, S. M., Leroith, D., and Levy, J. (1980). Rhythms in urine flow are not correlated with rhythmic secretion of antidiuretic hormone (ADH) in well hydrated men. *Hormones & Metabolic Research* **12**, 66–70.

Lavie, P., Oksenberg, A., Kedar, S., Suboshitzky, R., and Shen-Orr, Z. (1979). Nocturnal secretion of urine flow — peculiar relation with REM sleep. *Sleep Research* **8**, 63.

Lavie, P. and Scherson, A. (1981). Ultrashort sleep–wake schedule 1: Evidence of ultradian rhythmicity in 'Sleep Ability'. *Electroencephalography and Clinical Neurophysiology* **52**, 163–174.

Lewis, B. D., Kripke, D. F., and Bowden, D. M. (1977). Ultradian rhythms in hand mouth behavior in Rhesus monkey. *Physiology and Behavior* **18**, 283–286.

Loeb, M. and Alluisi, E. A. (1977). An update of findings regarding vigilance and a reconsideration of underlying mechanisms. In: *Vigilance: Theory, Operational Performance and Physiological Correlates*. R. R. Mackie (Ed.). New York, Plenum.

Lorenz, K. (1937). Uber die Bildung des Instinktbegriffs. *Die Naturwissenschaften* **25**, 289–300, 307–318, 324–331.

Lowenstein, O., Feinberg, R., and Lowenfeld, I. E. (1963). Pupillary movements during acute and chronic fatigue: A new test for the objective evaluation of tiredness. *Investigative Ophthalmology* **2**, 138–157.

Luboshitzky, R., Lavie, P., Sok, Y., Glick, S. M., Leroith, D., Shen-Orr, Z., and Barzilai, D. (1978). Antidiuretic hormone secretion and urine flow in aged catheterized patients. *T.I.T. J. Life Sciences* **8**, 99–103.

Lucas, E. A. and Harper, R. M. (1976). Periodicities in the rate of on-demand electrical stimulation of the mesencephalic reticular formation to maintain wakefulness. *Experimental Neurology* **51**, 444–456.

Mandell, A. J., Chaffey, B., Brill, P., Mandell, M. P., Rodnick, J., Rubin, R. T., and Sheff, R. (1966). Dreaming sleep in man: Changes in urine volume and osmolality. *Science* **151**, 1558–1560.

McGinty, D. J. and Siegel, J. M. (1977). Neuronal activity patterns during rapid-eye-movement sleep: Relation to waking patterns. In: *Neurobiology of Sleep and Memory*. New York, Academic Press.

McPortland, R. J. and Kupfers, D. J. (1978). Rapid eye movement sleep cycles, clock time and sleep onset. *EEG Clinics in Neurophysiology* **45**, 178–185.

Mealey, L. and Carman, G. J. (1978). REM sleep across 52 consecutive nights of a restricted sleep–wake regimen. *Sleep Research* **7**, 309.

Meier-Ewert, K. and Broughton, R. J. (1967). Photomyoclonic response of epileptic and non-epileptic subjects during wakefulness, sleep and arousal. *Electroencephalography and Clinical Neurophysiology* **23**, 142–151.

Moruzzi, G. (1969). Sleep and instinctual behavior. *Archives Italiennes de Biologie* **108**, 175–216.

Moses, J. M., Lubin, A., Johnson, L. C., and Naitoh, P. (1977). Rapid eye movement cycle is a sleep-dependent rhythm. *Nature* **265**, 360–361.

Moses, J., Lubin, A., Naitoh, P., and Johnson, L. C. (1978). Circadian variation in performance, subjective sleepiness, sleep and oral temperature during an altered sleep-wake schedule. *Biological Psychology* 6, 301–308.

Murrel, K. F. H. (1967). Performance differences in continuous tasks. In: *Activation and Long Term Performance. Proceedings of a Symposium on Attention and Performance*, pp.427–436. A. F. Sanders (Ed.). Amsterdam, North Holland Pub. Comp.

Orr, W., Hoffman, H., and Hegge, F. (1976). Ultradian rhythms in extended performance. *Aerospace Medicine* 45, 995–1000.

Oswald, I., Merrington, J., and Lewis, H. (1970). Cyclical 'on demand' oral intake in adults. *Nature* 225, 959–960.

Othmer, E., Hayden, M. P., and Segelbaum, R. (1969). Encephalic cycles during sleep and wakefulness in humans: A 24-hour pattern. *Science* 164, 447–449.

Rapoport, J. (1963). Massed practice and motion aftereffect. *Perceptual and Motor Skills* 17, 157–158.

Rechtschaffen, A. and Kales, A. (1968). *Manual of Standardized Terminology, Techniques and Scoring System for Sleep Stages of Human Subjects*, pp.1–62. NIH Publication No. 204. Washington, Superintendent of Documents.

Ruttenberg, A. (1968). The two arousal hypothesis: Reticular formation and limbic system. *Psychological Review* 75, 51–80.

Schulz, H., Dirlich, G., and Zulley, J. (1975). Phase shift in the REM sleep rhythm. *Pflugers Archives* 358, 201–212.

Scheibel, M. E. and Scheibel, A. B. (1965). Periodic sensory nonresponsiveness in reticular neurons. *Archives Italiennes de Biologie* 103, 300–316.

Sitaram, N., Wyatt, R. J., Dawson, S., and Gillin, J. C. (1976). REM sleep induction by physiostygmine infusion in normal volunteers. *Science* 191, 1281–1283.

Sterman, M. B. (1972). The basic rest-activity cycle and sleep: Developmental considerations in man and cat. In: *Sleep and the Maturing Nervous System*, pp.175–197. C. D. Clemente, D. P. Purpura, and F. E. Mayer (Eds.). New York, Academic Press.

Sterman, M. B., Lucas, E. A., and Macdonald, L. R. (1972). Periodicity within sleep and operant performance in the cat. *Brain Research* 38, 327–341.

Strumwasser, F. (1965). The demonstration and manipulation of a circadian rhythm in a single neuron. In: *Circadian Clocks*. J. Aschoff (Ed.). Amsterdam, North Holland Pub. Comp., pp.442–462.

Tassinari, C. A. Coccagna, G., Mantovani, M., Della Bernardina, B., Sprie, J. P., Mancia, D., Vela, A., and Vallicioni, P. (1973). Duodenal EMG activity during sleep in man. In: *The Nature of Sleep*, pp.55–58. U. J. Jovanovic (Ed.). Stuttgart, Gustave Fischer.

Thorndike, E. L. (1900). Mental fatigue. *Psychological Review* 7, 466–482.

Wada, T. (1922). An experimental study of hunger and its relation to activity. *Archives of Psychology* Monogr. 8.

Webb, W. B. and Agnew, H. W. Jr. (1977). Analysis of the sleep stages in sleep-wakefulness requirements of varied length. *Psychophysiology* 14, 445–450.

Webb, W., Agnew, H., and Sternthal, H. (1966). Sleep during the early morning. *Psychonomic Science* 6, 277–278.

Weitzman, E., Nogeire, C., Perlow, M., Fukushima, D., Sassin, J., McGregor, P., Gallagher, T., and Hellman, L. (1974). Effects of a prolonged 3-hour sleep wakefulness cycle on sleep stages, plasma cortisol, growth hormone and body temperature in man. *Journal of Clinical Endocrinology* 38, 1018–1030.

West, L. J., Janszen, H. H., Lester, B. K., and Cornelisoon, F. S. (1962). The psychosis of sleep deprivation. *Annals of the New York Academy of Science* 96, 66–70.

Yen, S. S. C., Vandenberg, G., Tsai, C. C., and Parker, D. C. (1974). Ultradian fluctuations of gonadotropins. In: *Biorhythms and Human Reproduction*, pp.203–218. M. Ferin *et al.* (Eds.). New York, Wiley & Sons.

Yoss, R. E., Mayer, N. J., and Hollenhorst, R. W. (1969). Pupil size and spontaneous pupillary waves associated with alertness, drowsiness and sleep. *Neurology* **20**, 545–554.

Zarcone, V., Gulevich, G., Pivik, T., *et al.* (1968). Partial REM phase deprivation and schizophrenia. *Archives of General Psychiatry* **18**, 194–202.

Chapter 10

Epilogue

Wilse B. Webb

In the early planning stages of this book, I agreed to write a final chapter. The purpose was to give perspective to the materials covered and to point prospectively toward the interaction between biological rhythms, sleep, and performance of the future. This was to be an effort to move from the trees to a view of the forest and to turn to the vistas beyond. That was a time of enthusiasm and visions unfettered by facts and reality. However, after reading (and rereading) each contribution and faced with the writing of this chapter, problems became apparent.

Each author, in fact, has conscientiously minded the perspectives of his contribution both historically and conceptually. A search for current wisdom beyond their expertise calls for more than I possess.

As for prospectives of the interactions of the research areas, a slight acquaintance with the history of ideas and science is properly discouraging. If the past is predictive of the future, and I believe that it is, the future lies in emergent insights and reconceptualizations, new technological breakthroughs, and countless efforts. To predict the future would require the predictions of the ideas of future Darwins, or Freuds, or Einsteins, of concepts equivalent to DNA, endomorphins, reinforcements, or relativity, of technologies like electroencephalograms, electron microscopes, computers, or cyclotrons. Specific to our concerns what seer was able to predict the impact of free running rhythm, the REM state or the correlation coefficient?

And yet, clearly, some coordinative statement was needed. The materials of this volume have ranged from psychophysics to personality tests, from microseconds to shift work schedules, from reaction time to complaints, from tendencies to Fourier transforms, from temperature to temperament, from EEGs to questionnaires. There is a plethora of details. Even the thematic schemes of biological rhythms, sleep, and performance seems to appear and disappear in unpredictable ways.

It was at least clear what the Editor and authors had in mind. They had attempted to bring together their lively enterprises—biological rhythms, sleep, and performance measurements—and appraise their current state of interaction. A question to be raised, however, was whether the effect has been blessed by the Grecian god, Proteus, who was capable of reshaping himself into many forms to accomplish his ends, or the character Procrusteus distorting his victims for his purposes.

As the time for writing the needed coordinative statement arrived, a hopeful solution emerged. I was reading a book review in the journal of book reviews, *Contemporary Psychology*. For that book the review gave me a comprehensive view of the book—a coordinative statement. Hopefully, the book review that follows will serve a similar purpose of our efforts.

Book Review: Biological Rhythms, Sleep, and Performance.

In the Henry Tizard Memorial Lecture, in 1965, Peter Medawar had a protagonist state:

> '. . . as science advances, the burden of factual information which it adds daily is becoming well nigh insupportable . . . the scientist avoids being crushed beneath this factual burden by taking refuge in specialization and the increase in specialization is the distinguishing mark of modern scientific growth. Because of it, scientists are becoming progressively less well able to communicate even with each other . . . we must look forward to an even finer fragmentation of knowledge, in which each specialist will live in a tiny world of his own . . .'

Medawar categorically denies that assertion. He states that the facts become amenable to generalization:

> '. . . particular facts are comprehended within, and therefore in a sense annihilated by, general statements of steadily increasing explanatory power and compass . . . we are progressively relieved of the burden of the particular. We need no longer record the fall of every apple.'

He further asserts the specialities are increasingly *interdependent:*

> 'As to the scientists becoming narrower and more specialized: the opposite is the case. One of the distinguishing marks of modern science is the disappearance of sectarian loyalties . . . Isolationism is over; we all depend upon and sustain each other . . . .'

The text under review is clearly an attempt to emulate Medawar's second tenet. Its purpose is, to quote the Editor, that of 'explicating the status and exciting presence of the healthy interaction occurring within each area'. The areas, in this instance, are biological rhythm, sleep, and performance research.

The book begins with two introductory chapters which present the backgrounds, variables, and research procedures of the three areas and detail the analytical procedures of chronobiology. Two chapters then review the variations in performance and in sleep associated with time of occurrence — in short, the chronobiology of performance and sleep. The following three chapters review the relationship between performance and major temporal variations in sleep: sleep loss, changes in sleep structure, and scheduled times of sleep and waking. A chapter details the limitations and potentials of performance while asleep. A final chapter considers ultradian rhythms within sleep and waking and their interrelations.

Certainly, a review of these chapters gives ample evidence that, while the areas may not 'depend upon' or 'sustain' each other, they can and do profit from each other.

The overall problem of the book is not: 'Is this trip necessary?' We admire the General Editor's decision to recognize the emerging data base indicating the relationships of sleep and biological rhythms and performance. The book presents abundant data to affirm that decision. The Editor of the volume has done extensive research in sleep with a strong performance bias and has become increasingly oriented toward biological rhythm considerations. From this background he asserts a belief that the time for a coordinative effort is called for. Our review of the book does not question this decision. The trip is necessary. One may ask, however, 'Did they schedule the trip too soon?' As an alternative one may inquire about the routing of the tour.

There are problems with the routing. Throughout the substantive chapters (III–IX) there are constant cross-referencings to other chapters. The details of this can be seen in the index where topic after topic, e.g., temperature, memory, REM sleep, deprivation, are scattered about. Or such generalized constructs as learning, 'fatigue', or motivation appear and disappear. Unfortunately, as one arrives at the cross-reference, matters are not often settled. One often has the fleeting picture of the Editor, like Laocoon, wrestling with a tangle of snakes, large and small, somewhat out of hand.

However, in the somewhat biased viewpoint of this reviewer, the problems of the book do not lie in the materials and their organization nor in the competence of the authors, but the level of development of the interrelations presented. An examination of each chapter reveals an expert and comprehensive portrayal of each area. Such an examination also often reveals that there has not yet been a full articulation of the three areas. A few examples will suffice. Chapter II outlines the highly sophisticated and complex analytical procedures of biological rhythm research. However, only Chapter III (Biological Rhythms and Performance) is referrant to some of the simpler design problems raised and only in the last chapter (IX) on ultradian rhythms does one find application of any of the more complex procedures. The separate authors provide little guidance as to whether one should lay down one's present tools and learn Fourier transforms. The authors dealing with the effect of sleep and performance (V–VIII) all give recognition to rhythmic effects, but one (VI) can only deplore the lack of data, one (VIII) must hypothesize an effect, and the remaining two (V and VII) struggle with unresolved complications.

To extend the trip analogy, one receives the impression of a number of seasoned travellers saying that, as you continue your journey into performance measurement, sleep, or biological rhythm research, you should carry along a travel guide from the other areas. That seems to be sound advice. I am sure, however, the authors (certainly the Editor) had intended that the reader follow the current advertising advice of a major credit card company; don't leave home without it (the associated disciplines).

This review began with Peter Medawar's reassurance that specialization is being overcome by facts becoming subservient to general principles and to increasing interdependence of research domains. The impression left by this book is indeed an increasing interdependence of these research areas .

This is, however, an interdependence burdened by 'facts' which have not yet yielded to principles and 'general statements of explanatory power'. The future interactions between the areas is less likely to be dependent upon recognized need or urging heard in this book than upon the ability to each area to coordinate their independent facts into more transferable principles.

Index